Methods in Molecular Biology

Series Editor
John M. Walker
School of Life and Medical Sciences
University of Hertfordshire
Hatfield, Hertfordshire, AL10 9AB, UK

For further volumes:
http://www.springer.com/series/7651

Inflammation and Cancer

Methods and Protocols

Edited by

Brendan J. Jenkins

Centre for Innate Immunity and Infectious Diseases, Hudson Institute of Medical Research
Clayton, VIC, Australia

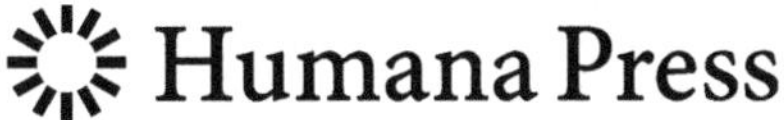

Editor
Brendan J. Jenkins
Centre for Innate Immunity and Infectious Diseases
Hudson Institute of Medical Research
Clayton, VIC, Australia

ISSN 1064-3745 ISSN 1940-6029 (electronic)
Methods in Molecular Biology
ISBN 978-1-4939-7567-9 ISBN 978-1-4939-7568-6 (eBook)
https://doi.org/10.1007/978-1-4939-7568-6

Library of Congress Control Number: 2017962419

Printed on acid-free paper

This Humana Press imprint is published by Springer Nature
The registered company is Springer Science+Business Media, LLC
The registered company address is: 233 Spring Street, New York, NY 10013, U.S.A.

Preface

Dysregulation of the immune system, both innate and adaptive, drives the pathogenesis of a plethora of chronic disease states, such as autoimmune and inflammatory disorders, infectious diseases, and cancer. With respect to cancer, it is now widely acknowledged that at least one third of all cancers are linked to chronic inflammatory responses, with cancer of the stomach, pancreas, colon, and lung, to name but a few, being prime examples. Accordingly, laboratory-based investigations using in vivo disease models and clinical samples, coupled with state-of-the-art molecular and cellular biological methodologies, along with next-generation sequencing, proteomics, and functional genomics technologies, underpin research efforts to understand the pathogenesis of disease.

This book, entitled *Methods in Molecular Biology: Inflammation and Cancer*, is the latest installment of the highly successful *Methods in Molecular Biology* laboratory protocol-based book series. As its name implies, the current book is designed to expose the reader to a broad spectrum of research models, techniques, and protocols, covered over 23 individual chapters, which are employed by basic and clinical research laboratories in the inflammation and cancer fields. Each chapter is divided into sections providing detailed information on the background and context for the chosen topic of interest, a list of the materials and reagents needed for each topic, a step-by-step methodology for the successful and reproducible execution of each topic, as well as notes to provide tips, troubleshooting advice, and elaborate further on specific materials or methods.

Considering the enormity of the vast number of research models (in vitro, ex vivo, and in vivo) and techniques that are collectively used by researchers, it is impossible to cover them all in detail in a single book. With this in mind, this edition has been divided into two parts: Part I, "Experimental Model Systems," provides an up-to-date snapshot of the generation and characterization of representative research models for chronic immune-based (i.e., infectious, autoimmune, inflammatory) diseases and inflammation-associated cancers. In Part II, "Experimental Techniques," experts in the inflammation and cancer fields cover a range of biochemical, molecular, and cellular biological techniques, which are commonly utilized to dissect the molecular mechanisms and cellular processes (including cell type(s)) that drive the pathogenesis of certain disease states.

With a heavy emphasis on practicality, *Methods in Molecular Biology: Inflammation and Cancer* will appeal to a readership with a very diverse range of laboratory-based experience, ranging from undergraduate students with limited research exposure to established basic and/or clinical researchers wishing to diversify their existing portfolio of practical knowledge. In addition, this book aims to supplement researchers with the necessary practical expertise and know-how to assist their efforts to publish their research findings, dissemination of which in the literature will enhance our collective knowledge of the processes that drive inflammation and cancer.

Clayton, VIC, Australia ***Brendan J. Jenkins***

Contents

Part II Experimental Techniques

Contributors

HELEN E. ABUD • *Cancer Program, Monash Biomedicine Discovery Institute, Monash University, Clayton, VIC, Australia; The Department of Anatomy and Developmental Biology, Monash University, Clayton, VIC, Australia*

REYHAN AKHTAR • *Cancer Program, Monash Biomedicine Discovery Institute, Monash University, Clayton, VIC, Australia; The Department of Anatomy and Developmental Biology, Monash University, Clayton, VIC, Australia*

GISELA MIR ARNAU • *Molecular Genomics, Peter MacCallum Cancer Centre, Melbourne, VIC, Australia*

MARIE-LIESSE ASSELIN-LABAT • *ACRF Stem Cells and Cancer Division, The Walter and Eliza Hall Institute of Medical Research, Parkville, VIC, Australia; Department of Medical Biology, The University of Melbourne, Parkville, VIC, Australia*

JEFFREY J. BABON • *The Walter and Eliza Hall Institute of Medical Research, Parkville, Melbourne, VIC, Australia; Department of Medical Biology, University of Melbourne, Melbourne, VIC, Australia*

WILLIAM BERRY • *Centre for Innate Immunity and Infectious Diseases, Hudson Institute of Medical Research, Clayton, VIC, Australia; Department of Molecular Translational Science, School of Clinical Sciences, Monash University, Clayton, VIC, Australia*

SARAH A. BEST • *ACRF Stem Cells and Cancer Division, The Walter and Eliza Hall Institute of Medical Research, Parkville, VIC, Australia; Department of Medical Biology, The University of Melbourne, Parkville, VIC, Australia*

MARNIE E. BLEWITT • *The Walter and Eliza Hall Institute, Parkville, VIC, Australia; Department of Medical Biology, University of Melbourne, Melbourne, VIC, Australia*

DAVE BOUCHER • *Institute for Molecular Bioscience and IMB Centre for Inflammation and Disease Research, The University of Queensland, St. Lucia, Australia*

STEVEN BOZINOVSKI • *School of Health and Biomedical Sciences, RMIT University, Bundoora, VIC, Australia*

AMY CHAN • *Institute for Molecular Bioscience and IMB Centre for Inflammation and Disease Research, The University of Queensland, St. Lucia, Australia*

LEONIE A. CLUSE • *Gene Regulation Laboratory, Peter MacCallum Cancer Centre, Melbourne, VIC, Australia*

KARLA J. COWLEY • *Victorian Centre for Functional Genomics, Peter MacCallum Cancer Centre, Melbourne, VIC, Australia*

DANIEL CROAGH • *Department of Surgery, School of Clinical Sciences at Monash Health, Monash University, Clayton, VIC, Australia*

VIRGINIE DESWAERTE • *Centre for Innate Immunity and Infectious Diseases, Hudson Institute of Medical Research, Clayton, VIC, Australia; Department of Molecular Translational Science, School of Clinical Sciences, Monash University, Clayton, VIC, Australia*

JAVIER UCEDA FERNANDEZ • *Division of Infection and Immunity, School of Medicine, Cardiff University, Cardiff, Wales, UK*

Richard L. Ferrero • *Centre for Innate Immunity and Infectious Diseases, Hudson Institute of Medical Research, Clayton, Melbourne, VIC, Australia; Department of Microbiology, Biomedicine Discovery Institute, Monash University, Clayton, VIC, Australia*

Ka Yee Fung • *Department of Medical Biology, University of Melbourne, Melbourne, VIC, Australia; Inflammation Division, The Walter and Eliza Hall Institute of Medical Research, Parkville, VIC, Australia*

Michael P. Gantier • *Centre for Innate Immunity and Infectious Diseases, Hudson Institute of Medical Research, Clayton, VIC, Australia; Department of Molecular and Translational Science, Monash University, Clayton, VIC, Australia*

Christoph Garbers • *Institute of Biochemistry, Kiel University, Kiel, Germany*

Tae-Su Han • *Division of Genetics, Cancer Research Institute, Kanazawa University, Kanazawa, Japan*

Elizabeth L. Hartland • *Department of Microbiology and Immunology, Peter Doherty Institute for Infection and Immunity, University of Melbourne, Melbourne, VIC, Australia; Centre for Innate Immunity and Infectious Diseases, Hudson Institute of Medical Research, Clayton, Australia; Department of Molecular and Translational Science, Monash University, Clayton, Australia*

Naoko Hattori • *Division of Epigenomics, National Cancer Center Research Institute, Tokyo, Japan*

David G. Hill • *Division of Infection and Immunity, Systems Immunity University Research Institute, School of Medicine, Cardiff University, Cardiff, Wales, UK*

Thierry Jardé • *Cancer Program, Monash Biomedicine Discovery Institute, Monash University, Clayton, VIC, Australia; The Department of Anatomy and Developmental Biology, Monash University, Clayton, VIC, Australia; Centre for Cancer Research, Hudson Institute of Medical Research, Clayton, VIC, Australia*

Brendan J. Jenkins • *Centre for Innate Immunity and Infectious Diseases, Hudson Institute of Medical Research, Clayton, VIC, Australia; Department of Molecular Translational Science, School of Clinical Sciences, Monash University, Clayton, VIC, Australia*

Ricky W. Johnstone • *Gene Regulation Laboratory, Peter MacCallum Cancer Centre, Melbourne, VIC, Australia; Sir Peter MacCallum Department of Oncology, University of Melbourne, Parkville, VIC, Australia*

Gareth W. Jones • *Division of Infection and Immunity, Systems Immunity University Research Institute, School of Medicine, Cardiff University, Cardiff, Wales, UK*

Simon A. Jones • *Division of Infection and Immunity, School of Medicine, Cardiff University, Cardiff, Wales, UK*

Andrew Keniry • *The Walter and Eliza Hall Institute, Parkville, VIC, Australia; Department of Medical Biology, University of Melbourne, Melbourne, VIC, Australia*

Catherine L. Kennedy • *Department of Microbiology and Immunology, Peter Doherty Institute for Infection and Immunity, University of Melbourne, Melbourne, VIC, Australia*

Genevieve Kerr • *Cancer Program, Monash Biomedicine Discovery Institute, Monash University, Clayton, VIC, Australia; The Department of Anatomy and Developmental Biology, Monash University, Clayton, VIC, Australia*

Ariena Kersbergen • *ACRF Stem Cells and Cancer Division, The Walter and Eliza Hall Institute of Medical Research, Parkville, VIC, Australia*

Deborah Knight • *Gene Regulation Laboratory, Peter MacCallum Cancer Centre, Melbourne, VIC, Australia*

NICHOLAS P. D. LIAU • *The Walter and Eliza Hall Institute of Medical Research, Parkville, Melbourne, VIC, Australia; Department of Medical Biology, University of Melbourne, Melbourne, VIC, Australia*
JENNII LUU • *Victorian Centre for Functional Genomics, Peter MacCallum Cancer Centre, Melbourne, VIC, Australia*
VICTORIA G. LYONS • *School of Biochemistry and Immunology, Trinity Biomedical Sciences Institute, Trinity College Dublin, Dublin 2, Ireland; Department of Molecular and Translational Science, Hudson Institute of Medical Research, Monash University Faculty of Medicine, Nursing and Health Sciences, Clayton, VIC, Australia*
PIYUSH B. MADHAMSHETTIWAR • *Victorian Centre for Functional Genomics, Peter MacCallum Cancer Centre, Melbourne, VIC, Australia*
ASHLEY MANSELL • *Centre for Innate Immunity and Infectious Diseases, Hudson Institute of Medical Research, Clayton, VIC, Australia; Department of Molecular Translational Science, School of Clinical Sciences, Monash University, Clayton, VIC, Australia*
MATTHEW P. MCCORMACK • *Australian Centre for Blood Diseases, Monash University, Melbourne, VIC, Australia*
CLAIRE E. MCCOY • *Department of Molecular and Translational Science, Hudson Institute of Medical Research, Monash University Faculty of Medicine, Nursing and Health Sciences, Clayton, VIC, Australia; Molecular and Cellular Therapeutics, Royal College of Surgeons in Ireland, Dublin 2, Ireland*
DAVID MILLRINE • *Division of Infection and Immunity, School of Medicine, Cardiff University, Cardiff, Wales, UK*
IVA NIKOLIC • *Victorian Centre for Functional Genomics, Peter MacCallum Cancer Centre, Melbourne, VIC, Australia*
MASANOBU OSHIMA • *Division of Genetics, Cancer Research Institute, Kanazawa University, Kanazawa, Japan*
GENEVIÈVE PÉPIN • *Centre for Innate Immunity and Infectious Diseases, Hudson Institute of Medical Research, Clayton, VIC, Australia; Department of Molecular and Translational Science, Monash University, Clayton, VIC, Australia*
NATALIE L. PAYNE • *Australian Regenerative Medicine Institute, Monash University, Clayton, VIC, Australia*
TRACY PUTOCZKI • *Department of Medical Biology, University of Melbourne, Melbourne, VIC, Australia; Inflammation Division, The Walter and Eliza Hall Institute of Medical Research, Parkville, VIC, Australia*
PHILLIP PYMM • *Infection and Immunity Program, Department of Biochemistry and Molecular Biology, Biomedicine Discovery Institute, Monash University, Clayton, VIC, Australia; Australian Research Council Centre of Excellence in Advanced Molecular Imaging, Monash University, Clayton, VIC, Australia*
STEFAN ROSE-JOHN • *Institute of Biochemistry, Kiel University, Kiel, Germany*
CONNIE ROSS • *Institute for Molecular Bioscience and IMB Centre for Inflammation and Disease Research, The University of Queensland, St. Lucia, Australia*
SALEELA M. RUWANPURA • *Centre for Innate Immunity and Infectious Diseases, Hudson Institute of Medical Research, Clayton, VIC, Australia; Department of Molecular Translational Science, School of Clinical Sciences, Monash University, Clayton, VIC, Australia*
MOHAMED SAAD • *Centre for Innate Immunity and Infectious Diseases, Hudson Institute of Medical Research, Clayton, VIC, Australia; Department of Molecular Translational Science, School of Clinical Sciences, Monash University, Clayton, VIC, Australia*

KATE SCHRODER • *Institute for Molecular Bioscience and IMB Centre for Inflammation and Disease Research, The University of Queensland, St. Lucia, Australia*
TIMOTHY SEMPLE • *Molecular Genomics, Peter MacCallum Cancer Centre, Melbourne, VIC, Australia*
BENJAMIN J. SHIELDS • *Australian Centre for Blood Diseases, Monash University, Melbourne, VIC, Australia*
JAKE SHORTT • *School of Clinical Sciences at Monash Health, Monash University, Clayton, VIC, Australia*
KATIE SIME • *Division of Infection and Immunity, Systems Immunity University Research Institute, School of Medicine, Cardiff University, Cardiff, Wales, UK*
KAYLENE J. SIMPSON • *Victorian Centre for Functional Genomics, Peter MacCallum Cancer Centre, Melbourne, VIC, Australia; Sir Peter MacCallum Department of Oncology, University of Melbourne, Parkville, VIC, Australia*
KATE D. SUTHERLAND • *ACRF Stem Cells and Cancer Division, The Walter and Eliza Hall Institute of Medical Research, Parkville, VIC, Australia; Department of Medical Biology, The University of Melbourne, Parkville, VIC, Australia*
MICHELLE D. TATE • *Centre for Innate Immunity and Infectious Diseases, Hudson Institute of Medical Research, Clayton, VIC, Australia; Department of Molecular Translational Science, School of Clinical Sciences, Monash University, Clayton, VIC, Australia*
TONY TIGANIS • *Department of Biochemistry and Molecular Biology, Biomedicine Discovery Institute, Monash University, Melbourne, VIC, Australia; Peter MacCallum Cancer Centre, Melbourne, VIC, Australia*
LE SON TRAN • *Centre for Innate Immunity and Infectious Diseases, Hudson Institute of Medical Research, Clayton, Melbourne, VIC, Australia; Department of Microbiology, Biomedicine Discovery Institute, Monash University, Clayton, VIC, Australia*
TOSHIKAZU USHIJIMA • *Division of Epigenomics, National Cancer Center Research Institute, Tokyo, Japan*
JULIAN P. VIVIAN • *Infection and Immunity Program, Department of Biochemistry and Molecular Biology, Biomedicine Discovery Institute, Monash University, Clayton, VIC, Australia; Australian Research Council Centre of Excellence in Advanced Molecular Imaging, Monash University, Clayton, VIC, Australia*
ROSS VLAHOS • *School of Health and Biomedical Sciences, RMIT University, Bundoora, VIC, Australia*
FLORIAN WIEDE • *Department of Biochemistry and Molecular Biology, Biomedicine Discovery Institute, Monash University, Melbourne, VIC, Australia; Peter MacCallum Cancer Centre, Melbourne, VIC, Australia*
ANWEN S. WILLIAMS • *Division of Infection and Immunity, Systems Immunity University Research Institute, School of Medicine, Cardiff University, Cardiff, Wales, UK*

Part I

Experimental Model Systems

Chapter 1

In Vivo Models of Inflammatory Bowel Disease and Colitis-Associated Cancer

Ka Yee Fung and Tracy Putoczki

Abstract

A single layer of epithelial cells separates luminal antigens from the host immune system throughout the gastrointestinal tract. A breakdown in the integrity of the epithelial barrier can lead to chronic inflammation, which is associated with numerous complications including cancer. Here we describe three experimental protocols to chemically induce acute and chronic inflammatory bowel disease (IBD) symptoms and colitis-associated colorectal cancer (CRC) progression. These in vivo mouse models are based on the induction of damage to the colonic epithelium, resulting in an inflammatory and wound healing response. In addition, we outline colonoscopy procedures to monitor the onset of disease in individual live mice.

Key words Colitis, Cancer, Endoscopy, Epithelial cell, Inflammation, Mucosa

1 Introduction

The gastrointestinal tract forms a tightly regulated barrier between the exterior environment, and the largest concentration of immune cells within our body. How the homeostatic regulation of this relationship is maintained is now a major area of research, since numerous gastrointestinal diseases are associated with the loss of epithelial barrier integrity and chronic inflammation. This is highlighted by ulcerative colitis (UC) patients, who have a greater risk of developing colitis-associated colon cancer (CAC) [1–3].

Mouse models highlight that colonic inflammation contributes to cancer progression. These models include the use of the polysaccharide Dextran Sulphate Sodium (DSS) [4, 5]. Unfortunately, the mechanism by which DSS triggers mucosal damage is not clear, and is thought to include inhibition of reverse transcriptase activities within cells, or the formation of nano-lipid complexes that fuse with the epithelial membrane [6, 7].

Azoxymethane (AOM) used in combination with DSS results in the induction of mutations in *β-catenin*, in parallel with an inflammatory microenvironment in the colon [8, 9]. AOM is a

Brendan J. Jenkins (ed.), *Inflammation and Cancer: Methods and Protocols*, Methods in Molecular Biology, vol. 1725,
https://doi.org/10.1007/978-1-4939-7568-6_1, © Springer Science+Business Media, LLC 2018

metabolite of the carcinogen 1,2-dimethylhydrazine that is hydrolyzed into methylazoxymethanol by the cytochrome isoform CYP2E1 in the liver, where AOM is conjugated with glucuronic acid and transported to the gastrointestinal tract through bile secretions [10]. In the colon, β-glucuronidase produced by the bacterium within the resident microflora creates the carcinogenic form of AOM, which induces DNA mutations in the epithelial cells [11].

Not dissimilar to clinical management of human gastrointestinal pathologies, colonoscopy can be used to monitor the health and progression of gastrointestinal pathologies in individual live mice. This provides a means to document changes to disease progression in real-time, and better monitor the health and welfare of experimental mice.

2 Materials

2.1 Mice

All animals should be bred in the same specific pathogen free (SPF) facility on the same genetic background, and age and gender matched.

2.2 Ethical Approval

All described procedures should only be performed following approval by the relevant Institute Animal Ethics or Welfare Committee.

2.3 Reagents

1. Dextran Sulfate Sodium (DSS), MW 36,000–50,000, store at room temperature.
2. Standard drinking water normally provided to mice.
3. Mouse food pellets, mashed into powder.
4. Protein shake powder, for example Vanilla Sustagen, store at room temperature.
5. Azoxymethane (AOM), store at −20 °C.
6. Phosphate buffered Saline (PBS), store at 4 °C.
7. Isoflurane.
8. 10% Neutral Buffered Formalin, store at room temperature.
9. 5 mL plastic storage tubes.
10. Water.
11. Paper towels.

2.4 Equipment

1. Class II down-flow recirculating laminar flow cabinet.
2. Pipettes, 0.100–0.200 mL, single channel.
3. Small petri dishes, 60 × 13 mm.

4. Anaesthetic machine, including an induction box and nose cone.
5. Karl Storz Coloview miniendoscopic system.
   (a) Endovision Tricam and 3-Chip camera head.
   (b) Xenon 175 light source with anti-fog pump.
   (c) HOPKINS straight forward Telescope, diameter 1.9 mm.
   (d) Examination and protection sheath.
   (e) Fibre Optic Light Cable and air hose.
6. Computer with media player software.
7. Scale for small animals.
8. Dissection kit, including scissors and forceps.
9. 50 mL syringe, and 0.100 mL pipette tip.
10. 20 gauge needles.
11. Standard bright-field microscope with 10× objective.
12. 500 mL Beaker.

3 Methods

3.1 Induction of Acute Mucosal Damage and Inflammation in the Colon

1. All experimental mice should be separated from stock mice and placed in boxes dedicated to the experiment (*see* **Notes 1** and **2**).
2. Weigh animals on Day 0 of the experiment and record the weights in a laboratory book.
3. On Day 1 of the experiment, prepare 1.5% (w/v) DSS solution using the drinking water routinely provided to the mice by the animal facility.
   (a) Dilute 1.5 g of DSS in 100 mL of drinking water, mix gently, and decant into a standard mouse drinking apparatus (*see* **Notes 3–5**).
4. Immediately return the drinking water apparatus to the cage, and leave for the mice to drink ad libitum for 5 continuous days (*see* **Note 6**) (Fig. 1a).

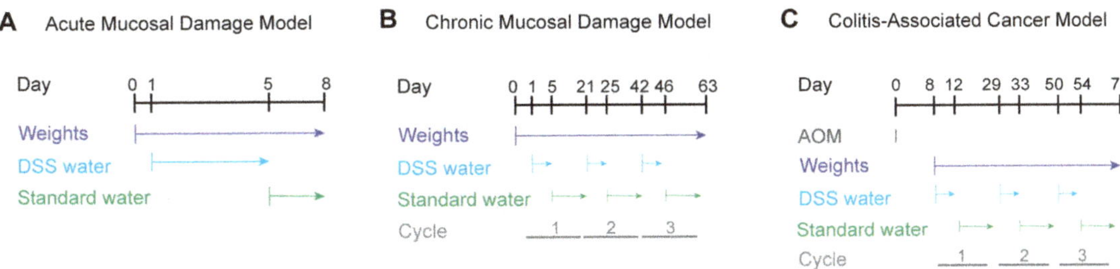

Fig. 1 Schematic illustration of the experimental procedures for (**a**) Acute DSS-induced Colitis, (**b**) Chronic DSS-induced Colitis, and (**c**) Colitis-Associated Cancer

5. Weigh each mouse daily and record the weights in a laboratory book.
6. At the end of Day 5 of DSS administration, remove the DSS water and provide standard mouse drinking water.
7. Place mashed food pellets and a protein supplement decanted into small petri dishes into each cage. Replace daily.
   (a) Combine 100 g of mashed (powdered) food pellets, 10 g protein shake, 10 mL mouse drinking water and stir with a sterile spoon to mix. Decant into small petri dishes, so that the petri dish is full (*see* **Notes** 7 and **8**). Add one petri dish to each cage of mice.
8. After 3 days of standard mouse drinking water, Day 8 of the experiment, euthanize mice by CO_2 intoxication and prepare the colonic tissue for histological analysis (*see* **Note 9**, and Subheading 3.3).
9. Calculate the change in body weight for each mouse on each day of the experiment, with Day 0 representing 100% of the body weight. Graph the results.

3.2 Induction of Chronic Mucosal Damage and Inflammation

1. Follow Procedure 3.1 (Induction of Acute Mucosal Damage and Inflammation in the Colon) **steps 1**–7.
2. Weigh the animals daily and record the weights in a laboratory notebook.
3. Place mashed food pellets and a protein supplement decanted into small petri dishes into each cage. Replace daily for 5 days.
   (a) Combine 100 g of mashed (powdered) food pellets, 10 g protein shake, 10 mL mouse drinking water and stir with a sterile spoon to mix. Decant into small petri dishes, so that the petri dish is full (*see* **Notes** 7 and **8**). Add one petri dish to each cage of mice.
4. Allow mice 16 days of standard mouse drinking water, finishing on Day 21 of the experiment. This is the 'first cycle' of the experiment (*see* **Note 9**) (Fig. 1b).
5. On Day 21 of the experiment, repeat Procedure 3.1 (Induction of Acute Mucosal Damage and Inflammation in the Colon) **steps 1**–**6**. This is the 'second cycle' of the experiment.
6. On Day 42 of the experiment, repeat Procedure 3.1 (Induction of Acute Mucosal Damage and Inflammation in the Colon) **steps 1**–**6**. This is the 'third cycle' of the experiment.
7. On Day 63 of the experiment, euthanize mice by CO_2 intoxication and prepare the colonic tissue for histological analysis (*see* **Note 11**, and Subheading 3.3).

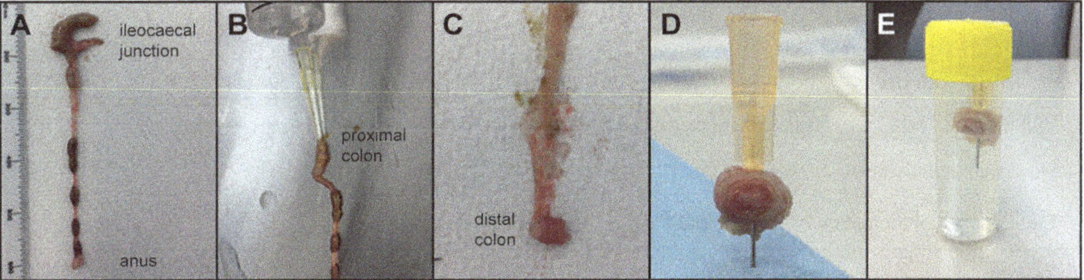

Fig. 2 Preparation of colon tissue for histological assessment. (**a**) Removal of the entire colon from the mouse. (**b**) Flushing fecal matter using PBS. (**c**) Preparation of a 'Swiss roll'. (**d**) A 'Swiss roll' that can then (**e**) be submitted for histological processing

8. Calculate the change in body weight for each mouse on each day of the experiment, with Day 0 representing 100% of the body weight. Graph the results.

3.3 Dissection of the Colon

1. Following ethical euthanasia of the mouse, remove the entire colon and measure the length from the ileocaecal junction to the anus (Fig. 2a) (*see* **Note 12**).
2. Insert a 50 mL syringe with a 0.100 mL pipette tip into the proximal end of the colon (Fig. 2b) and flush the colon with approximately 5 mL of cold PBS (*see* **Note 13**).
3. Lay the colon on a sheet of paper towel with the proximal end away from you, and cut the colon open longitudinally using scissors.
4. Using fine forceps, role the distal end of the colon towards the proximal end of the colon, creating a 'swiss roll' (Fig. 2c) (*see* **Note 14**).
5. Holding the 'swiss roll' with forceps, place a 20 gauge needle through the colon (Fig. 2d).
6. Transfer the 'swiss roll' to 10% neutral-buffered formalin for 24 h (Fig. 2e).
7. Send to a histology service for paraffin blocking and the generation of H&E sections (4 μm thick).

3.4 Histopathological Scoring of the Colon

1. Place slide under a microscope 10× objective, and orient the distal colon in the centre of the field of view (*see* **Note 15**).
2. Score each region of the colon of each individual mouse separately, meaning you will have a score for the distal colon, middle colon, and proximal colon, respectively. Score for epithelial damage, mucosal inflammation and submucosal inflammation as outlined in Fig. 3a. A guide with representative scores has been provided in Fig. 3b.
3. Graph the scores for epithelial damage, mucosal inflammation and submucosal inflammation separately.

A Histology Scoring Parameters

Score	0	1	2	3	4	5	TOTAL
Epithelial Damage	*Normal*	*Hyper-proliferative*	*<50% crypt loss*	*>50% crypt loss*	*100% crypt loss*	*Ulceration*	**0-5**
Mucosal Inflammation	*None*	*Mild*	*Moderate*	*Severe*			**0-3**
Submucosal Inflammation	*None*	*Mild*	*Moderate*	*Severe*			**0-3**

MAXIMUM SCORE 11

B

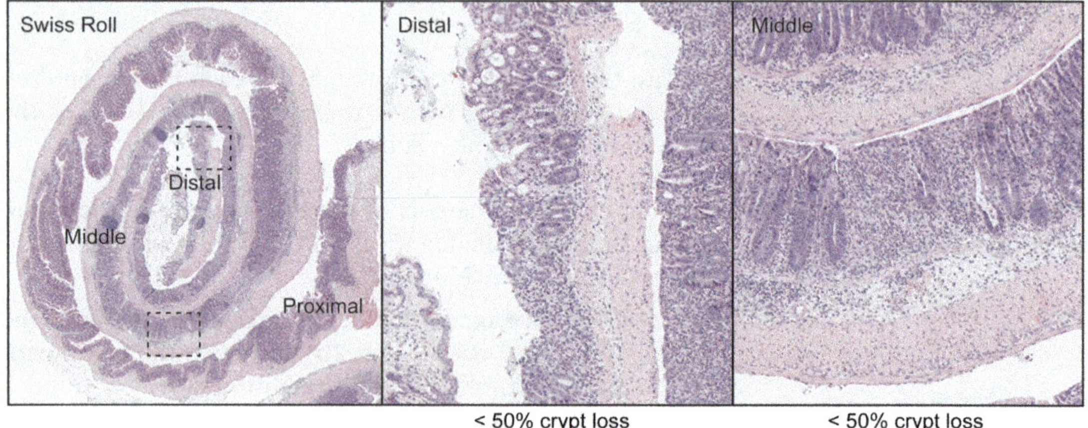

< 50% crypt loss
Moderate mucosal inflammation
Mild submucosal inflammation
SCORE of 5

< 50% crypt loss
Moderate mucosal inflammation
Moderate submucosal inflammation
SCORE of 6

Fig. 3 Severity of colitis can be determined by (**a**) histopathological scores of H&E sections. (**b**) Representative scores are shown

3.5 Induction of Colitis-Associated Cancer

1. All experimental mice should be separated from stock mice and placed in boxes dedicated to the experiment (*see* **Notes 1** and **2**).
2. Weigh animals on Day 0 of the experiment and record the weights in a laboratory book.
3. On Day 1, inject, intraperitoneally, each mouse with 10 mg/kg (w/w) Azoxymethane (AOM). All boxes should be handled according to cytotoxic policies.
   (a) Prepare stock solutions of AOM at a concentration of 1 mg/mL diluted in sterile PBS and store at −20 °C (*see* **Notes 16–19**).
4. On Day 7, all animal bedding should be changed following standard cytotoxic procedures. Animals are no longer considered cytotoxic.
5. On Day 8, prepare 1.5% (w/v) DSS solution and provide to the mice ad libitum.

(a) Dilute 1.5 g of DSS in 100 mL of drinking water, mix gently, and decant into a standard mouse drinking apparatus (*see* **Notes 3–5**).

6. On Day 8, resume daily weighing of the animals and record the weights in laboratory notes.
7. On Day 13, remove the DSS solution and replace with normal drinking water.
8. Place mashed food pellets and a protein supplement decanted into small petri dishes into each cage. Replace daily for 5 days.
   (a) Combine 100 g of mashed (powdered) food pellets, 10 g protein shake, 10 mL mouse drinking water and stir with a sterile spoon to mix. Decant into small petri dishes, so that the petri dish is full (*see* **Note** 7 and **8**). Add one petri dish to each cage of mice.
9. Allow mice 16 days of standard mouse drinking water, finishing on Day 28 of the experiment. This is the 'first cycle' of the experiment (Fig. 1c).
10. On Day 29 of the experiment, repeat **steps 5–8**. This is the 'second cycle' of the experiment.
11. On Day 50 of the experiment, repeat **steps 5–8**. This is the 'third cycle' of the experiment.
12. On Day 72 of the experiment, euthanize mice by CO_2 intoxication and prepare the colonic tissue for histological analysis (*see* Subheading 3.3).
13. In addition, count the number of macroscopically visible tumors in the colon, and measure their length and width (*see* **Note 20**).
14. Calculate the change in body weight for each mouse on each day of the experiment, with Day 0 representing 100% of the body weight (*see* **Note 21**). Graph the results.
15. Calculate the total macroscopically visible tumor burden for each mouse by adding the individual tumor area (length × width) together. Graph the results.
16. Graph the total number of macroscopically visible tumors for each mouse.

3.6 Monitoring of Mice by Colonoscopy

1. Turn on the Coloview Endoscopy Unit, air pump and computer.
2. Anesthetize live mice in an induction chamber with 3% isoflurane and 100% oxygen at a flow rate of 0.4 L/min.
3. Once breathing has stabilized to 1 breath per second, remove a mouse from the induction chamber and secure the head in a nose cone, with the mouse positioned ventral side up and the hind legs comfortably stretched out behind.

4. Maintain the isoflurane flow to the nose cone at 0.5–2% for the endoscopy procedure.
5. Insert the endoscope sheath up to 3 cm into the rectum (*see* **Notes 22** and **23**).
6. Initiate video recording at any stage of the endoscopy procedure using standard media software run by a computer.
7. On completion of endoscopy, return the mouse to its cage and monitor for recovery from anesthetic.
8. On completion, clean all equipment for storage.

3.7 Scoring Colonoscopy Videos for Colitis

1. Endoscopy (Subheading 3.6) is generally performed on day 0, 5 and 8 of the acute DSS model (Subheading 3.1).
2. Endoscopy (Subheading 3.6) is generally performed during the second week of water in each cycle of the chronic DSS model (Subheading 3.2).
3. Colitis severity should be determined following the Murine Endoscopic Index of Colitis Severity (MEICS [12]) guidelines. This allows documentation of changes in (1) the thickness of the colon wall, indicated by transparency, (2) stool consistency, (3) blood vessel integrity and presence, (4) ulcers and areas of epithelial regeneration that present as granular ridges, (5) bleeding indicated by fibrin. Scoring parameters are provided in Fig. 4a, b.

3.8 Scoring Colonoscopy Videos for Tumor Formation

1. Endoscopy (Subheading 3.6) is generally performed during the second week of water in each cycle of the CAC model (Subheading 3.5).
2. Record tumor number and size. Tumor size is determined by the diameter of the colon lumen occupied by a tumor [8]. Scoring parameters are provided in Fig. 5a, b.

4 Notes

1. The use of female mice will permit co-housing of mice from different lines, limit box numbers, and reduce cage-to-cage variation.
2. Variations in microflora between animal facilities should be taken into consideration when determining the appropriate control mice and genotypes for each experiment [13]. Only mice bred in the same animal facility should be compared.
3. When preparing DSS assume one mouse drinks 5 mL of water per day. This will assist with determining the volume of DSS water that is appropriate for each experiment. For example, 12 mice × 5 days = prepare 300 mL of DSS.

A MEICs Scoring Parameters for Colonoscopy

Score	0	1	2	3	TOTAL
Thickening of colon	*Transparent*	*Mild*	*Moderate*	*Thickened*	**0-3**
Stool consistency	*Normal*	*Soft*	*Loose*	*Runny*	**0-3**
Granularity	*Smooth*	*Mild*	*Moderate*	*Severe*	**0-3**
Vasculature	*None*	*Mild*	*Moderate*	*Severe*	**0-3**
Fibrin	*None*	*Mild*	*Moderate*	*Severe*	**0-3**

MAXIMUM SCORE 15

B

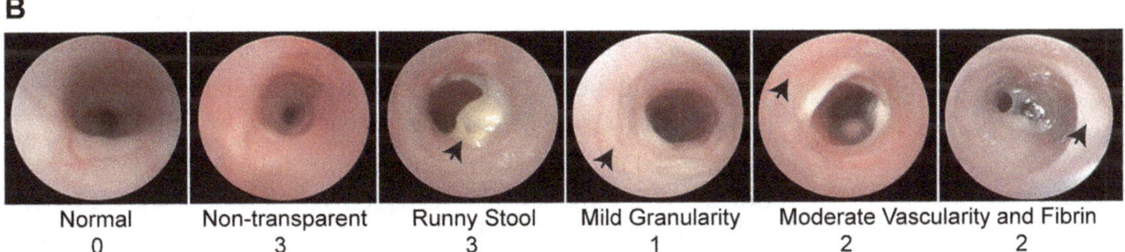

Fig. 4 Colitis severity can be monitored using the (**a**) Murine Endoscopic Index of Colitis Severity (MEICs) scoring parameters. (**b**) Representative scores

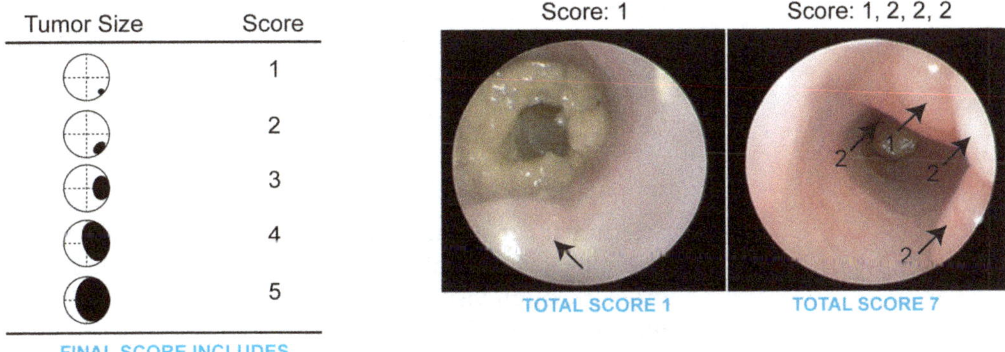

Fig. 5 Visible tumors can be scored by colonoscopy. (**a**) Scoring guidelines and (**b**) representative scores

4. DSS is an irritant and should be handled in accordance with MSDS instructions.
5. There can be batch-to-batch variations in DSS. On receipt of a new batch compare 1.5%, 2% and 2.5% DSS induction of clinical pathology in mice, and choose the best concentration

for use in all future studies. The appropriate dosage should be based on weight-loss (not greater than 20% of original weight) and confirmed colitis histopathology.

6. Once made up in solution, DSS degrades with time. If any of the drinking apparatuses leak, new DSS will need to be prepared for each cage of mice in order to ensure consistency in the experiment.
7. The provision of standard mouse food pellets, wet mashed, with a protein supplement ensures that mice do not suffer from dehydration, and assists with management of weight-loss. Weight-loss, diarrhea and bloody stools are all clinical features of this model. Lethargy, ruffled fur, hunching and reduced movement should be monitored, and animals euthanized if their welfare appears compromised.
8. Do not provide mashed food when the mice are receiving DSS in their drinking water, to ensure that the mice drink the water.
9. Mice should be euthanized if they experience ≥20% weight-loss for more than three consecutive days.
10. 5 days of DSS in the drinking water, followed by 16 days of normal drinking water is referred to as 'one cycle'. For the induction of chronic DSS induced mucosal damage 'three cycles' are performed.
11. All mice should be euthanized on Day 63, or when the mice experience ≥20% weight-loss for more than three consecutive days, whichever occurs first.
12. Most of the mucosal damage induced by DSS occurs at the most distal portion of the colon right down to the anus, meaning that it is essential to remove this portion of the colon for histological analysis.
13. Flushing the colon with PBS removes any fecal matter.
14. A "Swiss roll" allows for histological analysis of the entire colon on one slide.
15. Starting at the distal colon, using the skin around the anus as a guide to location, allows you to orient yourself. You can then move through visualizing the remaining colon, with the middle and proximal colon then easier to distinguish.
16. AOM is a carcinogen and should be handled in accordance with MSDS instructions.
17. AOM should not be freeze thawed. In general, each mouse will receive 250 μg of AOM based on the average weight of an 8 week old mouse, which equates to 0.250 mL per mouse at a 1 mg/mL stock concentration.
18. Routine batch testing of AOM is required to establish the appropriate AOM dosage in order to circumvent toxicity to

mice due to batch-to-batch variation. AOM is commonly used at 8–12 mg/kg.

19. During Days 1–7 following AOM administration, weights will be stable and do not need to be recorded to avoid handling animals that will excrete cytotoxic metabolites in their feces.
20. Generally, tumors are visible by Day 40 of the CAC model by colonoscopy and therefore the third cycle of DSS can be omitted if necessary.
21. All mice should be euthanized on Day 72, or when the mice experience $\geq$20% weight-loss for more than three consecutive days, whichever occurs first.
22. Confirm the rate of airflow through the endoscopy sheath by placing the tip of the endoscopy sheath in a beaker of water. One air bubble at a time should emerge from the sheath.
23. The airflow will permit the colon to inflate. If the airflow is too strong, air will be pumped into the stomach of the mouse.

Acknowledgment

We thank Paul Nguyen for provision of histology images.

References

1. Rutter M, Saunders B, Wilkinson K et al (2004) Severity of inflammation is a risk factor for colorectal neoplasia in ulcerative colitis. Gastroenterology 126:451–459
2. Eaden JA, Abrams KR, Mayberry JF (2001) The risk of colorectal cancer in ulcerative colitis: a meta-analysis. Gut 48:526–535
3. Lakatos PL, Lakatos L (2008) Risk for colorectal cancer in ulcerative colitis: changes, causes and management strategies. World J Gastroenterol 14:3937–3947
4. Perse M, Cerar A (2012) Dextran sodium sulphate colitis mouse model: traps and tricks. J Biomed Biotechnol 2012:718617
5. Rose WA 2nd, Sakamoto K, Leifer CA (2012) Multifunctional role of dextran sulfate sodium for in vivo modeling of intestinal diseases. BMC Immunol 13:41
6. Laroui H, Ingersoll SA, Liu HC et al (2012) Dextran sodium sulfate (DSS) induces colitis in mice by forming nano-lipocomplexes with medium-chain-length fatty acids in the colon. PLoS One 7:e32084
7. Miyazawa F, Olijnyk OR, Tilley CJ et al (1967) Interactions between dextran sulfate and Escherichia coli ribosomes. Biochim Biophys Acta 145:96–104
8. Neufert C, Becker C, Neurath MF (2007) An inducible mouse model of colon carcinogenesis for the analysis of sporadic and inflammation-driven tumor progression. Nat Protoc 2:1998–2004
9. Schwitalla S, Ziegler PK, Horst D et al (2013) Loss of p53 in enterocytes generates an inflammatory microenvironment enabling invasion and lymph node metastasis of carcinogen-induced colorectal tumors. Cancer Cell 23:93–106
10. Fiala ES (1977) Investigations into the metabolism and mode of action of the colon carcinogens 1,2-dimethylhydrazine and azoxymethane. Cancer 40:2436–2445
11. Chen J, Huang XF (2009) The signal pathways in azoxymethane-induced colon cancer and preventive implications. Cancer Biol Ther 8:1313–1317
12. Becker C, Fantini MC, Neurath MF (2006) High resolution colonoscopy in live mice. Nat Protoc 1:2900–2904
13. Ivanov I, Atarashi K, Manel N et al (2009) Induction of intestinal Th17 cells by segmented filamentous bacteria. Cell 139:485–498

Chapter 2

Combining Cell Type-Restricted Adenoviral Targeting with Immunostaining and Flow Cytometry to Identify Cells-of-Origin of Lung Cancer

Sarah A. Best, Ariena Kersbergen, Marie-Liesse Asselin-Labat, and Kate D. Sutherland

Abstract

Lung cancers display considerable intertumoral heterogeneity, leading to the classification of distinct tumor subtypes. Our understanding of the genetic aberrations that underlie tumor subtypes has been greatly enhanced by recent genomic sequencing studies and state-of-the-art gene targeting technologies, highlighting evidence that distinct lung cancer subtypes may be derived from different "cells-of-origin". Here, we describe the intra-tracheal delivery of cell type-restricted Ad5-Cre viruses into the lungs of adult mice, combined with immunohistochemical and flow cytometry strategies for the detection of lung cancer-initiating cells in vivo.

Key words Recombinant adenovirus, Intra-tracheal injection, Immunohistochemical staining, Tissue dissociation, Flow cytometry, Cells-of-origin

1 Introduction

Traditionally, lung cancers are broadly classified into two main histopathological groups, non-small cell lung cancer (NSCLC) and small cell lung cancer (SCLC). NSCLC constitutes approximately 80% of lung cancers, and is a heterogeneous group of diseases comprising of adenocarcinomas (ADC), squamous cell carcinoma (SCC) and large cell carcinoma. The remaining 20% of lung cancers exhibit features of neuroendocrine differentiation and are classified as SCLC. Interestingly, different tumor subtypes reside in distinct anatomical locations, consistent with the cell-of-origin hypothesis [1]. In addition to morphology and expression of histopathological markers, molecular profiling studies comparing the expression signatures of normal cellular subsets to cancer subtypes highlight a close association between cell-lineage and cancer phenotype [2]. However, it is becoming clear that histopathology is

Brendan J. Jenkins (ed.), *Inflammation and Cancer: Methods and Protocols*, Methods in Molecular Biology, vol. 1725,
https://doi.org/10.1007/978-1-4939-7568-6_2, © Springer Science+Business Media, LLC 2018

not always a true reflection of the cellular origins and ultimately a complex interplay between genetic/epigenetic alterations, the nature of the cell-of-origin and extrinsic factors culminate to influence the fate and resulting tumor phenotype [3].

The adult airway is a highly ordered branched structure that contains populations of regional stem and progenitor cells responsible for maintenance and repair of airway epithelia throughout adult life. In the proximal airways, elegant in vivo lineage tracing studies, combined with in vitro colony formation assays have shown that basal cells ($NGFR^+$, $K5^+$, $K14^+$) act as stem cells that have the ability to self-renew, and give rise to club, ciliated and goblet cells [4]. Club cells ($Scgb1a1/CC10^+$) line the bronchi and bronchioles and constitute a progenitor cell population that self-renew to give rise to differentiated ciliated cells ($FoxJ1^+$) [5], while pulmonary neuroendocrine cells ($CGRP^+$) are a rare terminally differentiated cell population located in the intrapulmonary airways, often at airway bifurcations. In response to injury, neuroendocrine cells proliferate, but fail to replenish cells of other epithelial lineages [6]. The alveolar compartment is composed of squamous alveolar type I (ATI; $T1\alpha^+$), and secretory alveolar type II (AT2; SPC^+) cells responsible for gas-exchange. AT2 cells exhibit progenitor cell activity, having the ability to self-renew and give rise to AT1 cells following lung injury [7]. The anatomical location and morphology, combined with the expression of specific cellular markers, allows us to identify distinct epithelial cell types by traditional immunohistochemical techniques. More recently, novel fluorescence-activated cell sorting (FACS) strategies have been developed that enable the isolation of epithelial cells ($EpCAM^+$; epithelial cell adhesion molecule) from mouse and human lung tissue [2, 8]. In the adult mouse lung, $EpCAM^+$ cells can be further subdivided based on their expression level of CD104 (β4 integrin) [8], defining alveolar ($EpCAM^+CD104^-$) and bronchiolar ($EpCAM^+CD104^+$) populations. Further division of the bronchiolar population using CD24 (heat-stable antigen) [8] enriches for ciliated ($CD24^+$) and club ($CD24^-$) cells generating multiple parameters for cell characterization in normal and tumor-bearing lungs.

To investigate the cellular origins of lung cancer, a series of recombinant adenoviruses with expression of Cre-recombinase under the control of apromoter specifically active in basal (Ad5-K5-Cre, Ad5-K14-Cre), club (Ad5-CC10-Cre), neuroendocrine (Ad5-CGRP-Cre), and AT2 cells (Ad5-SPC-Cre) have been generated [9, 10]. Importantly, intra-tracheal administration of these cell type-restricted Ad5-Cre viruses into $p53^{f/f}$;$Rb1^{f/f}$ mice demonstrated that neuroendocrine ($CGRP^+$) cells are the predominant cell-of-origin of SCLC [10], while both club and AT2 cells have the ability to give rise to adenocarcinoma formation following oncogenic $K\text{-}ras^{G12D}$ activation concomitant with *p53* loss [11].

The protocols described herein have been adapted for the in vivo targeting of distinct lung epithelial cell lineages, and their subsequent assessment as lung cancer-initiating cells utilizing powerful conditional targeting technology.

2 Materials

Prepare all solutions using ultrapure water (prepared by purifying deionized water to obtain a sensitivity of 18 ΩM-cm at 25 °C) and analytical grade reagents. Prepare and store all reagents at room temperature (RT; unless otherwise indicated).

2.1 Adenoviral Infection

1. Mice: Cre-reporter; *mT/mG* [12] and conditional mouse strains, $K\text{-}ras^{LSL\text{-}G12D/+}$;$p53^{f/f}$ [13] (*see* **Note 1**).
2. High titer Adenovirus-Cre (Ad5-Cre) viruses (University of Iowa, Gene Transfer Core) (*see* **Note 2**).
3. Phosphate-buffered saline (PBS): 2.85 g/L $NaHPO_4 \cdot 2H_2O$ (16 mM HPO_4), 0.625 g/L $NaH_2PO_4 \cdot 2H_2O$ (4 mM PO_4), 8.7 g/L NaCl (149 mM NaCl).
4. Intubation device (UNO Roestvrijstaal).
5. Light source (Zeiss KL1500 LCD).
6. 2 French (0.012″/0.3 mm ID × 0.025″/0.6 mm OD) × 25′ polyurethane catheter (Access Technologies).
7. Weighing scales.
8. 29G × ½ (0.33 × 12 mm) needle.
9. 1 mL insulin syringe.
10. Two curved tissue Forceps.
11. Warming pads.
12. Mouse anesthetic: 1 mg/mL Xylazil (Troy Laboratories), 5 mg/mL Ketamine (Hospira).
13. Eye lubricant.
14. Ruler.
15. Scissors.
16. Cotton thread.

2.2 Immunohistochemistry

1. 5 mL syringe.
2. 21G 1 ½ TW (0.8 mm × 38 mm) PrecisionGlide™ Needle.
3. 4% (w/v) Paraformaldehyde (PFA), pH 7.4. Add 4 g PFA in 90 mL of PBS, preheated to 60 °C. Dissolve, while stirring on a heat-block. Allow the solution to reach room temperature, and then adjust the pH to 7.4 with the addition of 1 M HCl (*see*

Note 3). Store in 10 mL aliquots in polypropylene tubes at −20 °C.

4. PBS.
5. PBS containing 0.2% Triton X-100 (PBST).
6. 3% hydrogen peroxidase (v/v) in deionized water (dH_2O).
7. Blocking solution: 5% normal goat serum in PBS.
8. Dako PAP pen.
9. Antibodies: anti-GFP (Abcam, ab6556), biotinylated goat anti-rabbit IgG antibody.
10. Humid Chamber.
11. Paper towels or Whatman™ paper.
12. Kimwipes™.
13. VECTASTAIN Elite ABC HRP Kit (Peroxidase, Standard) (Vector Laboratories). Stored at 4 °C.
14. ImmPACT DAB Peroxidase (HRP) Substrate (Vector Laboratories) (*see* **Note 4**). Stored at 4 °C.
15. 70%, 80%, 95% and 100% Ethanol in Wheaton glass Coplin staining jars.
16. Xylene/histolene in Wheaton glass Coplin staining jar.
17. Oven for baking slides at 60 °C.

2.3 Dissociation of Mouse Lung Tissue

1. McIlwain tissue chopper (Mickle Laboratory Engineering) (*see* **Note 5**).
2. Double edge shaving blades.
3. Dulbecco PBS (DPBS).
4. DPBS/glucose: 0.2 g/L glucose in DPBS. Filter sterilize with a 0.22 μm filter and store at 4 °C (*see* **Note 6**).
5. Fetal Bovine Serum (FBS), stored in 50 mL aliquots at −20 °C.
6. Collagenase I: 20 mg/mL collagenase I dissolved in DPBS/glucose and filter sterilized. Store as 1 mL aliquots at −20 °C.
7. Red blood cell lysis buffer: 8 g/L NH_4Cl in dH_2O. Filter sterilize with a 0.22 μm filter and store at 4 °C.
8. Wash buffer: DPBS, 2% FBS.
9. 40 μm cell strainer, sterile individually wrapped.
10. 18G and 21G needles.
11. 5 mL syringe.
12. 15 and 50 mL sterile polypropylene tubes.
13. Shaking incubator 160 rpm 37 °C.
14. 0.4% trypan blue solution.
15. Hemocytometer counting chamber.

2.4 Flow Cytometry

1. DPBS.
2. FBS, stored in 50 mL aliquots at −20 °C.
3. Antibodies and reagents for flow cytometry (diluted in wash buffer):
   (a) FcR blocking reagent (CD16/CD32).
   (b) Rat IgG.
   (c) 1/250 CD31-PE-Cy7.
   (d) 1/250 CD45-PE-Cy7.
   (e) 1/200 EpCAM-APC-Cy7.
   (f) 1/100 CD104-PE.
   (g) 1/200 CD24-APC.
4. Propidium Iodide (PI).
5. 5 mL round bottom FACS tubes with 35 μm cell strainer snap caps.
6. Tissue culture hood with a light that can be switched off (*see* **Note** 7).
7. Eppendorf 1.5 mL tubes.

3 Methods

3.1 Intra-tracheal Adenoviral Infection

Preparation and administration of adenoviruses should be carried out in a Class II biosafety hood, according to the guidelines for Biosafety Level 2 Research.

1. Preparation of cannula: Insert the ultra-fine 29G needle inside the catheter tubing and push all the way to the hilt of the needle. Using a ruler, measure 28 mm of the catheter from the tip of the needle (not the hilt) and cut the catheter with scissors (*see* **Note 8**) (Fig. 1a).
2. Anesthetize mice by intra-peritoneal injection of 400 units Xylazil/Ketamine (inject 0.4 mL per 20 g mouse weight) using an insulin syringe. Confirm the mice are fully anesthetized by ensuring that they lack a toe reflex. Apply eye lubricant to both eyes to maintain moisture.
3. To place the mouse in the intubation device, hold the mouse face up in your right hand. Loop the lasso end of the string around the top teeth of the mouse (Fig. 1b). Pull the mouse face up into the nose-cone area of the stand, making sure that only the front teeth are in the cone. Loop the string around the knob and secure it, using tape at the base of the stand. Direct a cold light source on the mouse's upper chest to aid in the visualization of the opening of the trachea.

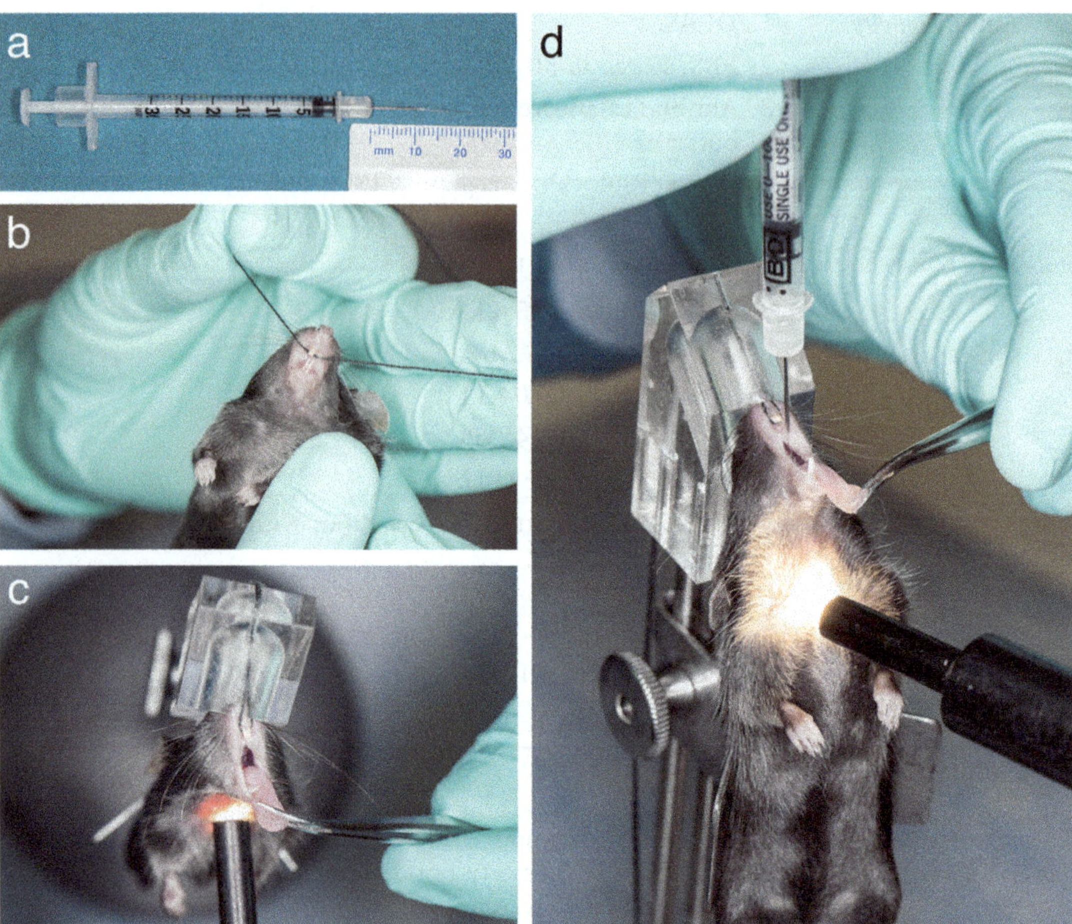

Fig. 1 Intra-tracheal injection of recombinant adenoviruses. (**a**) The cannula is prepared by inserting an ultra-fine needle inside catheter tubing. (**b**) String is looped around the top teeth of the anesthetized mice, and the mouse placed in the intubation device. (**d**) The mouth is opened and the tongue is gently pulled out using flat forceps. (**d**) The cannula is inserted and the virus is slowly injected via the trachea into the lungs

4. To prepare the needle, first fill the syringe with 100 μL of air, before taking up 20 μL of Ad5-Cre virus (*see* **Note 9**), then take up an additional 50 μL of air.
5. Pick up two curved forceps, one in each hand. Use the tweezers to open the mouth and fixate the tongue (Fig. 1c). When the vocal cords are clearly visible, insert the cannula in between the vocal cords into the trachea (Fig. 1d).
6. Inject the Ad5-Cre virus very slowly into the lung, without damaging the surrounding tissues.
7. Remove the cannula and carefully take the mouse out of the intubation device. Mice are placed back into their cage atop a warming pad and monitored until fully conscious.

3.2 Immuno-histochemistry

1. At the defined time-point following Ad5-Cre delivery (*see* **Note 10**), euthanize the mouse by CO_2 asphyxiation. This will avoid bleeding into the thoracic cavity. Expose the lung and trachea, and using a 5 mL syringe filled with PFA, insert the needle into the trachea and inflate the lungs with PFA. Store lungs in PFA for 24 h at 4 °C.
2. Prepare paraffin-embedded lungs (*see* **Note 11**; Fig. 2a) and cut 3 μm sections onto Superfrost Plus coated glass slides.

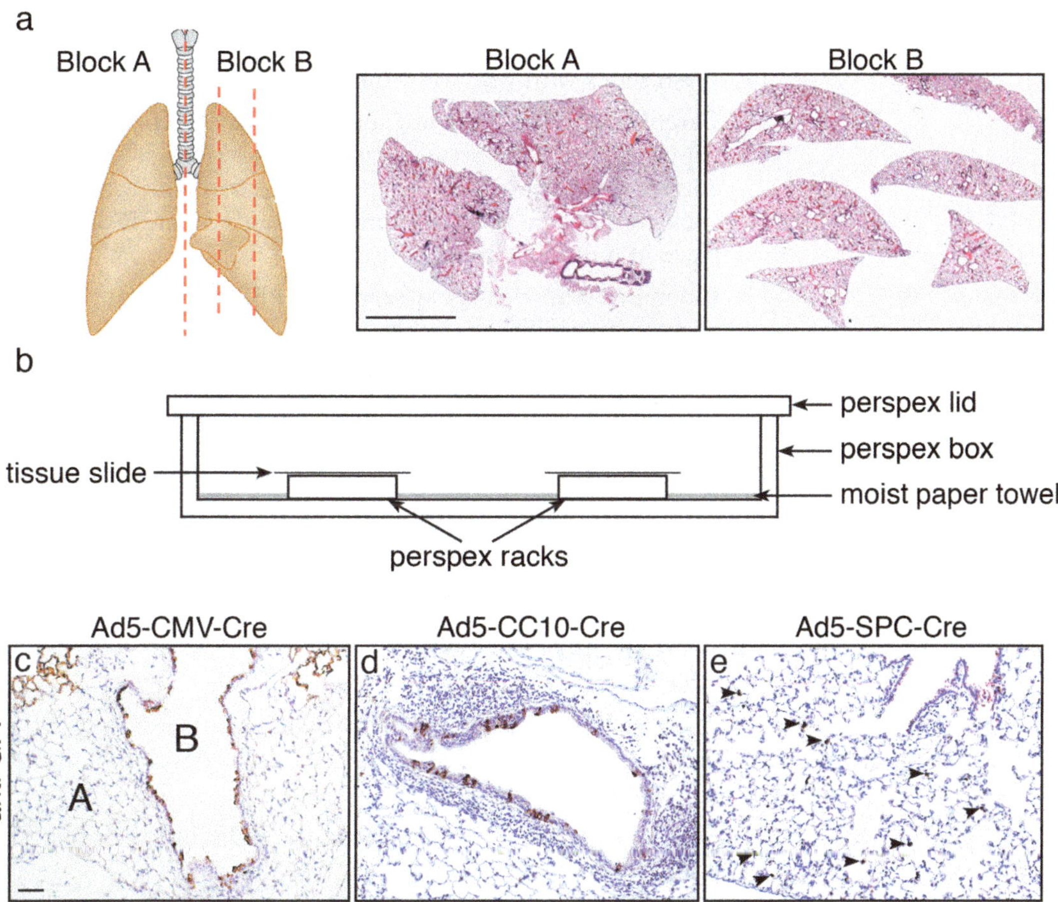

Fig. 2 Cre-recombined "switched" cells can be identified by immunohistochemical staining. (**a**) Schematic diagram of an adult mouse lung. Sagittal cuts as indicated by the red lines, are made in the right-hand lobe. H&E-stained lung sections following tissue processing. Scale bar; 5 mm. (**b**) Schematic representation of a humidified chamber. (**c–e**) Anti-GFP immunostaining of lung tissue sections from *mT/mG* reporter mice, 2 weeks following administration of cell type-restricted Ad5-Cre viruses, reveals distinct expression patterns. (**c**) GFP^+ cells can be detected lining the bronchioles (A) and within the alveolar epithelium (B) of *mT/mG* mice following Ad5-CMV-Cre-infection. (**d**) Switching was observed in the cells lining the bronchioles, but not in the alveolar epithelium of Ad5-CC10-Cre-infected *mT/mG* mice. (**e**) Following Ad5-SPC-Cre-infection, GFP^+ cells were observed in AT2 cells resident in the alveoli but not in bronchiolar epithelium. Arrows indicate GFP^+ "switched" AT2 cells. Scale bar (**c–e**); 50 μm

3. Dewax slides by baking at 60 °C for 1 h then hydrate in graded alcohols for 1–2 min each.
4. Wash slides with H_2O for 5 min.
5. Wash slides with PBS for 5 min.
6. Wash slides with PBST for 3 min.
7. Wash slides twice with PBS for 5 min.
8. Wash slides with H_2O for 5 min.
9. Quench endogenous peroxidase activity in 3% H_2O_2 for 10 min.
10. Wash slides with H_2O for 5 min.
11. Wash slides with PBS for 5 min.
12. Carefully dry the areas around each tissue section with Kimwipes. Drying the areas around the sections allows for the correct application of PAP pen, otherwise the wax will not stick to the wet slide. Outline sections with a PAP pen and place in humid chamber (Fig. 2b).
13. Block in 5% normal goat serum in PBS for 30 min at RT in perspex humidified chamber.
14. Apply primary antibody (1:400 anti-GFP) in 1% BSA/0.1% Triton X-100, incubate overnight at 4 °C in humidified chamber.
15. The following day, wash slides three times with PBS for 5 min.
16. Apply secondary antibody (biotinylated), diluted to 1:300 in blocking solution for 30 min at RT.
17. Wash slides three times with PBS for 5 min.
18. Apply peroxidase-conjugated Streptavidin for 30 min at RT.
19. Wash slides three times with PBS for 5 min.
20. Apply liquid DAB (one drop DAB per 1 mL buffer) and incubate for 30 s–5 min. Check for color development under a light microscope
21. Stop DAB reaction by immersing the slides in a slide box filled with tap water for 5 min.
22. Immuno counterstain in hematoxylin for 30 s and Scotts tap water for 1 min (clear in running tap water after each step), then dehydrate in graded alcohols for 1–2 min each, and clear in two changes of histolene and mount slides in DPX (coverslip).

3.3 Dissociation of Mouse Lung Tissue

1. At the defined time-point following Ad5-Cre delivery (*see* **Note 10**), euthanize the mouse by CO_2 asphyxiation. This will avoid bleeding into the thoracic cavity. Open the thoracic cavity and excise the lungs using standard dissection procedures.

2. Harvest lungs in DPBS on ice.
3. Transfer lungs onto plastic disc and install into McIlwain tissue chopper. Chop in three directions.
4. Transfer the finely minced tissue into a 50 mL Falcon tube containing 2.7 mL DPBS/glucose and 0.3 mL collagenase per lung (*see* **Note 12**). Place the tube in an orbital shaker and agitate (160 rpm) at 37 °C for 20 min.
5. Dissociate the sample by passing the cell suspension through an 18G needle attached to a 5 mL syringe three times. Place the tube in the orbital shaker and agitate (160 rpm) at 37 °C for 20 min. Pass the cell suspension once more through a 21G needle attached to a 5 mL syringe three times.
6. Wash the digestion with 20 mL of DPBS/2% FBS and centrifuge at 400 × *g* for 5 min at 4 °C.
7. Discard supernatant, being careful to remove all liquid without disrupting the pellet.
8. Resuspend the cell pellet in 1 mL DPBS/2% FBS. Add 4 mL of Red Blood Cell lysis buffer (pre-warmed to 37 °C) and swirl to mix. Incubate for 3 min at RT. To stop the lysis reaction, add 15 mL of 2% FCS/DPBS.
9. Filter the cell suspension into 40 μm cell strainer (*see* **Note 13**). Take aliquot of cells for cell counting and spin the cells at 400 × *g* for 5 min.
10. Count the cells using 1:1 mix of trypan blue on a hemocytometer. Calculate cell number using 20 mL total volume
11. Cells are now ready to be stained for flow cytometry.

3.4 Preparing Cells for Flow Cytometry

1. For blocking of non-specific binding, incubate cells with anti-FcR (1:80 CD16/CD32) and Rat IgG (stock 1 mg/mL, 1:10) in DPBS/2% FBS in a volume of 40 μL/1 × 10^6 cells for 15 min (*see* **Note 14**).
2. Generate antibody mixtures in eppendorf tubes. Remove 5 μL blocked cells for each control sample: unstained, single-stained controls, and Fluorescence Minus One (FMO) using CD24 as the excluded antibody (*see* **Note 15**).
3. Add antibody mixes directly to the blocked cells and incubate on ice in the dark for 25 min.
4. Wash labeled cells to remove unbound antibodies by adding 20 mL of DPBS/2% FBS.
5. Centrifuge at 400 × *g* for 5 min at 4 °C. Discard the supernatant.
6. Prepare 4 mL of PI (1/1000 of the stock solution in DPBS/2% FCS). Resuspend cells in PI at a concentration of 8–10 × 10^6 cells/mL (*see* **Note 16**).

7. Filter cells into FACS tube with cell strainer cap. Cells are now ready for flow cytometry analysis.

3.5 Flow Cytometry

1. Initiate flow cytometry machine and software.
2. Run unstained control sample to generate appropriate voltages for FSC (forward scatter) and SSC (side scatter) (*see* **Note 17**).
3. Run single stained control samples to identify appropriate voltages for each antibody. After voltages are set, re-run each control and save at least 1000 events to generate a compensation strategy (*see* **Note 18**).
4. Generate gating strategy (Fig. 3a), including:
   (a) FSC-A v SSC-A: gate large cells, remove small debris.
   (b) FSC-H v FSC-W: gate single cells.
   (c) PI v FSC-A: gate PI negative live cells.
   (d) PEcy7 v FSC-A: gate PEcy7 negative lineage negative cells (Fig. 3a, left panel).
   (e) APCcy7 v PE: gate alveolar and bronchiolar cells (Fig. 3a, middle panel)
   (f) APC histogram: gate ciliated and club cell-enriched populations (Fig. 3a, right panel)
5. Run FMO control sample to generate negative and positive CD24 gating strategy (*see* **Note 19**).
6. Run lung sample. Acquire at least 200,000 events in order to generate measurable populations in EpCAM and CD24 gates. For *mT/mG* mouse strain analysis, first gate on GFP positive cells, prior to EpCAM analysis (Fig. 3b). For tumor models, such as *K-ras*$^{\text{LSL-G12D/+}}$;*p53*$^{\text{f/f}}$, expanded tumor cell population is identified as the alveolar population using this analysis (Fig. 3c), consistent with the predominant cellular origin of this tumor [11, 14, 15].

4 Notes

1. All experiments performed with animals should be conducted in accordance with protocols approved by the Local Animal Ethics Committee. One of the most well-characterized mouse models of human lung adenocarcinoma is based on the activation of oncogenic *K-ras*$^{\text{G12D}}$ (*K-ras*$^{\text{LSL-G12D/+}}$) along with loss of *p53* (*p53*$^{\text{f/f}}$), herein referred to as *K-ras*$^{\text{LSL-G12D/+}}$;*p53*$^{\text{f/f}}$ mice [13]. The *mT/mG* reporter mouse strain expresses membrane-targeted tandem dimer Tomato (*mT*) in all cells, and membrane-targeted GFP (*mG*) in cells that have undergone Cre-mediated recombination [12].

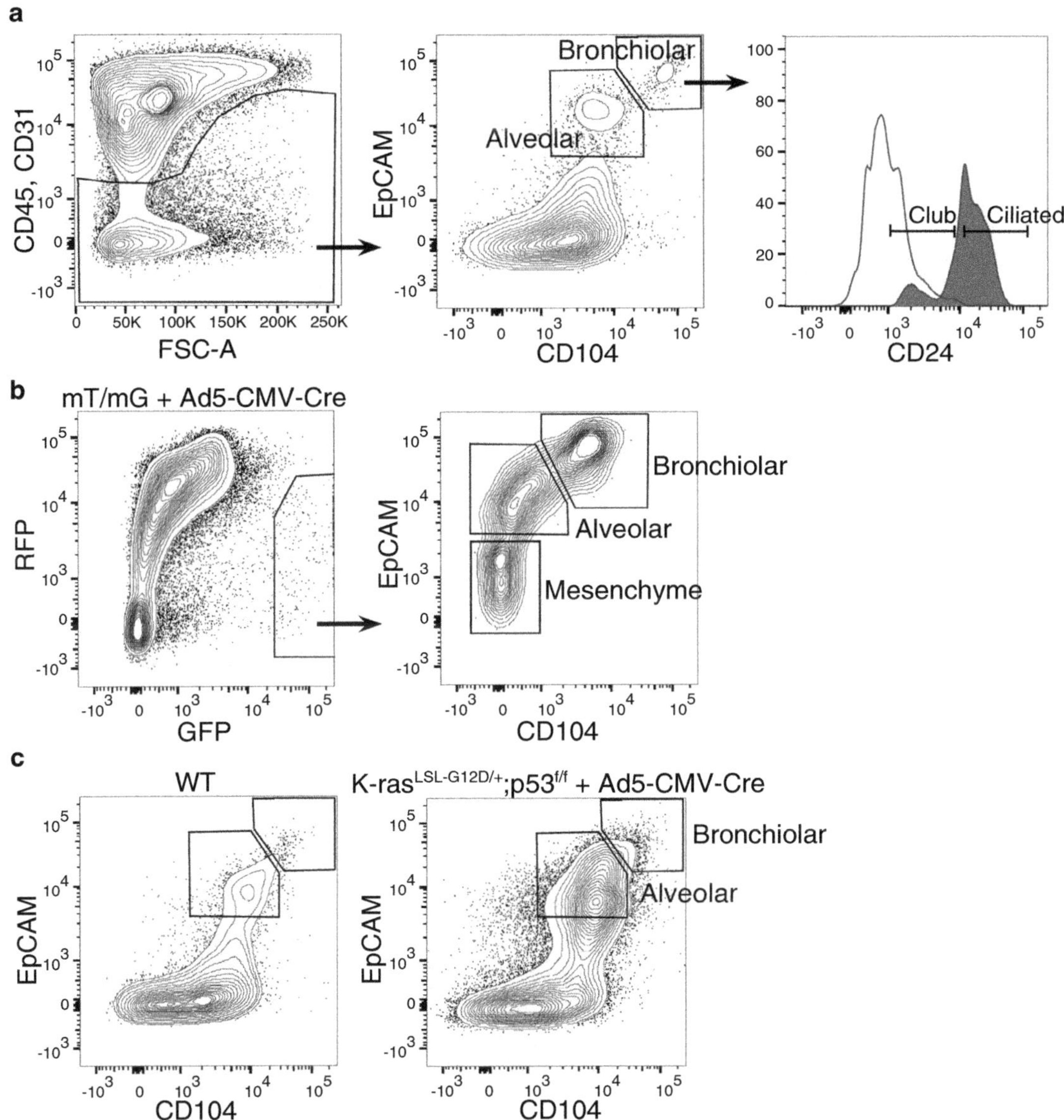

Fig. 3 Flow cytometry analysis of lung epithelial cells. (**a**) Schematic of flow cytometry to obtain alveolar ($EpCAM^+CD104^-$), bronchiolar ($EpCAM^+CD104^+$), club ($EpCAM^+CD104^+CD24^-$) and ciliated ($EpCAM^+CD104^+CD24^+$) cell populations. (**b**) Representative FACS plot of *mT/mG* reporter mice analyzed 2 weeks following Ad5-CMV-Cre infection. (**c**) Representative FACS plot of *Kras*$^{LSL\text{-}G12D/+}$;*p53*$^{f/f}$ mice following Ad5-CMV-Cre infection 2 months post adenovirus infection

2. A number of different titered Ad5-Cre viruses are available from the University of Iowa Gene Transfer Core. The Ad5-CMV-Cre virus, whereby *Cre*-recombinase is under the control of the ubiquitous CMV promoter, is used to direct *Cre*-mediated recombination in a variety of lung epithelial cell types. While *Cre*-recombinase expression can be limited to

club (Ad5-CC10-Cre), alveolar type 2 (Ad5-mSPC-Cre), neuroendocrine (Ad5-CGRP-Cre) and basal (Ad5-K5-Cre, Ad5-K14-Cre) cells through use of the respective cell type-restricted viruses as previously described [9, 10].

3. Paraformaldehyde is highly toxic and contact with the skin, eyes or mucous membrane should be avoided. Preparation should be carried out in a biosafety hood, while wearing a protective mask and safety glasses.
4. Diaminobezidene (DAB) is a carcinogen and should be handled with great care, using gloves and protective wear. Unused compound can be disposed of as a hazardous waste, neutralized using a potassium permanganate-sulfuric acid procedure.
5. The McIlwain tissue chopper is advised for mincing tissues. It is set up using four paper discs (generated using Whatman™ paper) and one plastic disc, inserted into the stand. A razor is attached loosely into the arm, and lowered onto the discs, to generate the ideal razor placement. Tighten the razor onto the arm at this point.
6. Tissue dissociation: It is critical to use DPBS that contains Ca^{2+} and Mg^{2+}. Standard PBS is Ca^{2+}/Mg^{2+}-free and the enzymatic digestion with collagenase will not work properly without these ions.
7. It is important that the tissue culture hood light is turned off when fluorescent antibodies are in use. Light exposure will decrease the efficacy of fluorescence which will impact the signal by flow cytometry.
8. The length of the cannula may need to be adjusted when using different viruses. For example, a shorter cannula length (18 mm) is used when injecting basal cell-restricted viruses (Ad5-K5-Cre, Ad5-K14-Cre), to ensure that basal cells located in the proximal airways of the adult mouse lung, are efficiently exposed to the injected virus. Adjustments to cannula length may also be required when injecting different mouse strains or mice of different sizes/sexes.
9. High (1.5–2.5 × 10^9 infectious particles) titers of Ad5-Cre viruses are administered in *Rosa26R-LacZ* or *mT/mG* reporter mice [12, 16], in order to visualize Cre-infected "switched" cells under homeostatic conditions. Intra-tracheal injection of 5 × 10^8 infectious particles of Ad5-Cre in *K-ras*$^{LSL\text{-}G12D/+}$ and *p53*$^{f/f}$;*Rb1*$^{f/f}$ mice is sufficient for the generation of sporadic lung tumors [10, 11]. Importantly, there is a direct correlation between adenoviral titer and tumor multiplicity. For example, infection of *K-ras*$^{LSL\text{-}G12D/+}$ mice with 5 × 10^6 PFU of Ad5-CMV-Cre virus resulted in an approximate sixfold increase in tumor number, compared *K-ras*$^{LSL\text{-}G12D/+}$ mice infected with 5 × 10^5 PFU of Ad5-CMV-Cre virus [17].

10. In general, to validate cell type-restricted targeting of Ad5-Cre viruses, *Cre*-reporter mice, (*mT/mG* [12] and *Rosa26R-LacZ* [16]), are sacrificed 2 weeks following Ad5-Cre infection. Collection of conditional tumor-prone strains following Ad5-Cre-infection is dependent upon the following factors: (a) the tumor latency, which differs between models, and is also influenced by the titer of adenovirus injected (*see* **Note 9**) and (b) whether you are interested in examining tumor initiation or tumor progression.
11. Paraffin embedding lung tissue is performed as routinely described [18]. Briefly, following fixation, the lung lobes (left, right and triangular) are separated. Sagittal cuts as outlined in Fig. 2a, are made to the right-hand lobe. The left and triangle lobe are laid flat into Block A, while each piece of cut right lobe, are placed, cut surface down, in Block B (Fig. 2a). Embed all tissue as it is placed for processing.
12. For analysis purposes, individual lungs should not be pooled. For bulk sorting up to five lungs can be pooled per 3 mL digestion mix for tissue dissociation. The efficiency of tissue dissociation is compromised if more than five lungs are pooled for digestion.
13. It is important not to pipette cells in the red blood cell lysis mixture. Pour the solution through the cell strainer to minimize cell loss.
14. For example, for 1×10^6 cells (final volume 40 μL) add: 0.5 μL of anti-FcR and 4 μL rat IgG. Incubate on ice for 10 min.
15. Example antibody mixes for 12.5×10^6 cells (500 μL blocked cells) are outlined in Table 1.
16. PI is toxic to cells. Add just before analysis/sort.
17. Lung epithelial cells are large, caution needs to be taken in the voltage settings in order to generate well-spread events, while keeping the larger cells in range.
18. Some flow cytometry machines (i.e. BD Canto) have software that automatically set the compensation based on the single stained controls. Otherwise, manually set the compensation by eye. It is important to seek the assistance of an experienced flow cytometry user to ensure the voltages and compensation are correct.
19. For initial gating strategy example and additional information, *see* McQualter et al. [8].

Table 1
An example of antibody mixes for 12.5 × 10[6] cells (500 μL blocked cells)

Antibody mix	Antibody (Ab)	Vol. Ab (μL)	Vol. cells (μL)	Vol. PBS (μL)
PEcy7 single stain	CD45 PEcy7	0.2	5	45
APCcy7 single stain	EpCAM APCcy7	0.25	5	45
PE single stain	CD104 PE	0.4	5	45
APC single stain	CD24 APC	0.25	5	45
FMO	CD31 PEcy7 CD45 PEcy7 EpCAM APCcy7 CD104 PE	0.2 0.2 0.25 0.4	5	20
Sample stain	CD31 PEcy7 CD45 PEcy7 EpCAM APCcy7 CD104 PE CD24 APC	2 2 2.5 4 2.5	475	25

Acknowledgement

We thank Ellen Tsui, Cary Tsui and Ji-Ying Song for their expert histological assistance. The intra-tracheal procedure is performed by highly-trained staff following protocols approved by the WEHI Animal Ethics Committee. K.D.S. is supported by the Peter and Julie Alston Centenary Fellowship, M.L.A.-L. is the recipient of The Viertel Charitable Foundation Senior Medical Research Fellowship, and S.A.B is supported by the Victorian Cancer Agency Early-Career Fellowship. This work was made possible through Victorian State Government Operational Infrastructure Support and Australian Government NHMRC IRIISS.

References

1. Sutherland KD, Berns A (2010) Cell of origin of lung cancer. Mol Oncol 4:397–403
2. Weeden CE, Chen Y, Ma SB et al (2017) Lung basal stem cells rapidly repair DNA damage using the error-prone nonhomologous end-joining pathway. PLoS Biol 15:e2000731
3. Sutherland KD, Visvader JE (2015) Cellular mechanisms underlying intertumoral heterogeneity. Trends Cancer 1:15–23
4. Rock JR, Onaitis MW, Rawlins EL et al (2009) Basal cells as stem cells of the mouse trachea and human airway epithelium. Proc Natl Acad Sci U S A 106:12771–12775
5. Rawlins EL, Okubo T, Xue Y et al (2009) The role of Scgb1a1+ Clara cells in the long-term maintenance and repair of lung airway, but not alveolar, epithelium. Cell Stem Cell 4:525–534
6. Song H, Yao E, Lin C et al (2012) Functional characterization of pulmonary neuroendocrine cells in lung development, injury, and tumorigenesis. Proc Natl Acad Sci U S A 109:17531–17536

7. Barkauskas CE, Cronce MJ, Rackley CR et al (2013) Type 2 alveolar cells are stem cells in adult lung. J Clin Invest 123:3025–3036
8. McQualter JL, Yuen K, Williams B et al (2010) Evidence of an epithelial stem/progenitor cell hierarchy in the adult mouse lung. Proc Natl Acad Sci U S A 107:1414–1419
9. Ferone G, Song JY, Sutherland KD et al (2016) SOX2 is the determining oncogenic switch in promoting lung squamous cell carcinoma from different cells of origin. Cancer Cell 30:519–532
10. Sutherland KD, Proost N, Brouns I et al (2011) Cell of origin of small cell lung cancer: inactivation of Trp53 and Rb1 in distinct cell types of adult mouse lung. Cancer Cell 19:754–764
11. Sutherland KD, Song JY, Kwon MC et al (2014) Multiple cells-of-origin of mutant K-Ras-induced mouse lung adenocarcinoma. Proc Natl Acad Sci U S A 111:4952–4957
12. Muzumdar MD, Tasic B, Miyamichi K et al (2007) A global double-fluorescent Cre reporter mouse. Genesis 45:593–605
13. Jackson EL, Olive KP, Tuveson DA et al (2005) The differential effects of mutant p53 alleles on advanced murine lung cancer. Cancer Res 65:10280–10288
14. Mainardi S, Mijimolle N, Francoz S et al (2014) Identification of cancer initiating cells in K-Ras driven lung adenocarcinoma. Proc Natl Acad Sci U S A 111:255–260
15. Xu X, Rock JR, Lu Y et al (2012) Evidence for type II cells as cells of origin of K-Ras-induced distal lung adenocarcinoma. Proc Natl Acad Sci U S A 109:4910–4915
16. Soriano P (1999) Generalized lacZ expression with the ROSA26 Cre reporter strain. Nat Genet 21:70–71
17. Jackson EL, Willis N, Mercer K et al (2001) Analysis of lung tumor initiation and progression using conditional expression of oncogenic K-ras. Genes Dev 15:3243–3248
18. Suvarna KS, Layton C, Bancroft JD (eds) (2013) Bancroft's theory and practice of histological techniques, 7th edn. London, Churchill Livingstone

Chapter 3

Utility of Endoscopic Ultrasound-Guided Fine-Needle Aspiration for Preclinical Evaluation of Therapies in Cancer

William Berry and Daniel Croagh

Abstract

Personalising cancer therapy is a way of improving treatment efficacy, by selecting specific treatments for patients with certain molecular changes to their tumour. This requires both molecular material to detect these targets and a preclinical disease model to demonstrate treatment efficacy. In pancreatic cancer this is problematic, as most patients present with advanced disease and are therefore ineligible for surgery. As a result, biological material derived from such patients has been excluded from all preclinical studies in personalised medicine. This chapter presents methodology to achieve both of the above-mentioned requirements using endoscopic ultrasound-guided fine-needle aspiration, which can be offered to nearly all patients with early or advanced disease.

Key words RNAseq, RNA, Xenograft, Target therapy, Personalised therapy, NOD-SCID mice, EUS-FNA, Pancreatic cancer, Oncology

1 Introduction

Pancreatic cancer (PC) is a highly lethal malignancy, and often patients will present late, with advanced disease. As such, only very few patients are eligible for surgical resection, and the overall 5-year survival remains low at 5%. PC and other malignancies are beginning to look towards personalised therapy, whereby treatments are designed to specifically target mutations unique to individual tumours. In terms of establishing viable therapeutic targets in a pre-clinical setting, two main points need to be addressed. (1) obtain genetic material from the tumour to detect molecular target; (2) demonstrate efficacy for targeted therapy against specific tumour phenotype. In PC, this presents a problem, as genetic material is often obtained from surgery, however, surgery is only offered to 20% of patients. Tissue can also be obtained from percutaneous biopsy of liver metastases but this is often of small volume and quality and thus the majority of patients are not potential candidates for personalised therapy [1].

Brendan J. Jenkins (ed.), *Inflammation and Cancer: Methods and Protocols*, Methods in Molecular Biology, vol. 1725,
https://doi.org/10.1007/978-1-4939-7568-6_3,

Endoscopic ultrasound-guided fine-needle aspirate (EUS-FNA) is a minimally invasive biopsy technique that is an important means of obtaining tissue in PC. It is the predominant method of obtaining tissue from patients with locally advanced PC [1] and with the increasing utilization of neoadjuvant chemotherapy it is likely that EUS-FNA will also be increasingly utilised in patients with resectable PC. This emphasizes the importance of maximizing the potential utility of this technique to guide personalised therapy in PC. However, to date there has been minimal use of EUS-FNA to characterize the genetic profile of PC.

Although DNA has been isolated from these samples in numerous studies [2–9], RNA has only been reported in two studies [10, 11]. Both of these studies performed RNAseq, a highly sensitive sequencing technology to analyse the entire transcriptome. To address this issue, this chapter presents methodology for utilizing EUS-FNA for molecular characterisation of PC based on the isolation of DNA and RNA from EUS-FNA samples.

Any novel personalised therapies will need to be assessed in preclinical models to establish their potential efficacy, prior to embarking on clinical trials. Patient-derived xenografts represent an excellent in vivo model for this purpose [12]. Patient-derived xenograft studies involve the growth of a cancer cells in an immune-deficient mouse, whereby the cancer cells for the xenografts are derived directly from the patient. Xenografted tumours have been shown to retain the characteristics of the original patient tumour in terms of histological architecture and molecular profiles [13–15], which makes xenograft models an ideal tool to demonstrate a biological response to personalised therapies designed to target specific tumour molecular profiles [16]. However, patient-derived xenograft models in PC have been largely restricted to utilizing surgical resection specimens that are only available in approximately 20% of patients. Importantly, there have only been two reports of the use of EUS-FNA samples to create patient-derived xenograft models [10, 17]. Here we present the methodology for using EUS-FNA to develop patient-derived xenograft models in PC and thus allow preclinical trials of targeted therapy in this setting.

2 Materials

2.1 Human Specimen Collection

1. EUS-FNA needle used by Endoscopist to collect tissue for diagnostic, molecular and xenograft purposes (*see* **Note 1**).
2. Microscope, glass slides and *Diff-Quik* stain, used by cytopathologist to confirm adequate cellularity and provide a provisional diagnosis.

3. 1 × 2 mL plastic collection tube with lockable lid labeled with de-identified sample code to collect research sample for molecular studies.
4. 1× specimen jar with 5 mL cell culture medium for collecting research sample for xenograft studies.
5. 2 mL sterile 0.9% saline, used to flush the EUS-FNA needle.
6. Liquid nitrogen in insulated container for snap freezing sample for molecular analyses.
7. Wet ice in insulated container for transporting sample for xenografting.

2.2 Molecular Analyses

1. *Qiagen Universal Allprep kit* (*see* **Note 2**).
2. Supplement *Allprep* lysis buffer with 5% beta-mercaptoethanol.

2.3 Xenograft

1. Cell culture sterile fume hood.
2. Wet ice for transporting samples at ~4 °C.
3. Sterile cell culture petri-dish and scalpel for preparing the sample.
4. 100 μm cell strainer.
5. 15 and 50 mL conical centrifuge tubes for washing and re-suspending the sample.
6. Centrifuge.
7. 1:1 ratio (v/v) of 300 μL of *Matrigel* diluted in cell culture medium (*see* **Note 3**).
8. 4 × 1 mL syringe (for xenograft and analgesic drug delivery).
9. 2 × 27 gauge needles (for xenograft and analgesic drug delivery).
10. 2 × 6 week-old female (preferred for housing logistics) NOD-SCID or NOD-SCID Gamma mice (Non-obese diabetic, severe combined immune deficiency).
11. Isoflurane for light anesthesia with anesthetic chamber.
12. Heat mat and sterile sheet for operating field
13. Caprofen and bupivacaine for peri-operative analgesia for the mice.
14. Recovery cage.
15. Cell culture medium (serum free): RPMI (Roswell Park Memorial Institute) medium supplemented with 1% Penicillin-Streptomycin, 1% L-Glutamine, 1% HEPES (4-(2-hydroxyethyl)-1-piperazineethanesulfonic acid), 1% Non-essential amino acids. Store at 4 °C (*see* **Note 4**).

2.4 Passage of Xenografts

1. Donor NOD-SCID mouse with grafted tumour.
2. Recipient NOD-SCID mice (up to $n = 8$ per 1000 mm^3 tumour).
3. Sterile cell culture petri dish.
4. Thawed 1:1 (v/v) *Matrigel* diluted with cell culture medium.
5. Wet ice in insulated container.
6. Specimen pot with formalin.
7. 1 × 2 mL plastic collection tube with lockable lid.
8. Liquid nitrogen in insulated container.
9. Isoflurane and anesthesia induction chamber, with nose cone and maintenance flow (or injectable anesthesia equipment).
10. Hair clippers.
11. Antiseptic solution (betadine or 80% ethanol).
12. Surgical kit (with dissection scissors, forceps and scalpel).
13. Suturing material or surgical staples for wound closure.
14. Heat mat and sterile sheet for surgical field.
15. Caprofen and bupivacaine for peri-operative analgesia for the mice.
16. 3 × 1 mL syringes for local anaesthesia, analgesia and blood collection.
17. 3 × 27 gauge needles for local anaesthesia, analgesia and blood collection.
18. Recovery cage.

3 Methods

3.1 Human Specimen Collection

1. PC samples were collected from patients undergoing EUS FNA for investigation of a pancreatic mass. Initial diagnostic aspirates from the pancreatic mass were collected using 22 gauge *Procore* needles with 10 cc of suction for immediate cytological assessment (*see* **Note 1**).
2. Cytopathologist confirms the cellular quantity and provides a provisional diagnosis based on the initial passes and diagnostic material is obtained for the cell block, which is then processed according to local pathology service protocol.
3. Additional 1–2 passes were taken from the same position as the diagnostic passes and then either snap-frozen in liquid nitrogen or placed into 5 mL of cell culture medium pot to be kept on wet ice (*see* **Note 5**).
4. To expel samples from the needle stylus replacement was followed by 1 mL flush with 0.9% saline and 5 mL of air (*see* **Note 6**).

3.2 Molecular Analyses

1. Snap frozen EUS-FNA samples are transferred into double the recommended volume of lysis buffer provided in the *Allprep* kit (*see* **Notes 2** and 7).
2. Samples are homogenised and then processed according to the manufacturer's instructions (*see* **Note 8**).

3.3 Xenograft

1. EUS-FNA samples appear as a "worm" of tissue, which is carefully transferred to a sterile petri dish in a cell culture hood.
2. The sample (worm) is minced with a scalpel blade.
3. This slurry of sample and 5 mL cell culture medium is then passed through the 100 μm cell strainer into a 50 mL conical centrifuge tube. This is done with a 1 mL pipette and then gently pressed through the 100 μm strainer with the flat plunger end of a 2–5 mL sterile syringe.
4. Once the majority of the slurry has been strained, invert the strainer and "back-wash" with cell culture medium into the same conical centrifuge tube (*see* **Note 9**).
5. Centrifuge the slurry at 800 × *g* for 5 min (at 4 °C if possible).
6. Remove supernatant.
7. Re-suspend pellet in 5 mL cell culture medium.
8. Centrifuge the slurry at 800 × *g* for 5 min (at 4 °C if possible) to wash sample.
9. Re-suspend pellet in 5 mL cell culture medium.
10. Centrifuge the slurry 800 × *g* for another 5 min (at 4 °C if possible) for final wash.
11. Re-suspend pellet in 300 μL 1:1 (v/v) of *Matrigel* and cell culture medium (*see* **Notes 3** and **4**).
12. Mix gently by slowly pipetting up and down ten times.
13. Draw up 150 μL of slurry into 2 × 1 mL syringes and carefully place on ice (*see* **Note 10**).
14. Maintaining sterility and sample temperature ~4 °C, by keeping all samples on wet ice in a closed container, transport all materials to animal housing facility (*see* **Note 11**).
15. Prepare heat mat, sterile field and a spare recovery cage for mice to rise from sedation.
16. Prepare isoflurane anesthesia chamber.
17. Induce isoflurane anesthesia by placing mouse in induction chamber, then move mouse into position for maintenance dose (onto nose cone with low flow isoflurane) (*see* **Notes 12–14**).
18. Check for adequate sedation using toe or tail pinch and corneal reflex.

19. Once the animal is sedated inject a small volume (10–50 μL) of bupivacaine into the site of the graft (flank) intradermally (*see* **Note 15**).
20. Inject 150 μL of sample slurry into the flank subcutaneously.
21. Inject 50 μL of caprofen into another site subcutaneously (*see* **Notes 12** and **16**).
22. Cease isoflurane flow and administer oxygen or room air until animal wakes.
23. Place animal into recovery cage and monitor.
24. Repeat above steps with second animal.
25. Monitor both animals until effects of anesthesia have worn off.
26. Return 24 h later to administer second dose of caprofen subcutaneously.
27. Monitor mice twice weekly for tumour growth using palpation and digital calipers (*see* **Notes 17** and **18**).

3.4 Passage of Xenografts

1. Prepare surgical equipment and surgical field in animal house fume hood (*see* **Note 11**).
2. Euthanize donor mouse using carbon dioxide induced asphyxiation (*see* **Note 12**).
3. Collect blood for serum if desired via cardiac puncture of venipuncture using a 1 mL syringe and 27 gauge needle.
4. Make a midline incision in the skin on the abdomen of the mouse using surgical scissors and expand this up the midline of the mouse, taking care to only cut the skin and not pierce the abdominal wall.
5. Expose the tumour by creating a large mobile skin flap with the tumour still attached to the skin, but dissected away from the abdominal wall.
6. Dissect away tumour using blunt dissection.
7. Take photos of the tumour with a ruler or measuring device and weigh the tumour.
8. Cut the tumour into quarters.
9. Place one quarter into specimen pot with 5 mL formalin for histology (*see* **Note 19**).
10. Place one quarter into a plastic 2 mL capped tube and then into liquid nitrogen for subsequent molecular analyses.
11. The remaining half (i.e. two quarters) will be used for passaging.
12. In the sterile petri dish, use the scalpel to shave off 2 mm pieces of the fleshy outer layer of the tumour (*see* **Note 20**).
13. Place these into the diluted *Matrigel* and leave on wet ice

14. Anaesthetize one recipient mouse using inhaled isofluorane (*see* **Notes 12** and **13**).
15. Shave the flank of the mouse where the graft will be implanted.
16. Clean the graft sight with antiseptic solution (betadine or 80% ethanol).
17. Make a 2 mm incision in the flank of the animal using surgical scissors.
18. Using blunt dissection create a larger subcutaneous pocket.
19. Carefully implant 2 × 2 mm slices of grafted tumour coated with diluted *Matrigel* into the pocket.
20. Oppose wound edges with forceps and close wound with either sutures or surgical staples.
21. Inject 50 μL bupivacaine intradermally into the wound and surrounding skin (*see* **Note 15**).
22. Inject 50 μL caprofen subcutaneously in a site separate to graft site (*see* **Notes 12** and **16**).
23. Monitor animal until complete recovery from anesthesia.
24. Return in 24 h for a second dose of 50 μL caprofen injected subcutaneously.
25. Repeat this process with all remaining recipient mice
26. Monitor tumour growth in new cohort of mice twice weekly with palpation and digital calipers (*see* **Notes 17**, **18** and **21**).

4 Notes

1. Collection needle will be determined by Endoscopist.
2. It is likely that the RNA or DNA extraction kit is immaterial, however, it is important to use more than the recommended volume of lysis buffer as the amount of sample and type of tissue can result in low or degraded yields if the lysis buffer volume is inadequate.
3. Matrigel needs to be stored at −80 °C and thawed at 4 °C overnight to become a viscous liquid. At room temperature this will set and become solid, therefore care must be taken to ensure Matrigel is kept on ice at 4 °C and needles, syringes and cell culture medium that will come into contact with Matrigel should be kept on ice also.
4. Additional growth factors can be added to supplement cell growth and facilitate grafting, however many of these are already present in *Matrigel.*

5. Number of passes and amount of material available to researchers will be determined by the Endoscopist, local ethical research governance and patient factors.
6. Caution should be taken when expelling samples from needles as this requires handling of the sharp needle. In addition, the flushing of saline and air can result in a splash, eye protection should be worn and care taken to avoid the sample splashing out of the collection tube or pot.
7. Ensure lysis buffer is supplemented with beta-mercaptoethanol to stabilize RNA throughout the process.
8. Make sure extraction process is performed in an RNAase free environment and performed in an efficient manner, as contamination and prolonged time at room temperature can lead to RNA degradation.
9. The purpose of the cell strainer is not to create a single-cell suspension, but to finely break up sample into small enough pieces so that the slurry that can be injected. As such, the "back-wash" step is used to capture any cells that didn't pass through the strainer, but they are still able to be used.
10. It is important that these needles remain sterile and that the contents are not accidentally expelled when they are placed on ice.
11. NOD-SCID and NOD-SCID Gamma mice are severely immunocompromised. Animal housing facility needs to maintain diligent pathogen free environment and all animal handling needs to be performed in a sterile fume hood with sterile surgical gown and gloves.
12. Anesthesia, analgesia and euthanasia protocols should be used in accordance with the local practices of the animal facility, the training of the researcher and the approval of relevant ethical governing bodies.
13. When administering general anesthesia or sedation to animals it is best if two researchers are present, one to monitor the animal's breathing and conscious state, while the other researcher performs the xenograft.
14. High flow oxygen aids recovery and minimizes sedation time, the availability of high flow oxygen on inhaled anesthetic machines is also an important tool to prevent overdose as rapid reversal can be achieved.
15. Bupivicaine is a local anesthetic agent that works for 4–8 h and provides relief as there is a significant stretch of the skin at the site of injection.
16. Caprofen is a non-steroidal anti-inflammatory drug that acts systemically to minimize inflammation, this should be

administered at the time of injection and 24 h later to prevent pain and excessive inflammation.

17. Once tumours reach a maximum size (defined as an ethical end point in ethics approval document), then tumours must be passaged or cryopreserved and the animal humanely sacrificed.
18. Tumour volume calculated using the following formula: $(2 \times \text{Width} \times \text{Length})/2 = V\,\text{mm}^3$.
19. Histology staining should be performed at each passage to confirm cell type and tumour architecture. Xenografts of upper gastrointestinal tumours can commonly grow lymphoma, rather than the desired adenocarcinoma, therefore immunostaining for epithelial markers should be performed.
20. It is important to only use the fleshy out layers of the tumour, as the hard inner layer is fibrotic and paucicellular, as can be seen on the histology studies of the formalin fixed samples. In addition, some larger tumours will have a liquefied core, this is necrosis and therefore not viable grafting tissue.
21. Tumours tend to grow much faster in subsequent passages, therefore care should be taken to monitor these tumours closely.

References

1. Wade TP, Halaby IA, Stapleton DR, Virgo KS, Johnson FE (1996) Population-based analysis of treatment of pancreatic cancer and Whipple resection: Department of Defense hospitals, 1989-1994. Surgery 120:680–687
2. Fuccio L, Hassan C, Laterza L, Correale L, Pagano N, Bocus P, Fabbri C, Maimone A, Cennamo V, Repici A, Costamagna G, Bazzoli F, Larghi A (2013) The role of K-ras gene mutation analysis in EUS-guided FNA cytology specimens for the differential diagnosis of pancreatic solid masses: a meta-analysis of prospective studies. Gastrointest Endosc 78:596–608
3. Bournet B, Souque A, Senesse P, Assenat E, Barthet M, Lesavre N, Aubert A, O'Toole D, Hammel P, Levy P, Ruszniewski P, Bouisson M, Escourrou J, Cordelier P, Buscail L (2009) Endoscopic ultrasound-guided fine-needle aspiration biopsy coupled with KRAS mutation assay to distinguish pancreatic cancer from pseudotumoral chronic pancreatitis. Endoscopy 41:552–557
4. Maluf-Filho F, Kumar A, Gerhardt R, Kubrusly M, Sakai P, Hondo F, Matuguma SE, Artifon E, Monteiro da Cunha JE, Cesar Machado MC, Ishioka S, Forero E (2007) Kras mutation analysis of fine needle aspirate under EUS guidance facilitates risk stratification of patients with pancreatic mass. J Clin Gastroenterol 41:906–910
5. Pellise M, Castells A, Gines A, Sole M, Mora J, Castellvi-Bel S, Rodriguez-Moranta F, Fernandez-Esparrach G, Llach J, Bordas JM, Navarro S, Pique JM (2003) Clinical usefulness of KRAS mutational analysis in the diagnosis of pancreatic adenocarcinoma by means of endosonography-guided fine-needle aspiration biopsy. Aliment Pharmacol Ther 17:1299–1307
6. Tada M, Komatsu Y, Kawabe T, Sasahira N, Isayama H, Toda N, Shiratori Y, Omata M (2002) Quantitative analysis of K-ras gene mutation in pancreatic tissue obtained by endoscopic ultrasonography-guided fine needle aspiration: clinical utility for diagnosis of pancreatic tumor. Am J Gastroenterol 97:2263–2270
7. Takahashi K, Yamao K, Okubo K, Sawaki A, Mizuno N, Ashida R, Koshikawa T, Ueyama Y, Kasugai K, Hase S, Kakumu S (2005) Differential diagnosis of pancreatic cancer and focal pancreatitis by using EUS-guided FNA. Gastrointest Endosc 61:76–79
8. Wang X, Gao J, Ren Y, Gu J, Du Y, Chen J, Jin Z, Zhan X, Li Z, Huang H, Lv S, Gong Y

(2011) Detection of KRAS gene mutations in endoscopic ultrasound-guided fine-needle aspiration biopsy for improving pancreatic cancer diagnosis. Am J Gastroenterol 106:2104–2111

9. Ogura T, Yamao K, Hara K, Mizuno N, Hijioka S, Imaoka H, Sawaki A, Niwa Y, Tajika M, Kondo S, Tanaka T, Shimizu Y, Bhatia V, Higuchi K, Hosoda W, Yatabe Y (2013) Prognostic value of K-ras mutation status and subtypes in endoscopic ultrasound-guided fine-needle aspiration specimens from patients with unresectable pancreatic cancer. J Gastroenterol 48:640–646
10. Berry W, Algar E, Kumar B, Desmond C, Swan M, Jenkins BJ, Croagh D (2017) Endoscopic ultrasound-guided fine-needle aspirate-derived preclinical pancreatic cancer models reveal panitumumab sensitivity in KRAS wild-type tumors. Int J Cancer 140:2331–2343
11. Rodriguez SA, Impey SD, Pelz C, Enestvedt B, Bakis G, Owens M, Morgan TK (2016) RNA sequencing distinguishes benign from malignant pancreatic lesions sampled by EUS-guided FNA. Gastrointest Endosc 84:252–258
12. Morton CL, Houghton PJ (2007) Establishment of human tumor xenografts in immunodeficient mice. Nat Protoc 2:247–250
13. Daniel VC, Marchionni L, Hierman JS, Rhodes JT, Devereux WL, Rudin CM, Yung R, Parmigiani G, Dorsch M, Peacock CD, Watkins DN (2009) A primary xenograft model of small-cell lung cancer reveals irreversible changes in gene expression imposed by culture in vitro. Cancer Res 69:3364–3373
14. Fichtner I, Rolff J, Soong R, Hoffmann J, Hammer S, Sommer A, Becker M, Merk J (2008) Establishment of patient-derived non--small cell lung cancer xenografts as models for the identification of predictive biomarkers. Clin Cancer Res 14:6456–6468
15. Whiteford CC, Bilke S, Greer BT, Chen Q, Braunschweig TA, Cenacchi N, Wei JS, Smith MA, Houghton P, Morton C, Reynolds CP, Lock R, Gorlick R, Khanna C, Thiele CJ, Takikita M, Catchpoole D, Hewitt SM, Khan J (2007) Credentialing preclinical pediatric xenograft models using gene expression and tissue microarray analysis. Cancer Res 67:32–40
16. Rangarajan A, Weinberg RA (2003) Opinion: Comparative biology of mouse versus human cells: modelling human cancer in mice. Nat Rev Cancer 3:952–959
17. Jang SY, Bae HI, Lee IK, Park HK, Cho CM (2015) Successful xenograft of endoscopic ultrasound-guided fine-needle aspiration specimen from human extrahepatic cholangiocarcinoma into an immunodeficient mouse. Gut Liver 9:805–808

Chapter 4

Modelling Intestinal Carcinogenesis Using In Vitro Organoid Cultures

Thierry Jardé, Genevieve Kerr, Reyhan Akhtar, and Helen E. Abud

Abstract

Mouse models of intestinal carcinogenesis are very powerful for studying the impact of specific mutations on tumour initiation and progression. Mutations can be studied both singularly and in combination using conditional alleles that can be induced in a temporal manner. The steps in intestinal carcinogenesis are complex and can be challenging to image in live animals at a cellular level. The ability to culture intestinal epithelial tissue in three-dimensional organoids in vitro provides an accessible system that can be genetically manipulated and easily visualised to assess specific biological impacts in living tissue. Here, we describe methodology for conditional mutation of genes in organoids from genetically modified mice via induction of Cre recombinase induced by tamoxifen or by transient exposure to TAT-Cre protein. This methodology provides a rapid platform for assessing the cellular changes induced by specific mutations in intestinal tissue.

Key words Intestinal organoids, Conditional mutation, Cre recombinase

1 Introduction

The establishment of intestinal organoids was initially described by Sato and colleagues in 2009 [1]. With this method, isolated intestinal crypts, or isolated single stem cells cultured in a cocktail of growth factors in Matrigel, develop into complex organised three dimensional epithelial structures. These structures recapitulate the cellular composition, including the stem cell niche, and closely resemble in vivo intestinal epithelium. This powerful system permits mouse intestinal epithelial cells to be studied, visualised and genetically manipulated in vitro. The specific effects on intestinal stem cells can be studied by isolating single cells and using fluorescent activated cell sorting (FACS) sorting protocols to isolate stem cells by reference to GFP in the case of the Lgr5GFP mouse model or using a combination of cell surface markers [1, 2]. Organoid models can be used to examine the effects of specific environmental signals including immune cells and cytokines [3].

Brendan J. Jenkins (ed.), *Inflammation and Cancer: Methods and Protocols*, Methods in Molecular Biology, vol. 1725, https://doi.org/10.1007/978-1-4939-7568-6_4,

Intestinal organoid culture provides an opportunity to introduce specific mutations and observe their immediate effect in culture [4, 5]. Tissue from conditional mouse models can be used to generate organoid cultures. Specific mutations can be introduced by using inducible Cre recombinase models or generating knockout organoids by introduction of TAT-Cre [6, 7]. Organoid models can be used to confirm intestinal phenotypes, and mutation of tumour suppressor genes commonly found in bowel cancer can be induced in vitro [8, 9]. The accessibility of the organoid cultures permits examination of the interaction between specific mutations and environmental regulators [10]. Here, we describe the steps involved in tamoxifen inducible expression of recombinase driven by VillinCre in intestinal organoids that acts to promote recombination of specific floxed alleles. We also describe an alternative approach of transfection of TAT-Cre which can be utilised in organoid cultures containing floxed alleles without the requirement of an endogenous Cre recombinase allele. FACS sorting of positive cells within organoids permits the establishment of purified cultures containing specific mutations.

2 Materials

All reagents should be prepared using ultrapure water from Milli-Q Advantage A10 water purification system.

2.1 Isolation of Crypts from Tissue and Organoid Culture

1. Wildtype mice or mice containing desired floxed or Cre recombinase alleles (males and females 6–12 weeks old).
2. 1× Phosphate buffered Saline (PBS) pH 7.4, use ice cold.
3. 4 mM Ethylenediaminetetraacetate (EDTA) pH 8.0 in PBS, keep on ice.
4. 70 μm cell strainer.
5. Growth factor reduced, phenol red free Matrigel (*see* **Note 1**).
6. 15 and 50 mL tubes, 9 cm Petri dishes, 10 mL Serological pipettes.
7. Bench top centrifuge.
8. Automatic P1000 pipette, P200 and P100 manual pipettes.
9. Crypt culture medium reagents: DMEM/F12, GlutaMax, Hepes, Penicillin/Streptomycin, N2 supplement, B27 supplement, retinoic acid free, Fungizone, Mouse recombinant EGF, Mouse recombinant Noggin, Mouse recombinant R-spondin-1 or 5% R-spondin-1 conditioned media. Aliquot all reagents at stock concentration and store them at −20 °C (*see* **Note 2**).
10. Test tube rotating wheel in a 4 °C fridge.
11. CO_2 incubator.
12. 24 well plates (*see* **Note 3**).

2.2 Isolation of Single Cells from Intestinal Tissue and Organoids, FACS Sorting and Single Cell Seeding

1. Fetal bovine serum.
2. Reagents for dissociation medium, TrypLE Express, Y-27632, DNAse 1.
3. Jagged-1.
4. 96 well plates.
5. Single cell culture medium: DMEM/F12, GlutaMax, Hepes, Penicillin/Streptomycin, N2 supplement, retinoic acid free B27 supplement, Fungizone, CHIR (GSK-3 inhibitor), Mouse recombinant EGF, Jagged-1, Mouse recombinant Noggin, Mouse recombinant R-spondin-1, Wnt-3a, and Y-27632. Aliquot all reagents at stock concentration and store them at −20 °C.

2.3 Induction of Cre Recombinase and Transfection Using TAT-Cre

1. Tamoxifen. Make 0.5 mM stock by dissolving 1.86 mg in 10 mL DMSO.
2. TAT-Cre recombinase.

2.4 Analysis of Cell Viability

1. PrestoBlue solution.
2. Black 96 well plates.

3 Methods

3.1 Crypt Isolation and Organoid Culture

1. Make basal medium by adding the following stock solutions: 46.9 mL DMEM/F12, 500 μL N2, 1 mL B27, 500 μL glutamax, 500 μL Penicillin Streptomycin, 500 μL 1 M HEPES, 100 μL Fungizone (*see* **Note 4**).
2. Make the crypt culture medium by adding the following reagents to 948 μL basal medium: 5% R-spondin-1 conditioned media (or 500 ng/mL recombinant R-spondin-1), 1 μL 50 μg/mL EGF (final concentration 50 ng/mL), 1 μL 100 μg/mL Noggin (final concentration 100 ng/mL).
3. Euthanise mouse and dissect out small intestine (about 20 cm). Flush twice with cold PBS using a 25 mL syringe to remove faeces.
4. Remove any fragments of adipose tissue by dissecting them away. Cut the intestine longitudinally with small scissors and gently scrape with a glass coverslip to remove villi (*see* **Note 5**).
5. Cut the intestine into small pieces (5 mm) and transfer into a 50 mL tube containing 25 mL ice cold PBS (*see* **Note 6**).
6. Wash the tissue pieces by inverting the tube 20 times to remove unattached epithelial fragments, mucus and faeces. After the pieces settle to the base of the tube, discard supernatant. Repeat this step five times.

7. Incubate the intestinal tissues in 4 mM EDTA in PBS in a 50 mL tube on a tube rotator machine at 10 rpm at 4 °C for 30 min.
8. Discard the supernatant and wash the tissue pieces with 25 mL cold PBS by gently inverting the tube 20 times. Discard the supernatant (this fraction is enriched for villus fragments), and re-suspend in 20 mL PBS.
9. Mechanically pipette tissue samples vigorously ten times (using a 10 mL pipette and an automatic pipettor, force the tissue fragments to go through the pipette) and collect the crypt enriched supernatant. Repeat this process a total of three times and combine the three fractions in a 50 mL tube.
10. Centrifuge the sample for 3 min ($453 \times g$) at 4 °C and discard the supernatant.
11. Re-suspend the cell pellet with 20 mL PBS and transfer in a new 50 mL tube containing a 70 μm cell strainer to remove cell clumps and mucus. Wash the tube and strain with another 20 mL of PBS. Centrifuge the pool for 3 min (1500 rpm) at 4 °C.
12. Discard the supernatant, re-suspend the cell pellet in 10 mL PBS and transfer into a 15 mL tube. Centrifuge the tube for 3 min (1500 rpm) at 4 °C (*see* **Note 7**).
13. Discard the supernatant and re-suspend with 400 crypts per 30 μL of Matrigel.
14. Seed 30 μL of Matrigel to each well of a pre-warmed 24 well plate (spread out the Matrigel as much as possible to form a thin layer of Matrigel without touching the edge of the well) (*see* **Note 8**), and incubate at 37 °C for 10 min until Matrigel has solidified.
15. Add 500 μL of pre-warmed crypt culture medium in each well and incubate at 37 °C and 5% CO_2 in a humidified atmosphere (*see* **Note 9**).
16. Typically, the organoids start to form after 1–2 days in culture and start budding after 3–4 days (Fig. 1a). Replace crypt culture medium every 2–3 days.
17. 7–10 days after initial culture (Fig. 1b), the organoids need to be passaged. Discard culture medium, add 500 μL PBS and mechanically dissociate the Matrigel with a P1000 pipette (20–30 times up and down). Transfer the dissociated Matrigel and organoids into a 15 mL tube. Wash the well again with 500 μL PBS and transfer into the 15 mL tube.
18. Centrifuge the tube for 3 min (1500 rpm) at 4 °C. Discard the supernatant and re-suspend with Matrigel (1/3–1/6 split ratio).

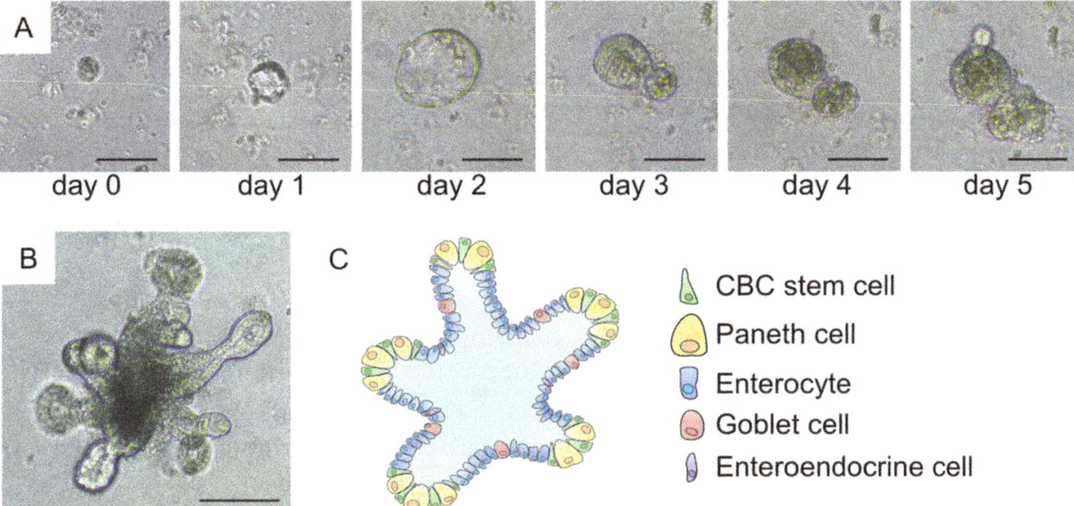

Fig. 1 Crypt isolation and organoid culture. (**a**) Small intestinal organoid growth over 5 days from a single isolated crypt. (**b**) Mature small intestinal organoid maintained in culture for 8 days with several protruding buds. (**c**) Schematic diagram of an intestinal organoid. Scale bars = 100 μm

19. Seed 50 μL of Matrigel on pre-warmed 24 well plate (spread out the Matrigel as much as possible to form a thin layer of Matrigel without touching the edge of the well), and incubate at 37 °C for 10 min until Matrigel has solidified.
20. Add 500 μL of pre-warmed crypt culture medium in each well and incubate at 37 °C and 5% CO_2.

3.2 Isolation of Single Cells from Tissue

1. Make basal medium as per Subheading 3.1, **step 1**.
2. Make the single cell culture medium by adding the following reagents to 984 μL basal medium: 1 μL 50 μg/mL EGF (final concentration 50 ng/mL), 1 μL 100 μg/mL Noggin (final concentration 100 ng/mL), 10 μL 100 μg/mL R-spondin-1 (final concentration 100 ng/mL), 1 μL 10 mM Y-27632 (final concentration 10 μM), 1 μL 100 μg/mL Wnt-3a (final concentration 100 ng/mL), 2 μL 500 μM Jagged-1 (final concentration 1 μM) and 0.25 μL 10 mM CHIR (final concentration 2.5 μM).
3. Complete **steps 1–11** according the crypt isolation method.
4. Discard supernatant, resuspend the pellet in 10 mL DMEM/F12 containing 10% FBS (this step is required to improve cell viability) and place at 4 °C for 30 min.
5. Add 30 mL PBS to the 50 ml tube, invert 20 times and centrifuge for 3 min (1500 rpm) at 4 °C.
6. Discard supernatant, resuspend the pellet in PBS, invert 20 times and centrifuge the tube for 3 min (1500 rpm) at 4 °C.

7. Discard the supernatant and resuspend the cell pellet in dissociating solution (1 mL TrypLE Express supplemented with 10 μM Y-27632 and 50 units DNAse 1) for 4 min at 37 °C.
8. Add 100 μL FBS, mix 20 times with a P1000 pipette, and resuspend in 20 mL PBS.
9. Transfer to a new 50 mL tube through a 70 μm cell strainer. Wash the tube and strain with another 20 mL of PBS. Centrifuge the tube for 5 min (1500 rpm) at 4 °C.
10. Discard supernatant, resuspend the pellet in PBS, invert 20 times and centrifuge the tube for 5 min (1500 rpm) at 4 °C. Cells are then ready for antibody labelling for FACS sorting.
11. In order to sort cells with organoid-forming capacities, a recent paper has described a new cell surface marker mediated strategy (combining six markers) that allows isolation of pure intestinal stem cells [2]. All antibody labelling steps are carried out in a 500 μL volume for 15 min on ice. After each antibody labelling step, cells are washed with 10 mL cold PBS and pelleted at 1500 rpm for 5 min. The cells are then resuspended in a final volume of 1 mL, passed through a 40 μm strainer and transferred into appropriate FACS tubes and propidium iodide (PI) added to a concentration of 2 μg/mL.
12. Cell sorting is carried out by selectively removing aggregates, debris, dead cells (PI+), and selecting specific sub-populations based on cell surface marker expressions [2].
13. Following FACS isolation, collect single epithelial stem cells in DMEM/F12 supplemented with 10% serum and 10 μM Y-27632. Centrifuge at 4 °C for 5 min at 1500 rpm.
14. Discard the supernatant and resuspend the cell pellet in growth-factor reduced Matrigel (1000 cells per μL,) containing 10 μM jagged-1. 5000 cells in 5 μL Matrigel are seeded per well in a 96 well plate. Spread out the Matrigel as much as possible to form a thin layer of Matrigel without touching the edge of the well.
15. Following Matrigel polymerisation, overlay 100 μL of pre-warmed single cell culture medium per well.
16. Maintain intestinal stem cells in a 37 °C humidified atmosphere under 5% CO_2. After 3 days, replace the entire culture medium with freshly made culture medium without Y-27632 and WNT-3A.

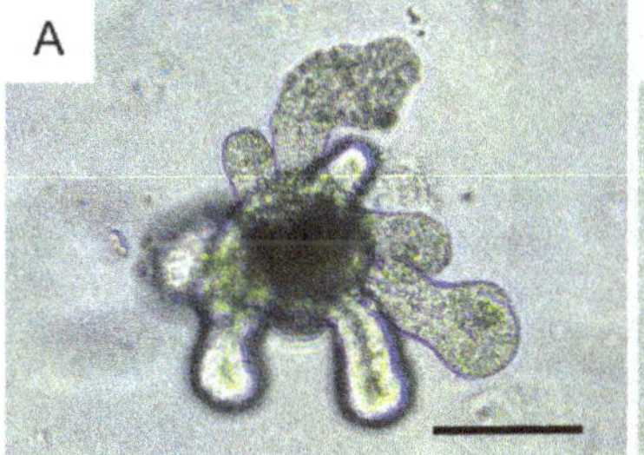

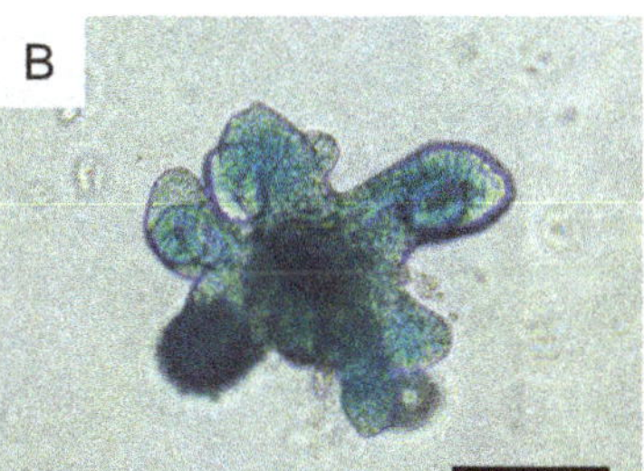

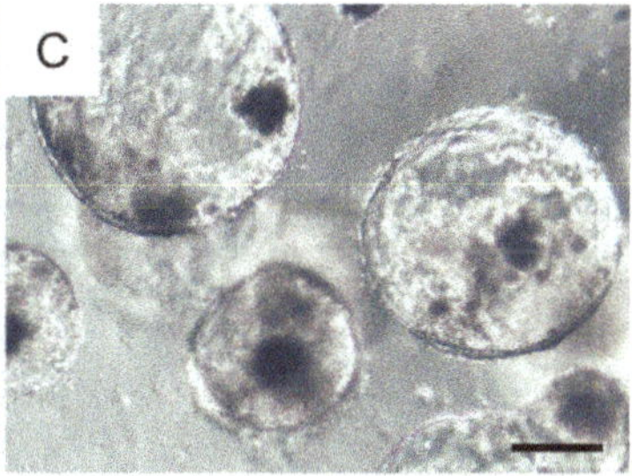

Fig. 2 Induction of tamoxifen-mediated Cre recombination in intestinal organoid culture. Organoids generated from Villlin-CreERT2-Rosa26-LacZ mice untreated (**a**) or treated with 0.5 μM tamoxifen for 1 day (**b**). Scale bars = 100 μm. Organoids were fixed and stained to reveal beta-galactosidase activity using the protocol described in [14]. Cells staining blue indicate successful recombination. (**c**) Small intestinal organoids showing loss of typical budding architecture 5 days after inducible loss of Apc

3.3 Induction of Cre Recombinase Using VillinCre and Floxed Alleles

1. Following organoid passaging (*see* Subheading 3.1, **steps 17** and **18**), 150 crypt fragments in 20 μL Matrigel are seeded per well in a 48 well plate. Alternatively, organoids generated from freshly isolated crypts or single cells maintained for 5 days in culture can be used.
2. Add tamoxifen to the culture medium at 0.5 μM for 1 day to induce recombination. In Fig. 2a, b, organoids were generated from isolated intestinal crypts of a Villin-CreERT2-Rosa26-LacZ transgenic mouse [6, 11]. This mouse model contains a loxP-flanked STOP cassette preventing transcription of a LacZ protein, which is expressed following Cre-mediated recombination. After a 1 day incubation with tamoxifen, the stop cassette is excised by the tamoxifen-induced Cre recombinase, which leads to LacZ expression and visualisation of recombined LacZ+ blue cells in these organoids. Fig. 2c depicts an organoid established from $Apc^{fl/fl}$ intestinal tissue [12].
3. After tamoxifen treatment, discard media and replace with normal culture medium. The resulting phenotype is generally analysed at day 4.

3.4 Transfection of TAT-Cre to Induce Recombination

1. Grow organoids for 5 days from crypts or single cells in 24 well plate. As an example, organoids were generated from isolated intestinal crypts of a Rosa26-ZsGreen1 transgenic mouse (Fig. 3) [13]. This mouse model contains a loxP-flanked STOP cassette preventing transcription of an enhanced green fluorescent protein (ZsGreen1), which is expressed following Cre-mediated recombination.
2. Harvest organoids from six wells by first discarding the culture medium, adding 500 μL PBS to each well and mechanically dissociating the Matrigel with a P1000 pipette (20–30 times up and down). Transfer the dissociated Matrigel and organoids

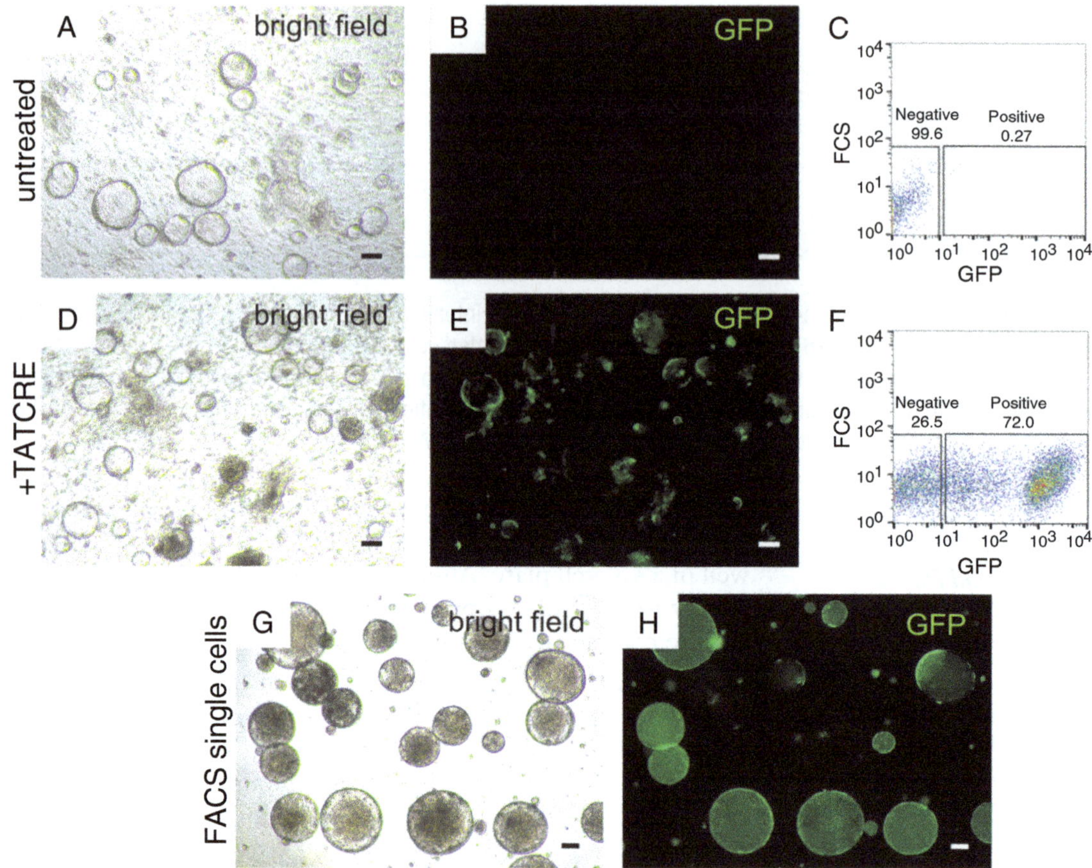

Fig. 3 Induction of TAT-Cre mediated recombination in intestinal organoids. Rosa26-ZsGreen1 organoids untreated (**a**, **b**) or treated with 8 μM TAT-Cre (**d**, **e**) showing TAT-Cre mediated recombined GFP+ organoids. Flow cytometry analysis of Rosa26-ZsGreen1 organoids untreated (**c**) or treated with 8 μM TAT-Cre (**f**) showing efficient GFP expression induced by TAT-Cre recombination in organoids. (**g**, **h**) Organoids generated from FACS sorted single GFP+ cells. Scale bars = 100 μm

into a 15 mL falcon tube placed on ice. Wash the wells again with 500 μL PBS and transfer to same 15 mL falcon tube.

3. Centrifuge the tubes for 5 min (1500 rpm) at 4 °C. Discard the supernatant and re-suspend cells in 500 μL culture media in a 1.5 mL eppendorf tube (approx. 300,000 cells per tube) with 8 μM TAT-Cre (*see* **Note 10**). Incubate tube at 37 °C for 4 h.
4. Centrifuge the cells at 1500 rpm at 4 °C for 5 min. Resuspend pellet in 100 μL of Matrigel and plate into 5 wells in a 48 well plate. Add crypt culture medium and incubate for at least 5 days changing the media every other day.
5. After 5 days in culture, the TAT-Cre activated fluorescent reporter gene can be visualised by microscopy (Fig. 3a, b, untreated Rosa26-ZsGreen1 organoids; Fig. 3d–e, TAT-Cre treated Rosa26-ZsGreen1 organoids).

6. Transfected organoid cultures can be analysed by reference to GFP expression by mechanically dissociating the Matrigel with a P1000 pipette (20–30 times up and down) in each well. Transfer the dissociated Matrigel and organoids of three wells into a 15 mL tube. Wash each well again with 500 μL PBS and add to the tube.
7. Centrifuge at 1500 rpm for 5 min at 4 °C. Re-suspend pellet in 1 mL TrypLE Express supplemented with 10 μM Y-27632 and 50 units DNAse 1 by pipetting up and down (10–15 times). Incubate at 37 °C for 3 min.
8. Pipette up and down for (15–20 times) to allow dissociation of organoids into single cells. Add 9 mL of cold DMEM to tube to stop the dissociation process and centrifuge cells at 1500 rpm for 5 min at 4 °C.
9. Re-suspend pellet in 500 μL of FACS buffer (DMEM/F12 + 10% FBS + 10 μM Y-27632). Proceed with flow cytometry analysis. Measuring the percentage of GFP+ cells gives a measure of successful transfection and TAT-Cre efficiency (Fig. 3c, f). In our hands, 8 μM TAT-CRE induced a high degree of recombination (72% recombined GFP+ cells) and higher concentrations of TAT-Cre did not increase this percentage.
10. Transfected organoid cells can also be FACS sorted by reference to GFP expression and single recombined GFP+ stem cells cultured (*see* Subheading 3.2, **steps 11–16**) (Fig. 3g, h).

3.5 Analysis of Cell Viability

One potential readout after genetic manipulation in organoids (gene loss or over-expression) is to analyse cell viability using the PrestoBlue assay.

1. Make up PrestoBlue working solution by diluting ten times using basal medium in a falcon tube. Wrap tube in aluminium foil and incubate at 37 °C for 5 min (*see* **Note 11**).
2. Remove culture media from organoid plate and add 200 μL PrestoBlue working solution to each well (48 well plate). Start with blank wells and then proceed to wells with organoids whilst working in triplicate.
3. Incubate organoids with PrestoBlue for 20–40 min depending on organoid density. For higher density, incubate for 20 min. If organoid density is low, incubate for 30 or 40 min.
4. After incubation, transfer PrestoBlue solution from blank and organoid wells (90 μL per well) into a new fluorescence-grade black 96 well plate working in duplicates and protect from light.
5. Measure PrestoBlue fluorescence using a fluorescence plate reader (excitation: 540 nm; emission: 590 nm) (*see* **Note 12**).

4 Notes

1. Bottles of Matrigel should be stored at −20 °C to −80 °C for long term storage. To make up smaller working stocks, warm Matrigel to 4 °C in fridge overnight then aliquot. Smaller (i.e. 1 mL) stocks can be store at −20 °C. Avoid multiple freeze thaw cycles where possible. Keep Matrigel on ice prior to use. Do not allow Matrigel to warm to room temperature as it will solidify and this process cannot be reversed.
2. Make up working stocks to the following recommended concentrations: 100 μg/mL Noggin: 50 μg/mL EGF: 500 μM Jagged: 100 μg/mL R-spondin: 100 μg/mL Wnt3a: 10 mM CHIR: 10 mM Y-27632.
3. We recommend using NUNC plates. Matrigel does not adhere as well to some other plate brands making seeding more difficult.
4. Organoid basal media can be prepared and stored at 4 °C for 2–3 weeks. Complete crypt or single cell media should be prepared on the day of use.
5. When scraping the epithelial surface of the intestine with a glass coverslip, do not apply too much pressure. Only light pressure is required to remove mucus and villi. Scraping too firmly may compromise crypt structure.
6. All reagents and samples should be kept on ice at all times during organoid isolation. Cell viability and therefore organoid forming ability will be compromised if samples are allowed to warm to room temperature.
7. Do not centrifuge samples at higher speeds. This will cause more single cell contamination and will not yield a pure crypt culture.
8. There are numerous Matrigel seeding methods described in the literature. More Matrigel can be used per well when passaging and maintaining lines (i.e. 50 μL per well of a 24 well plate). However, when seeding organoids directly from crypts or isolated single cells, a thinner layer of Matrigel facilitates organoid growth. This allows for optimal diffusion of the required growth factors to cells.
9. Do not allow cells to sit in Matrigel for extended periods of time (>30 min) without media as organoid viability may be compromised.
10. TAT-Cre recombinase protein (EMD Millipore) is sold as units. To calculate the amount of TAT-Cre required follow the example below. A standard of 100 units is defined as the amount of TAT-Cre (μg) in 1 mL of tissue culture medium that is required

to induce 50% GFP expression in a HEK293T reporter cell line assay. Hence EC50 = 100 units. If EC50 value is 127 μg/mL, the amount of TAT-Cre protein in 1 unit is equal to 1.27 μg/mL (this value is different for every batch of TAT-Cre). Therefore, a TAT-Cre stock solution at a concentration (10,000 units) is prepared by adding 12.7 g/L and can be converted to μM by dividing by 41,000 (molecular mass of TAT-Cre protein). Molarity of TAT-Cre stock solution = 12.7 g/1 L × 1 mol/41,000 g = 309.6 μM. In this case, to obtain a final concentration of 8 μM, use 25.6 μL TAT-Cre stock in 1 mL culture media.

11. Both the resazurin dye and resorufin product in PrestoBlue are light sensitive leading to increased background fluorescence. Store the reagent in the dark where possible. If exposure to light is unavoidable (i.e. during assay setup) ensure a no cell control well is included to correct for background fluorescence.
12. If the PrestoBlue plate is unable to be read immediately after assay completion, the black plate can be store at 4 °C protected from light for up to 48 h.

Acknowledgements

This work was supported by NHMRC project grants 3156594 to H.A. and 1129600 to T.J. Authors wish to acknowledge support from the Monash Flowcore and Monash Microimaging platform facilities.

References

1. Sato T, Vries RG, Snippert HJ et al (2009) Single Lgr5 stem cells build crypt-villus structures in vitro without a mesenchymal niche. Nature 459:262–265
2. Nefzger CM, Jarde T, Rossello FJ et al (2016) A versatile strategy for isolating a highly enriched population of intestinal stem cells. Stem Cell Rep 6:321–329
3. Lindemans CA, Calafiore M, Mertelsmann AM et al (2015) Interleukin-22 promotes intestinal-stem-cell-mediated epithelial regeneration. Nature 528:560–564
4. Holik AZ, Krzystyniak J, Young M et al (2013) Brg1 is required for stem cell maintenance in the murine intestinal epithelium in a tissue-specific manner. Stem Cells 31:2457–2466
5. Horvay K, Jarde T, Casagranda F et al (2015) Snai1 regulates cell lineage allocation and stem cell maintenance in the mouse intestinal epithelium. EMBO J 34:1319–1335
6. El Marjou F, Janssen KP, Chang BH et al (2004) Tissue-specific and inducible Cre-mediated recombination in the gut epithelium. Genesis 39:186–193
7. Peitz M, Pfannkuche K, Rajewsky K et al (2002) Ability of the hydrophobic FGF and basic TAT peptides to promote cellular uptake of recombinant Cre recombinase: a tool for efficient genetic engineering of mammalian genomes. Proc Natl Acad Sci U S A 99:4489–4494
8. Jarde T, Evans RJ, Mcquillan KL et al (2013) In vivo and in vitro models for the therapeutic targeting of Wnt signaling using a Tet-ODeltaN89beta-catenin system. Oncogene 32:883–893
9. Morin PJ, Sparks AB, Korinek V et al (1997) Activation of beta-catenin-Tcf signaling in colon cancer by mutations in beta-catenin or APC. Science 275:1787–1790

10. Hill DR, Spence JR (2017) Gastrointestinal organoids: understanding the molecular basis of the host-microbe interface. Cell Mol Gastroenterol Hepatol 3:138–149
11. Soriano P (1999) Generalized lacZ expression with the ROSA26 Cre reporter strain. Nat Genet 21:70–71
12. Shibata H, Toyama K, Shioya H et al (1997) Rapid colorectal adenoma formation initiated by conditional targeting of the Apc gene. Science 278:120–123
13. Madisen L, Zwingman TA, Sunkin SM et al (2010) A robust and high-throughput Cre reporting and characterization system for the whole mouse brain. Nat Neurosci 13:133–140
14. Shorning BY, Jarde T, Mccarthy A et al (2012) Intestinal renin-angiotensin system is stimulated after deletion of Lkb1. Gut 61:202–213

Chapter 5

Protocols to Evaluate Cigarette Smoke-Induced Lung Inflammation and Pathology in Mice

Ross Vlahos and Steven Bozinovski

Abstract

Cigarette smoking is a major cause of chronic obstructive pulmonary disease (COPD). Inhalation of cigarette smoke causes inflammation of the airways, airway wall remodelling, mucus hypersecretion and progressive airflow limitation. Much of the disease burden and health care utilisation in COPD is associated with the management of its comorbidities and infectious (viral and bacterial) exacerbations (AECOPD). Comorbidities, in particular skeletal muscle wasting, cardiovascular disease and lung cancer markedly impact on disease morbidity, progression and mortality. The mechanisms and mediators underlying COPD and its comorbidities are poorly understood and current COPD therapy is relatively ineffective. Many researchers have used animal modelling systems to explore the mechanisms underlying COPD, AECOPD and comorbidities of COPD with the goal of identifying novel therapeutic targets. Here we describe a mouse model that we have developed to define the cellular, molecular and pathological consequences of cigarette smoke exposure and the development of comorbidities of COPD.

Key words COPD, Cigarette smoke, Comorbidities, AECOPD, Emphysema, Lung inflammation

1 Introduction

Chronic Obstructive Pulmonary Disease (COPD) is a major incurable global health burden and is the fourth leading cause of death worldwide [1]. COPD is a "disease characterized by airflow limitation that is not fully reversible. The airflow limitation is usually progressive and associated with an abnormal inflammatory response of lungs to noxious particles and gases" [1]. Cigarette smoking is the major cause of COPD and accounts for more than 95% of cases in industrialized countries, but other environmental pollutants are important causes in developing countries [1]. COPD is heterogeneous and encompasses chronic obstructive bronchiolitis with fibrosis and obstruction of small airways, leading to closure of small airways. Emphysema caused by enlargement of airspaces due to destruction of lung parenchyma and loss of lung elasticity can subsequently develop. Most patients with COPD have multiple

Brendan J. Jenkins (ed.), *Inflammation and Cancer: Methods and Protocols*, Methods in Molecular Biology, vol. 1725,
https://doi.org/10.1007/978-1-4939-7568-6_5,

pathologic conditions (chronic obstructive bronchiolitis, emphysema and mucus plugging), but the relative extent of emphysema and obstructive bronchiolitis within individual patients can vary. As the disease worsens, patients experience progressively more frequent and severe exacerbations, which are due in greatest part to viral and bacterial chest infections [2–5]. Patients are also increasingly disabled by disease comorbidities, such as skeletal muscle wasting and cardiovascular disease, which further reduce their quality of life [6–8]. In addition, respiratory infections can worsen these comorbidities and further impact on the patient's life [7].

Current forms of therapy for COPD are relatively ineffective and the development of effective treatments for COPD have been severely hampered as the mechanisms and mediators that drive the induction and progression of chronic inflammation, emphysema, altered lung function, defective lung immunity, musculoskeletal derangement and markedly worsened cardiovascular risk remain only poorly understood. Given that cigarette smoke is the major cause of COPD, "smoking mouse" models, using either nose only or whole body smoke exposure systems, that accurately reflect disease pathophysiology have been developed and have made rapid progress in identifying candidate pathogenic mechanisms and new therapies (reviewed in [9–18]). To date, many species have been used including rodents, dogs, guinea-pigs, monkeys and sheep [16, 19]. However, mice have been the most popular choice by many investigators given the enormous information about the mouse genome, the abundance of antibody and gene probes, the ability to produce animals with genetic modifications that shed light on specific processes within COPD, the availability of numerous mouse strains with different responses to smoke and ultimately the low cost. It has been established that there is excellent concordance between biological pathways initiated by cigarette smoke exposure in the lungs of humans and mice [20].

Regardless of the method of cigarette smoke exposure, many of the of the characteristic features of human COPD, namely (1) chronic lung inflammation, (2) impaired lung function; (3) emphysema; (4) mucus hypersecretion; (5) small airway wall thickening and remodeling; (6) vascular remodeling; (7) lymphoid aggregates and (8) pulmonary hypertension can be mimicked in the "smoking mouse model". Acute and chronic cigarette smoke exposure protocols have been developed where acute protocols (1–4 days) are typically used to explore the mediators and mechanisms involved in the induction of cigarette smoke-induced lung inflammation [16, 19]. Chronic cigarette smoke exposure protocols have largely been used to explore the mechanisms that drive chronic inflammation, impaired lung function, emphysema, small airway wall thickening and remodeling and vascular remodeling [16, 19].

2 Materials

Prepare all solutions described below using ultrapure water (prepared by purifying deionized water, to attain a sensitivity of 18 MΩ-cm at 25 °C) and analytical grade reagents. Prepare and store all reagents at room temperature (RT, unless indicated otherwise). Diligently follow all waste disposal regulations when disposing waste materials.

2.1 Cigarette Smoke Exposure

1. 18 L perspex chamber.
2. Specific pathogen-free male mice (e.g. BALB/c, C57BL/6).
3. Winfield Red cigarettes (16 mg of tar, 1.2 mg of nicotine, and 15 mg of CO).

2.2 Characterization of Cigarette Smoke Exposure: Total Suspended Particulate Mass Concentration

1. Polytetrafluoroethylene filters (47 mm Teflon, 2 μm pore size).
2. Microbalance with a resolution of 0.0001 mg.

2.3 Bronchoalveolar Lavage and Lung Collection

1. 240 mg/kg sodium pentobarbital anesthetic.
2. Phosphate-buffered saline (PBS): 2.85 g/L $NaHPO_4{\cdot}2H_2O$ (16 mM HPO_4), 0.625 g/L $NaH_2PO_4{\cdot}2H_2O$ (4 mM PO_4), 8.7 g/L NaCl (149 mM NaCl).
3. Weighing scales.
4. 27 gauge × ½ in. (0.43 × 13 mm) needle.
5. 1 and 5 mL insulin syringe.
6. Tracheotomy needle 21 gauge × 1 in. (0.80 × 25 mm).
7. Two curved tissue forceps.
8. Scissors.
9. Liquid nitrogen.
10. 1.7 mL Eppendorf tube.

2.4 Total and Differential Cell Counts

1. Ethidium bromide and acridine orange.
2. Neubauer hemocytometer.
3. Shandon CytoSpin 3 centrifuge.
4. Merck Microscopy Hemacolor and Kwik™ Diff Solution.
5. Microscope glass slides.
6. Glass cover slips.
7. Entellan® mounting medium.

2.5 Carboxyhemoglobin Measurements

1. 240 mg/kg sodium pentobarbital anesthetic.
2. 27 gauge × ½ in. (0.40 × 13 mm) needle.
3. 1 mL heparinized blood gas syringe.

2.6 RNA Extraction, cDNA Synthesis and qPCR

1. Liquid nitrogen.
2. 1.7 mL Eppendorf tube.
3. RLT Lysis buffer (RNeasy® Mini Kit 250).
4. β-Mercaptoethanol.
5. 21 gauge × 1 in. (0.80 × 25 mm) needle.
6. 1 mL syringe.
7. RNeasy Mini Kit 250.
8. NanoDrop 2000 spectrophotometer.
9. Taqman primers.

2.7 Histology

1. 240 mg/kg sodium pentobarbital anesthetic.
2. 27 gauge × ½ in. (0.40 × 13 mm) needle.
3. 10% neutral buffered formalin.
4. Hematoxylin and eosin stain.

2.8 Acute Exacerbations of COPD

1. Influenza A virus (H3N1, Mem 71 strain).

3 Methods

3.1 Animals

Specific pathogen-free male mice (e.g. BALB/c, C57BL/6) aged 7 weeks and weighing ~20 g are obtained from an animal resource centre. The mice are then housed at 20 °C on a 12:12 h day-night cycle in sterile microisolators and fed a standard sterile diet of Purina mouse chow with water allowed ad libitum. The experiments need to be approved by an institutional animal experimentation ethics committee and be conducted in compliance with the guidelines of the country's governmental bodies that regulate animal experimentation (*see* **Note 1**).

3.2 Cigarette Smoke Exposure

Mice are placed in an 18 L perspex chamber in a chemical hood and exposed to cigarette smoke generated from one cigarette for 15 min (*see* **Note 2**). The lid of the perspex chamber is then opened for 5 min before being closed and the mice exposed again to cigarette smoke generated from one cigarette for 15 min. This is repeated such that mice are exposed to three cigarettes for 1 h, three times a day for 4 days, delivered at 9 AM, 12 noon, and 3 PM. Cigarette smoke is generated in 50 mL tidal volumes over 10 s, by use of timed draw-back mimicking normal smoking inhalation volume and cigarette burn rate. Mice are then are killed by an intraperitoneal (ip) overdose of anesthetic (240 mg/kg sodium pentobarbital; *see* **Note 3**) on day 5 and the lungs lavaged with PBS as described below. For chronic cigarette smoke exposure protocols, mice are exposed to cigarette smoke generated as described above but for up to 6 months, 5 days/week. Sham-exposed mice are placed in an 18 L perspex chamber and do not receive cigarette smoke. Commercially available filter-tipped cigarettes of the following composition are used: 16 mg of tar, 1.2 mg of nicotine, and 15 mg of CO.

3.3 Characterization of Cigarette Smoke Exposure: Total Suspended Particulate Mass Concentration

Total suspended particulate (TSP) matter is collected on a polytetrafluoroethylene filter with a PMP support ring (47 mm Teflon, 2 μm pore size) enclosed in a polypropylene holder (47 mm holder), using a low-flow miniature diaphragm pump. The pump is calibrated to a volumetric flow rate of 50 mL/min using a National Association of Testing Authorities-certified soap bubble flowmeter. The unexposed and cigarette smoke-exposed filter is then equilibrated at a relative humidity of 50 ± 5% and a temperature of 21 ± 1 °C and weighed with a microbalance with a resolution of 0.0001 mg. The TSP mass concentration, reported in milligrams per cubic meter, is determined by dividing the difference in mass between the cigarette exposed and unexposed filter by the volume of air sampled through the filter. The mean TSP mass concentration in the chamber containing cigarette smoke generated from one cigarette, measured from 3 min 13 s to 15 min, is typically about 420 mg/m^3 for our set up [21].

3.4 Characterization of Cigarette Smoke Exposure: Particle Number Concentration

Particle number concentration is measured in the chamber immediately after injection of cigarette smoke into the chamber and again at the end of the 15 min period. Number concentration for a particle size range of 0.01 to >1.0 μm was measured with a handheld condensation particle counter. The particle number concentration dropped from 458,192 particles/cm^3 at 4 min 51 s to 373,987 particles/cm^3 at 15 min. The total particle number loss was 84,205 particles/cm^3, which was predominantly due to dilution during a 3 min sampling period with the condensation particle counter at 700 particles/cm^3/min.

3.5 Bronchoalveolar Lavage and Lung Collection

Euthanize mice with an intraperitoneal anesthetic overdose (240 mg/kg sodium pentobarbital) administered via a 27 gauge needle (*see* **Note 4**). Make a mid-line incision in the neck to expose the trachea and perform a tracheotomy using a blunt 21 gauge needle inserted into the trachea (*see* **Note 5**). Lavage the lungs in situ with 0.4 mL of chilled PBS followed by three aliquots of 0.3 mL of PBS with ~1 mL of bronchoalveolar lavage fluid (BALF) recovered from each animal. Clear the lungs of blood via right ventricular perfusion of the heart with 5 mL of PBS. Rapidly excise the lungs, rinse in PBS, snap-freeze in liquid nitrogen (*see* **Note 6**) and store at −80 °C until required.

3.6 Total and Differential Cell Counts

To determine the total viable cell numbers in BALF, take a 50 μL aliquot of BALF and dilute 1:2 with the fluorophores ethidium bromide/acridine orange (*see* **Note 7**) and count on a standard hemocytometer with a fluorescence microscope. Take 5×10^4 cells from the BALF samples and cytospin at 15 × *g* for 10 min at room temperature to produce a single layer of cells on a glass slide for differential cell counts. Allow cytospins to dry for 24 h and then stain with Merck Microscopy Hemacolor and Kwik™ Diff as stated by the manufacturer's instructions, mount with Entellan® medium and cover slip. Count the number of macrophages, lymphocytes and neutrophils (count at least 500 cells per slide) using standard morphological criteria on a microscope equipped with a digital camera. Centrifuge the remaining BALF at 660 × *g* for 5 min at 4 °C, and then collect the supernatant and store at −80 °C until required for analyses of proteins by standard ELISAs.

3.7 Carboxy-hemoglobin Measurements

To ensure that cigarette smoke exposure levels are comparable to those experienced by human smokers, measure the carboxyhemoglobin (CoHb) in the blood of mice. Immediately after removal from the smoke chamber, euthanize the mouse with an intraperitoneal anesthetic overdose (240 mg/kg sodium pentobarbital) administered via a 27 gauge needle and collect the blood in a heparinized blood gas syringe from the abdominal vena cava. Inject 85 μL of blood into a Radiometer ABL520 blood gas analyzer, which measures COHb across a range of 0–100%.

3.8 RNA Extraction, cDNA Synthesis and qPCR

The whole lung from each mouse is crushed into a powder using a mortar and pestle under liquid nitrogen to avoid thawing. Ground tissue powder (15 mg) is then transferred into a 1.7 mL Eppendorf tube containing 600 μL RLT Lysis buffer (RNeasy® Mini Kit 250) supplemented with a 1:100 dilution of β-Mercaptoethanol (*see* **Note 8**). The tissue is then homogenized by passing it through a 21 g needle and 1 mL syringe 5–10 times, following which centrifuge at 16,000 × *g* for 3 min. Collect the supernatant and purify total RNA using the RNeasy Mini Kit 250 according to the manufacturer's instructions. Determine the concentration, quality and purity of the extracted RNA using a NanoDrop 2000 spectrophotometer to generate absorbance 260/280 ratios. A ratio of ~2.0 is generally accepted as "pure" for RNA and should generally fall within the generally accepted ratios of 1.8 and 2.0. Synthesize single strand cDNA by reverse transcription using 1 μg of RNA for downstream qPCR application using Taqman primers (*see* **Note 9**) as previously published [21–23].

3.9 Histology

Histology should be performed to determine whether acute and chronic cigarette smoke exposure can affect the lung architecture.

To ensure consistent morphological preservation of lungs, mice are killed by intraperitoneal anesthesia (240 mg/kg sodium pentobarbital) overdose and then perfusion fixed via a tracheal cannula with 10% neutral buffered formalin (NBF) at exactly 200 mmH_2O pressure (*see* **Note 10**). After 15 min the trachea is ligated, and the lungs removed from the thorax and immersed in 10% NBF for a minimum period of 24 h. After fixation of the lung tissue and processing in paraffin wax, 3–4 μm thick section are cut longitudinally through the left and right lung so as to include all lobes. Sections are stained with hematoxylin and eosin for general histopathology as previously published [21]. Lung sections can also be investigated for signs of emphysema using the mean linear intercept method as previously published [24–27].

3.10 Acute Exacerbations of COPD

Given the important role of viruses in COPD, we have developed in vivo models to investigate the impact of viral infection on cigarette smoke-exposed mice [16]. The advantage of these models is the use of live, replication competent viruses rather than replication deficient adenovirus. Briefly, mice are exposed to cigarette smoke as described above but they are then infected with influenza A virus (H3N1, Mem71 strain). Mice are then culled 3–10 days post IAV infection and endpoints including lung inflammation, viral titers, lung pathology, body weight, BALF cytokine/protease expression and whole lung proinflammatory gene expression assessed as previously published [23, 28].

3.11 Modelling Systemic Comorbidities of COPD

COPD is often associated with systemic comorbidities that can impact on the patient's functional capacity, quality of life, and also increase the risk of hospitalization and mortality in COPD patients [1]. These comorbidities include skeletal muscle wasting, cardiovascular disease and lung cancer [1, 7]. Given that comorbidities have a profound impact on COPD patients, much research has now focused on developing preclinical mouse models of systemic comorbidities associated with COPD to elucidate the mechanisms underlying these conditions and to ultimately identify novel therapeutic options for these patients. We have developed in vivo models to investigate the mechanisms underlying skeletal muscle wasting in cigarette smoke-exposed mice [16, 19]. Briefly, mice are chronically exposed to cigarette smoke (8 weeks) as described above but they are then infected with influenza A virus (H3N1, Mem71 strain). Mice are then culled 3–10 days post influenza A virus infection and endpoints including lung inflammation, viral titers, lung pathology, body weight, BALF cytokine/protease expression and whole lung pro-inflammatory gene expression assessed as previously published [23, 28]. Using these models we have shown that mice exposed chronically to cigarette smoke had reduced body weight, hind limb skeletal muscles mass (gatrocnemius, tibialis anterior, soleus), grip strength (index of muscle strength) and aerobic endurance

[29–34]. Moreover, cigarette smoke altered the mRNA expression of a number of genes associated with the regulation of skeletal muscle mass including insulin-like growth factor-I, atrogin-1, MuRF-1 and IL-6 [33, 34]. Thus, chronic cigarette smoke exposure results in systemic features that closely resemble extrapulmonary manifestations observed in patients with COPD.

4 Notes

1. All experiments performed with mice need to be approved by an institutional animal experimentation ethics committee and be conducted in compliance with the guidelines of the country's governmental bodies that regulate animal experimentation.
2. All smoking procedures must be performed in a chemical fume hood. Personal protective equipment (PPE) (e.g. gloves, laboratory coat, safety glasses) must be worn at all time. Ensure all flammable chemicals and substances are kept away from ignited cigarettes. After completion of the smoking procedure, cigarettes should be extinguished into a commercial ashtray located within the chemical fume hood.
3. When working with the mouse anesthetic sodium pentobarbital ensure you wear a gown, gloves (irritant to skin), protective glasses (highly irritant to eyes), and closed shoes. Also note that working with and restraining mice involves risks as a result of bites, scratches and the development of animal allergies. It is necessary that all staff and students undergo an animal handling course prior to commencing animal experimentation.
4. Working with needles and syringes involves risks to personnel as a result of needle stick injury. Ensure appropriate safety techniques are used.
5. For the BAL procedure, use a 21 gauge needle that has been cut to a length of ½ an inch and overlaid it with a plastic cannula. This will ensure that the tracheotomy needle fits snuggly into the trachea and will not damage the trachea (i.e. pierce the tracheal wall causing the lavage fluid to leak). Clamp the trachea and tracheotomy needle together with a bulldog clamp.
6. Liquid nitrogen is a colourless, odourless, extremely cold liquid and gas under pressure. It can cause rapid suffocation when concentrations are sufficient to reduce oxygen levels below 19.5%. Contact with liquid nitrogen can cause severe frostbite. Ensure appropriate PPE is used when handling liquid nitrogen, especially cold resistant gloves, face shield and lab coat.
7. Ethidium bromide (EtBr) is toxic, a potent mutagen and the powder form irritant to skin and the upper respiratory tract.

Wear appropriate PPE and nitrile disposable gloves when working with EtBr.

8. Buffers used for qPCR are toxic, corrosive and flammable. Appropriate PPE (e.g. gloves, safety glasses, lab coat) must be worn when working with the solutions. All work must be conducted in a chemical hood. Waste solutions must be placed in a chemically-inert bottle for removal by contracted waste management company later. Do not work near ignition sources.
9. The Taqman Gene Expression Assay probes contain some mild carcinogens. Wear PPE such as gloves and lab coat while performing the procedure. Place used plates, tubes and reagents into a biohazard container. Electrical equipment is involved and must be checked yearly and tagged.
10. Neutral buffered formalin is highly toxic and contact with the skin, eyes or mucous membrane should be avoided. Preparation should be carried out in a chemical hood, while wearing gloves, safety glasses and a protective.

Acknowledgement

This work was supported by NHMRC Project Grants 1084627 and 1067547.

References

1. Vogelmeier CF, Criner GJ, Martinez FJ, Anzueto A, Barnes PJ, Bourbeau J, Celli BR, Chen R, Decramer M, Fabbri LM, Frith P, Halpin DM, Lopez Varela MV, Nishimura M, Roche N, Rodriguez-Roisin R, Sin DD, Singh D, Stockley R, Vestbo J, Wedzicha JA, Agusti A (2017) Global Strategy for the diagnosis, management, and prevention of chronic obstructive lung disease 2017 report: GOLD executive summary. Am J Respir Crit Care Med 195:557–582
2. Rohde G, Wiethege A, Borg I, Kauth M, Bauer TT, Gillissen A, Bufe A, Schultze-Werninghaus G (2003) Respiratory viruses in exacerbations of chronic obstructive pulmonary disease requiring hospitalisation: a case-control study. Thorax 58:37–42
3. Sethi S (2004) Bacteria in exacerbations of chronic obstructive pulmonary disease: phenomenon or epiphenomenon? Proc Am Thorac Soc 1:109–114
4. Seemungal T, Harper-Owen R, Bhowmik A, Moric I, Sanderson G, Message S, Maccallum P, Meade TW, Jeffries DJ, Johnston SL, Wedzicha JA (2001) Respiratory viruses, symptoms, and inflammatory markers in acute exacerbations and stable chronic obstructive pulmonary disease. Am J Respir Crit Care Med 164:1618–1623
5. Hurst JR, Vestbo J, Anzueto A, Locantore N, Mullerova H, Tal-Singer R, Miller B, Lomas DA, Agusti A, Macnee W, Calverley P, Rennard S, Wouters EF, Wedzicha JA (2010) Evaluation of CLtIPSEI. Susceptibility to exacerbation in chronic obstructive pulmonary disease. N Engl J Med 363:1128–1138
6. Barnes PJ, Celli BR (2009) Systemic manifestations and comorbidities of COPD. Eur Respir J 33:1165–1185
7. Cavailles A, Brinchault-Rabin G, Dixmier A, Goupil F, Gut-Gobert C, Marchand-Adam S, Meurice JC, Morel H, Person-Tacnet C, Leroyer C, Diot P (2013) Comorbidities of COPD. Eur Respir Rev 22:454–475
8. Maltais F, Decramer M, Casaburi R, Barreiro E, Burelle Y, Debigare R, Dekhuijzen PN, Franssen F, Gayan-Ramirez G, Gea J, Gosker HR, Gosselink R, Hayot M, Hussain SN,

Janssens W, Polkey MI, Roca J, Saey D, Schols AM, Spruit MA, Steiner M, Taivassalo T, Troosters T, Vogiatzis I, Wagner PD, ATS/ERS Ad Hoc Committee on Limb Muscle Dysfunction in COPD (2014) An official American Thoracic Society/European Respiratory Society statement: update on limb muscle dysfunction in chronic obstructive pulmonary disease. Am J Respir Crit Care Med 189: e15–e62

9. Stevenson CS, Birrell MA (2011) Moving towards a new generation of animal models for asthma and COPD with improved clinical relevance. Pharmacol Ther 130:93–105
10. Vlahos R, Bozinovski S, Gualano RC, Ernst M, Anderson GP (2006) Modelling COPD in mice. Pulm Pharmacol Ther 19:12–17
11. Stevenson CS, Belvisi MG (2008) Preclinical animal models of asthma and chronic obstructive pulmonary disease. Expert Rev Respir Med 2:631–643
12. Churg A, Cosio M, Wright JL (2008) Mechanisms of cigarette smoke-induced COPD: insights from animal models. Am J Physiol Lung Cell Mol Physiol 294:L612–L631
13. Wright JL, Cosio M, Churg A (2008) Animal models of chronic obstructive pulmonary disease. Am J Physiol Lung Cell Mol Physiol 295: L1–15
14. Wright JL, Churg A (2010) Animal models of cigarette smoke-induced chronic obstructive pulmonary disease. Expert Rev Resp Med 4:723–734
15. Goldklang MP, Marks SM, D'Armiento JM (2013) Second hand smoke and COPD: lessons from animal studies. Front Physiol 4:30
16. Vlahos R, Bozinovski S (2014) Recent advances in pre-clinical mouse models of COPD. Clin Sci 126:253–265
17. Fricker M, Deane A, Hansbro PM (2014) Animal models of chronic obstructive pulmonary disease. Expert Opin Drug Discov 9:629–645
18. Mercer PF, Abbott-Banner K, Adcock IM, Knowles RG (2015) Translational models of lung disease. Clin Sci 128:235–256
19. Vlahos R, Bozinovski S (2015) Preclinical murine models of chronic obstructive pulmonary disease. Eur J Pharmacol 759:265–271
20. Morissette MC, Lamontagne M, Berube JC, Gaschler G, Williams A, Yauk C, Couture C, Laviolette M, Hogg JC, Timens W, Halappanavar S, Stampfli MR, Bosse Y (2014) Impact of cigarette smoke on the human and mouse lungs: a gene-expression comparison study. PLoS One 9:e92498
21. Vlahos R, Bozinovski S, Jones JE, Powell J, Gras J, Lilja A, Hansen MJ, Gualano RC, Irving L, Anderson GP (2006) Differential protease, innate immunity, and NF-kappaB induction profiles during lung inflammation induced by subchronic cigarette smoke exposure in mice. Am J Physiol Lung Cell Mol Physiol 290:L931–L945
22. Vlahos R, Bozinovski S, Chan SP, Ivanov S, Linden A, Hamilton JA, Anderson GP (2010) Neutralizing granulocyte/macrophage colony-stimulating factor inhibits cigarette smoke-induced lung inflammation. Am J Respir Crit Care Med 182:34–40
23. Oostwoud LC, Gunasinghe P, Seow HJ, Ye JM, Selemidis S, Bozinovski S, Vlahos R (2016) Apocynin and ebselen reduce influenza A virus-induced lung inflammation in cigarette smoke-exposed mice. Sci Rep 6:20983
24. Ruwanpura SM, McLeod L, Miller A, Jones J, Bozinovski S, Vlahos R, Ernst M, Armes J, Bardin PG, Anderson GP, Jenkins BJ (2011) Interleukin-6 promotes pulmonary emphysema associated with apoptosis in mice. Am J Respir Cell Mol Biol 45:720–730
25. Ruwanpura SM, McLeod L, Miller A, Jones J, Vlahos R, Ramm G, Longano A, Bardin PG, Bozinovski S, Anderson GP, Jenkins BJ (2012) Deregulated Stat3 signaling dissociates pulmonary inflammation from emphysema in gp130 mutant mice. Am J Physiol Lung Cell Mol Physiol 302:L627–L639
26. Ruwanpura SM, McLeod L, Brooks GD, Bozinovski S, Vlahos R, Longano A, Bardin PG, Anderson GP, Jenkins BJ (2014) IL-6/Stat3-driven pulmonary inflammation, but not emphysema, is dependent on interleukin-17A in mice. Respirology 19:419–427
27. Ruwanpura SM, McLeod L, Dousha LF, Seow HJ, Alhayyani S, Tate MD, Deswaerte V, Brooks GD, Bozinovski S, MacDonald M, Garbers C, King PT, Bardin PG, Vlahos R, Rose-John S, Anderson GP, Jenkins BJ (2016) Therapeutic targeting of the IL-6 trans-signaling/mechanistic target of rapamycin complex 1 axis in pulmonary emphysema. Am J Respir Crit Care Med 194:1494–1505
28. Gualano RC, Hansen MJ, Vlahos R, Jones JE, Park-Jones RA, Deliyannis G, Turner SJ, Duca KA, Anderson GP (2008) Cigarette smoke worsens lung inflammation and impairs resolution of influenza infection in mice. Respir Res 9:53
29. Chen H, Hansen MJ, Jones JE, Vlahos R, Bozinovski S, Anderson GP, Morris MJ (2006) Cigarette smoke exposure reprograms the hypothalamic neuropeptide y axis to promote weight loss. Am J Respir Crit Care Med 173:1248–1254

30. Chen H, Vlahos R, Bozinovski S, Jones J, Anderson GP, Morris MJ (2005) Effect of short-term cigarette smoke exposure on body weight, appetite and brain neuropeptide Y in mice. Neuropsychopharmacology 30:713–719
31. Hansen MJ, Gualano RC, Bozinovski S, Vlahos R, Anderson GP (2006) Therapeutic prospects to treat skeletal muscle wasting in COPD (chronic obstructive lung disease). Pharmacol Ther 109:162–172
32. Chen H, Hansen MJ, Jones JE, Vlahos R, Anderson GP, Morris MJ (2007) Detrimental metabolic effects of combining long-term cigarette smoke exposure and high-fat diet in mice. Am J Physiol Endocrinol Metab 293: E1564–E1571
33. Hansen MJ, Chen H, Gualano RC, Jones JE, Vlahos R, Morris MJ, Anderson GP (2007) The balance of atrogin-1 and insulin-like growth factor-1 mRNA expression may contribute to wasting after long-term cigarette smoke exposure in mice. Am J Resp Crit Care Med 175:A649
34. Hansen MJ, Chen H, Jones JE, Langenbach SY, Vlahos R, Gualano RC, Morris MJ, Anderson GP (2013) The lung inflammation and skeletal muscle wasting induced by subchronic cigarette smoke exposure are not altered by a high-fat diet in mice. PLoS One 8:e80471

Chapter 6

Tracking Competent Host Defence to Chronic Inflammation: An In Vivo Model of Peritonitis

Javier Uceda Fernandez, David Millrine, and Simon A. Jones

Abstract

Anti-microbial host defence is dependent on the rapid recruitment of inflammatory cells to the site of infection, the elimination of invading pathogens, and the efficient resolution of inflammation so as to minimise damage to the host. The peritoneal cavity provides an easily accessible and physiologically relevant system where the delicate balance of these processes may be studied. Here, we describe murine models of peritoneal inflammation that enable studies of both competent anti-microbial immunity and inflammation associated tissue damage as a consequence of recurrent bacterial challenge. The inflammatory hallmarks of these models reflect the clinical and molecular features of peritonitis episodes seen in renal failure patients on peritoneal dialysis. Development of these models relies on the preparation of a cell-free supernatant derived from an isolate of *Staphylococcus epidermidis* (termed SES). Intraperitoneal administration of SES induces a TLR2-driven acute inflammatory response that is characterised by an initial transient influx of neutrophils that are replaced by a more sustained recruitment of mononuclear cells and lymphocytes. Adaptation of this model using a repeated administration of SES allows investigations into the development of adaptive immunity and memory responses, and the hallmarks associated with tissue remodelling and fibrosis. These models are therefore clinically relevant and provide exciting opportunities to study both innate and adaptive immune responses in the control of bacterial infection and pathogenesis.

Key words Peritonitis, Inflammation, Cytokine, Fibrosis

1 Introduction

Bacterial infections of the peritoneal membrane and the ensuing inflammation, termed peritonitis, is a major cause of treatment failure in patients undergoing peritoneal dialysis in response to renal failure. Using bacterial isolates derived from a patient with clinical peritonitis we have generated a cell free supernatant of *Staphylococcus epidermidis,* a gram-positive bacterium typically associated with the commensal microflora. Administration of this cell-free isolate to the peritoneal cavity triggers an acute inflammatory reaction [1]. This model has proven remarkably versatile and provides insights into cytokine/chemokine signalling networks, the tracking of immune cell recruitment, activation and survival within

Brendan J. Jenkins (ed.), *Inflammation and Cancer: Methods and Protocols*, Methods in Molecular Biology, vol. 1725, https://doi.org/10.1007/978-1-4939-7568-6_6,

a site of local infection, and mechanisms of inflammatory resolution [2–6]. These investigations have enabled the generation of new hypotheses that may be applied to a range of inflammatory settings or model systems. For instance, the requirement for interleukin-6 (IL-6) signalling in the recruitment and maintenance of leukocyte populations at the site of infection, originally observed in SES-induced peritonitis [5, 7], was readily translated into murine models of inflammatory arthritis [8, 9], where blockade of this pathway was seen to prevent synovitis, and the development of cartilage and bone damage [10, 11]. Insights have also been gained into the molecular events leading to fibrosis, an untreatable condition that is currently the subject of intense research interest [12]. By modifying the protocol of SES delivery we have developed a model that allows monitoring of adaptive immune memory and the underlining mechanisms responsible for peritoneal tissue damage and fibrosis [12]. Taken together, these studies support the broad relevance of SES-induced murine peritonitis as a model for understanding inflammatory activation and maintenance, and how recurrent bacterial infections may contribute to pathogenesis.

Studies have characterised many of the temporal events associated with acute inflammatory activation following SES administration. These include the rapid influx of neutrophils (within 24 h), their apoptotic clearance, and replacement with a population of mononuclear leukocytes (2–4 days post administration) that include inflammatory monocytes and effector $CD4^+$ T-cell subsets [13]. The model has also been applied to the understanding of immune homeostasis, and proliferative regulation of resident tissue monocytic cells [1, 12, 14]. The very nature of the peritoneal cavity allows analysis of the inflammatory infiltrate (e.g., multi-parameter flow cytometry), the generation of inflammatory mediators (e.g., ELISA; mass spectrometry), and studies of the stromal compartment (e.g., immuno-blotting, electrophoretic mobility shift assays, immunocytochemistry). Thus, the SES-induced model of peritoneal inflammation is highly versatile and amenable to manipulation to allow mechanistic insight into the working of acute inflammation. In this regard, the model shows a number of features reflecting the clinical context in end-stage renal failure patients of peritoneal dialysis, and provides opportunities to examine anti-microbial host defence and tissue damage.

2 Materials

Prepare all solutions using deionized water and analytical grade reagents. Store all reagents at room temperature (unless otherwise specified). Ensure all re-useable glassware is autoclaved before starting. Where appropriate use sterile disposable plastic ware, and good aseptic technique.

2.1 Preparation of Staphylococcus epidermidis Cell Free Supernatant

1. Bacterial Specimen. Slope of *S. epidermidis* dormant bacteria stored in glycerol at −80 °C (A clinical strain may be used or an ATCC derived *S. epidermidis* isolate; ATCC-12228).
2. Nutrient Broth No. 2 (OXOID): Dissolve 25 g of nutrient broth No. 2 per 1 L of deionized H_2O to a total volume of 2 L (2 × 1 L bottles). Autoclaved media might be stored at room temperature for approximately 1 week.
3. DST Agar (OXOID): Dissolve 40 g of DST agar in 1 L of deionized H_2O. Autoclave and cool the bottle sufficiently to allow handling. Ensure the agar is fully liquefied. Pour the molten agar broth into petri dishes to an approximate depth of 1 cm. This should be performed in a laminar flow hood using appropriate aseptic techniques. Allow the molten agar to solidify. Wipe any moisture for the petri dish lids with an alcohol swab and seal the petri dishes with parafilm. Plates may be stored at 4 °C for approximately 1 week.
4. Tyrode's salts (Sigma-Aldrich): Tyrode's salt, 0.012 M $NaHCO_3$. Dissolve a vial of Tyrode's salt powder (9.6 g) in 1 L of deionized H_2O. Add 1 g $NaHCO_3$ and filter in a Stericup filter bottle (Millipore). Store in the fridge at 4 °C and use within 1 month.
5. Petri dishes 90 mm.
6. 500 mL centrifuge tubes.
7. 125, 250 and 500 mL Erlenmeyer flasks.
8. Dialysis tubing MWCO 12–14,000 Da (Medicell International Ltd).
9. Plastic clips for dialysis tubing.
10. Graduated 25 mL sample tubes (universals).
11. MillexGP 0.22 μm filter unit (Millipore).
12. PBS, sterile.

2.2 SES Bioassay

1. Nuclon 24 well plates.
2. RPMI 1640 supplemented media (RPMI-complete; RPMIc): RPMI 1640, 10% (v/v) FCS, 0.002 M L-glutamine, 0.001 M sodium pyruvate, 100 U/mL penicillin, 100 mg/mL streptomycin, 0.055 M β-Mercaptoethanol.

2.3 Acute Resolving Inflammatory Challenge

1. Syringes (1 and 5 mL).
2. Needle (21 and 25 Gauge).

3 Methods

Perform the following procedure in a sterile hood using standard aseptic technique. A schematic flow chart summarising the experimental protocol required for the generation of SES is presented in Fig. 1.

3.1 Isolation and Culture of S. epidermidis Single Colonies

Allow all agar petri dishes to reach room temperature before bacterial inoculation.

1. Inoculate agar plate with a loop of dormant *S. epidermidis* bacteria (Fig. 2). Streaking of bacteria will ensure isolation of single colonies for subsequent expansion. Incubate at 37 °C for 48 h (*see* **Note 1**).
2. Using a flamed or disposable inoculation loop, capture a single bacterial colony of *S. epidermidis* and transfer it into a 250 mL Erlenmeyer flask bottle containing 50 mL of nutrient broth No. 2. Incubate at 37 °C overnight with agitation at 170 rpm (*see* **Note 2**).
3. Transfer 2 mL of the *S. epidermidis* liquid culture into 500 mL Erlenmeyer flask bottle containing 400 mL of nutrient broth No. 2 and incubate overnight at 37 °C with agitation at 170 rpm (*see* **Note 3**).

3.2 Preparation of S. epidermidis Cell Free Supernatant (SES)

1. Visibly check the turbidity of the bacterial culture medium. Transfer the *S. epidermidis* liquid culture into 500 mL centrifuge tubes. Centrifuge at 1800 × *g* for 20 min at 20 °C.
2. Decant supernatant and fully suspend the bacterial pellet in 50 mL Tyrode's salt. This can be achieved by gentle agitation using an automatic pipette. Centrifuge at 1800 × *g* for 20 min at 20 °C. Decant the supernatant and re-suspend Tyrode's salt solution as before. Check the optical density (OD) of the suspension on a spectrophotometer at 560 λ. Dilute the bacterial suspension in Tyrode's salt solution to an optical density of 0.5–0.6 at 560 nm (corresponding to 5×10^8 cfu/mL) (*see* **Note 4**).
3. Incubate the re-suspended culture for 18–24 h at 37 °C. Centrifuge at 5000 × *g* for 30 min at 20 °C. Collect the supernatant and filter using a 0.2 μm Stericup filter bottle system (*see* **Note 5**).
4. Microbiology check 1. SES is a cell free supernatant that is used to induce sterile, resolving inflammation. To ensure that no living bacteria remains in the suspension after the incubation with Tyrode's salt solution, streak a DST agar plate with a 50 μL sample of the filtered suspension. Incubate at 37 °C for 48 h and assess bacterial growth. The culture should be negative for any microorganism.

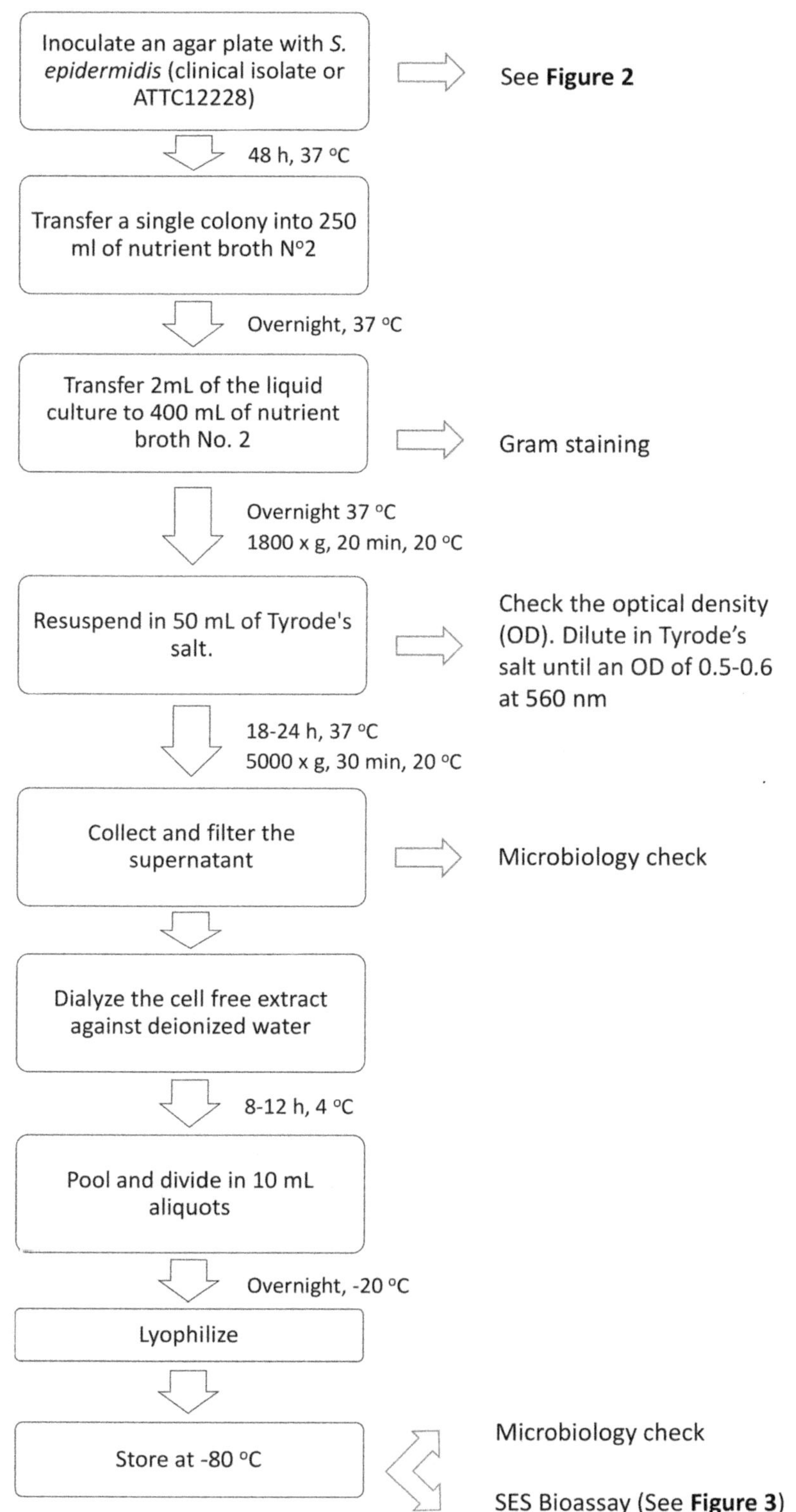

Fig. 1 Schematic flow chart summarising the experimental protocol required for the generation of SES

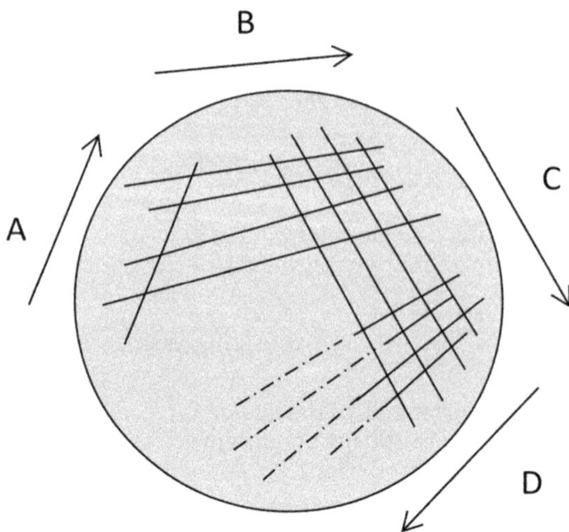

Fig. 2 Schematic representation of how to inoculate an agar plate to obtain single bacterial colonies. (**A**) Streak one line in the direction indicated by the arrow with a sterile loop of dormant *S. epidermidis* from the glycerol stock. (**B–D**) Streak four lines in the direction indicated by the arrow using a new sterile loop for each B, C and D

5. Dialyze the cell-free extract using deionized water in a ratio of 100 mL/5 L in a cold room at 4 °C (*see* **Note 6**). Prepare the dialysis tubing as instructed by the manufacturer. Knot one end of the dialysis tubing, then pour approximately 50 mL of the cell-free extract into the dialysis tubing and knot the other end. Clip one end so that the tube floats and place it in the water (*see* **Note 7**).
6. Leave for 8–12 h, then change water after 8–12 h and repeat a total of three times. Pool the dialyzed extract and divide into 10 mL aliquots in sterile universals. Remove the lids of the universal tubes, and replace with a Parafilm cover. Freeze the samples at −20 °C overnight (*see* **Note 8**).
7. Lyophilize the SES. Freeze dry the samples overnight or until the water has sublimated completely. Replace the lids of the sterile universals and store at −80 °C. Vials maybe stored for approximately 1 year.
8. Microbiology check 2. To ensure that the lyophilized SES is free of any viable bacteria, reconstitute one aliquot of SES in 400 μL of sterile PBS; pass through a MillexGP 0.22 μm filter unit and streak on a DST agar plate. Incubate at 37 °C for 48 h and assess the growth of *S. epidermidis* in the plate by eye. The culture should be negative for any microorganism.

3.3 Test Validation: SES Bioassay

(Optional): It is recommended that bioactivity of each SES batch is tested prior to use in vivo. Murine peritoneal mononuclear cells will generate inflammatory cytokines (e.g., IL-1β, IL-6, CXCL8, TNFα) in response to SES stimulation, and can be used as a reliable bioassay system. As SES triggers the activation of TLR2 [15, 16], PAM3CSK4 may be used as positive control.

1. Isolate resident peritoneal mononuclear cells. Perform a peritoneal lavage of C57Bl/6 mice with 5 mL of RPMIc using a 5 mL syringe and a 25 gauge needle. Centrifuge at 350 × *g* for 5 min to pellet the cell isolate, remove the supernatant and re-suspend the cells to a concentration of 2×10^6 cells/mL (*see* **Note 9**).
2. Plate 1×10^6/0.5 mL cells in 24 well tissue culture microtitre plates (Nuclon).
3. SES titration. Reconstitute SES at the ratio of 1 mL/vial in RPMIc and pass through a MillexGP 0.22 μm filter unit. Prepare serial dilutions of SES (neat, 1/2, 1/4, 1/8, 1/16, 1/32 and 1/64) in RPMIc.
4. Add 0.5 mL of each dilution of SES to each well containing 1×10^6 of resident peritoneal mononuclear cells (*see* **Note 10**).
5. Incubate the culture at 37 °C 5% CO_2 overnight. Transfer carefully the culture media to Eppendorf tubes and render cell free by centrifugation (2000 × *g*, 5 min).
6. Transfer the supernatant carefully to a new clean tube. Supernatants can be stored at −80 °C until needed.
7. Detection of cytokines in the culture supernatant. Cytokine production is quantified using a commercial ELISA (Fig. 3).

3.4 In Vivo Administration of SES and Assessment of Acute Resolving Inflammation

1. Reconstitute the SES in sterile PBS at ratio of 0.75 mL PBS/vial of SES.
2. Filter the reconstituted SES with a MillexGP 0.22 μm filter unit to a new, sterile tube. Load the 1 mL syringes with the required volume of SES (*see* **Note 11**).
3. Each mouse is treated with a 0.5 mL intra-peritoneal administration of SES.
4. Time points (0–96 h) can be selected to conduct analysis of the leukocyte infiltrate (e.g., flow cytometry, differential cell count), production of inflammatory mediators (e.g., ELISA, mass spectrometry), and stromal tissue responses (*see* **Note 12**). Peritoneal tissue can be harvested to determine gene expression or protein activation within the stromal compartment (e.g., immunohistochemistry, real-time PCR, electrophoretic mobility shift assays, immuno-blotting) (*see* **Note 13**). In wild type mice, a single episode of acute resolving inflammation is characterised by a rapid influx of neutrophils

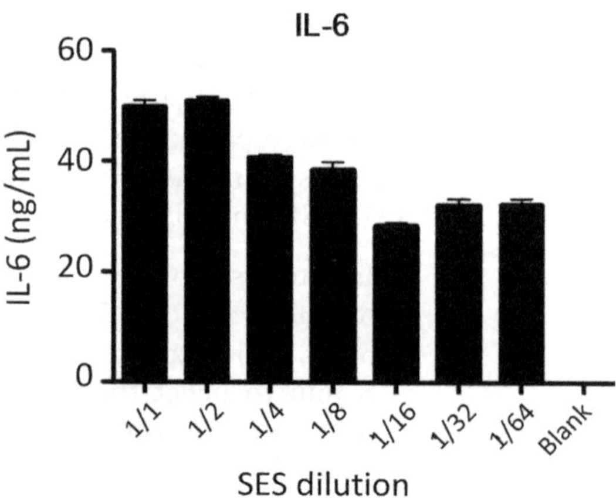

Fig. 3 Representative plot of the levels of IL-6 produced by murine peritoneal resident cells as a response of different concentrations of SES. SES was reconstitute with 1 mL of RPMIc per vial and filtered (0.22 μm). SES serial dilutions (neat 1/1, 1/2, 1/4, 1/8, 1/16, 1/32 and 1/64) were prepared with RPMIc as specified in Subheading 3.3. Blank corresponds to RPMIc alone. For positive control, murine peritoneal resident cells can be stimulated with 10–100 pg/mL of IL-1β or 1–10 ng/mL of TNFα

that peaks at 3–6 h and it is sustained until 24 h post stimulation. A more sustained monocytic cell population (24–36 h) replaces this initial neutrophil influx, and effector lymphocytes populate the peritoneal cavity at 24–48 h after SES treatment [1].

3.5 Repeated Administration of SES and Profiling of Recurrent Inflammatory Challenge

This model can be adapted to investigate the cellular and molecular events that lead to the development of memory responses and the onset of inflammation-induced tissue damage. Here, SES administration (i.p.) can be delivered at 7 day intervals (Day 0, 7, 14 and 21). This allows sufficient time for the resolution of inflammation between each SES treatment, and promotes a subsequent development of peritoneal fibrosis (Day 42–49 after the first SES injection) [12].

In summary, the SES model provides an adaptable means of investigating the molecular mechanisms of leukocyte recruitment and clearance, and provides opportunities to explore the relationships between innate and acquire immunity [13].

3.6 Live Model of S. epidermidis Infection

SES-driven peritonitis provides an extremely versatile model of sterile inflammation. This approach allows investigations of inflammatory regulation without the complications arising from live bacterial infections. However, this model may not be suitable for addressing other questions relevant to the control of infections—e.g., mechanisms of bacterial clearance and dissemination, or systemic responses to local infection. Thus, a modification of the SES acute resolving inflammatory challenge can be achieved using live *S. epidermidis* [17–20].

1. Inoculate an agar plate as before with a loop of dormant *S. epidermidis* bacteria (ATTC 12228 strain). Incubate for 48 h at 37 °C.
2. Using a sterile loop, capture a single colony of *S. epidermidis* and transfer it to an Erlenmeyer Flask (125 mL) containing 10 mL of nutrient broth No. 2. Incubate for 6 h at 37 °C and 170 rpm agitation. Transfer 60 μL of the liquid culture into a 250 mL Erlenmeyer flask with 60 mL of fresh nutrient broth No. 2. Incubate for 18 h at 37 °C and 170 rpm agitation.
3. Assess the desired inoculum size of bacteria (CFU) by spectrometry. Dilute the bacteria culture to an optical density of 1.1–1.15 at 600 nm (corresponding to 1×10^9 cfu/mL).
4. Wash three times in sterile PBS in order to remove the excess of nutrient broth No. 2, and reconstitute to the initial volume.
5. Administer mice with 5×10^8 cfu of *S. epidermidis* (delivered in a volume of 0.5 mL PBS). This bacterial dose is non lethal and causes no advice changes in body weight. Acute infection is resolved within 24–36 h.
6. Collect samples at different time points as before. Here, the model can be used to track dissemination of infection into the bloodstream and other organs, and can be adapted to investigate the acute phase response and systemic inflammatory outcomes including changes in body temperature.

4 Notes

1. The colonies should have a creamy and rounded aspect.
2. The suspension should have substantial turbidity.
3. It is suggested to prepare 4 × 400 mL of culture for each batch in order to obtain around 200 vials of SES at the end of the procedure. At this step, it is recommended to perform a Gram staining to characterise our culture. *Staphylococcus epidermidis* is a Gram-positive cocci. Under the microscope they should appear as rounded cells stained in dark blue following treatment with crystal violet.
4. The spectrophotometer is calibrated against Tyrode's salt solution. Experience shows that a 1/32 dilution gives an OD of 0.5–0.6 at 560 λ. However, it is advisable to perform serial dilutions until the OD required is achieved.
5. Due to the composition of the SES, the filter may become blocked. If so, replace as necessary.

6. The dialysis is performed to remove the Tyrode's salt from the SES suspension. The semi-permeable membrane (MWCO 12–14,000 Da) allows Tyrode's salt solute diffusion into dialysis solution.
7. To facilitate the handling of the dialysis membranes, wet them in deionized water before pouring the SES into them. Note that that preparation of dialysis membrane sometimes requires preparation in an EDTA solution. Check manufacturer instructions before commencing.
8. Make a hole in the Parafilm to allow sublimation of the frozen water during the lyophilisation process.
9. Approximately, $2.5–3 \times 10^6$ resident peritoneal tissue macrophages are isolated from each mouse lavage. Resuspend the cells in 1 mL of RPMIc and count them prior to adjustment to 2×10^6 cells/mL.
10. It is advised to prepare a non-stimulated control with 1×10^6 cells by adding 0.5 mL of RPMIc alone to 0.5 mL of cells.
11. It is essential to ensure that no bubbles remain in the syringe or the needle before injection. To eliminate this concern always draw more SES suspension than is required for administration.
12. To ensure optimal cell recovery by peritoneal lavage after SES stimulation, we recommend to lavage the cavity with 5 mL of RPMI. However, in order to assess the levels of inflammatory mediators, we recommend that the lavage is no bigger than 2 mL of PBS so as to avoid extreme dilution.
13. The peritoneum is an asymmetrical membrane consisting of different cell types and extracellular matrix components. Therefore, different sample processing is required depending on the downstream applications. For example, a correct orientation of the peritoneal membrane is essential for immunohistochemistry analysis; for protein quantification or gene expression analysis, it is recommended to snap-freeze the sample in liquid nitrogen immediately after collection.

References

1. Hurst SM, Wilkinson TS, McLoughlin RM, Jones S, Horiuchi S, Yamamoto N, Rose-John S, Fuller GM, Topley N, Jones SA (2001) Il-6 and its soluble receptor orchestrate a temporal switch in the pattern of leukocyte recruitment seen during acute inflammation. Immunity 14:705–714
2. Fielding CA, McLoughlin RM, McLeod L, Colmont CS, Najdovska M, Grail D, Ernst M, Jones SA, Topley N, Jenkins BJ (2008) IL-6 regulates neutrophil trafficking during acute inflammation via STAT3. J Immunol 181:2189–2195
3. McLoughlin RM, Hurst SM, Nowell MA, Harris DA, Horiuchi S, Morgan LW, Wilkinson TS, Yamamoto N, Topley N, Jones SA (2004) Differential regulation of neutrophil-activating chemokines by IL-6 and its soluble receptor isoforms. J Immunol 172:5676–5683
4. McLoughlin RM, Jenkins BJ, Grail D, Williams AS, Fielding CA, Parker CR, Ernst M, Topley N, Jones SA (2005) IL-6 trans-

signaling via STAT3 directs T cell infiltration in acute inflammation. Proc Natl Acad Sci U S A 102:9589–9594

5. McLoughlin RM, Witowski J, Robson RL, Wilkinson TS, Hurst SM, Williams AS, Williams JD, Rose-John S, Jones SA, Topley N (2003) Interplay between IFN-gamma and IL-6 signaling governs neutrophil trafficking and apoptosis during acute inflammation. J Clin Invest 112:598–607
6. Hams E, Colmont CS, Dioszeghy V, Hammond VJ, Fielding CA, Williams AS, Tanaka M, Miyajima A, Taylor PR, Topley N, Jones SA (2008) Oncostatin M receptor-beta signaling limits monocytic cell recruitment in acute inflammation. J Immunol 181:2174–2180
7. Jones GW, McLoughlin RM, Hammond VJ, Parker CR, Williams JD, Malhotra R, Scheller J, Williams AS, Rose-John S, Topley N, Jones SA (2010) Loss of CD4+ T cell IL-6R expression during inflammation underlines a role for IL-6 trans signaling in the local maintenance of Th17 cells. J Immunol 184:2130–2139
8. Nowell MA, Richards PJ, Horiuchi S, Yamamoto N, Rose-John S, Topley N, Williams AS, Jones SA (2003) Soluble IL-6 receptor governs IL-6 activity in experimental arthritis: blockade of arthritis severity by soluble glycoprotein 130. J Immunol 171:3202–3209
9. Richards PJ, Nowell MA, Horiuchi S, McLoughlin RM, Fielding CA, Grau S, Yamamoto N, Ehrmann M, Rose-John S, Williams AS, Topley N, Jones SA (2006) Functional characterization of a soluble gp130 isoform and its therapeutic capacity in an experimental model of inflammatory arthritis. Arthritis Rheum 54:1662–1672
10. Nowell MA, Williams AS, Carty SA, Scheller J, Hayes AJ, Jones GW, Richards PJ, Slinn S, Ernst M, Jenkins BJ, Topley N, Rose-John S, Jones SA (2009) Therapeutic targeting of IL-6 trans signaling counteracts STAT3 control of experimental inflammatory arthritis. J Immunol 182:613–622
11. Jones GW, Greenhill CJ, Williams JO, Nowell MA, Williams AS, Jenkins BJ, Jones SA (2013) Exacerbated inflammatory arthritis in response to hyperactive gp130 signalling is independent of IL-17A. Ann Rheum Dis 72:1738–1742
12. Fielding CA, Jones GW, McLoughlin RM, McLeod L, Hammond VJ, Uceda J, Williams AS, Lambie M, Foster TL, Liao CT, Rice CM, Greenhill CJ, Colmont CS, Hams E, Coles B, Kift-Morgan A, Newton Z, Craig KJ, Williams JD, Williams GT, Davies SJ, Humphreys IR, O'Donnell VB, Taylor PR, Jenkins BJ, Topley N, Jones SA (2014) Interleukin-6 signaling drives fibrosis in unresolved inflammation. Immunity 40:40–50
13. Jones SA (2005) Directing transition from innate to acquired immunity: defining a role for IL-6. J Immunol 175:3463–3468
14. Jenkins BJ, Grail D, Nheu T, Najdovska M, Wang B, Waring P, Inglese M, McLoughlin RM, Jones SA, Topley N, Baumann H, Judd LM, Giraud AS, Boussioutas A, Zhu HJ, Ernst M (2005) Hyperactivation of Stat3 in gp130 mutant mice promotes gastric hyperproliferation and desensitizes TGF-beta signaling. Nat Med 11:845–852
15. Colmont CS, Raby AC, Dioszeghy V, Lebouder E, Foster TL, Jones SA, Labeta MO, Fielding CA, Topley N (2011) Human peritoneal mesothelial cells respond to bacterial ligands through a specific subset of Toll-like receptors. Nephrol Dial Transplant 26:4079–4090
16. Strunk T, Power Coombs MR, Currie AJ, Richmond P, Golenbock DT, Stoler-Barak L, Gallington LC, Otto M, Burgner D, Levy O (2010) TLR2 mediates recognition of live Staphylococcus epidermidis and clearance of bacteremia. PLoS One 5:e10111
17. Raby AC, Le Bouder E, Colmont C, Davies J, Richards P, Coles B, George CH, Jones SA, Brennan P, Topley N, Labeta MO (2009) Soluble TLR2 reduces inflammation without compromising bacterial clearance by disrupting TLR2 triggering. J Immunol 183:506–517
18. Raby AC, Holst B, Le Bouder E, Diaz C, Ferran E, Conraux L, Guillemot JC, Coles B, Kift-Morgan A, Colmont CS, Szakmany T, Ferrara P, Hall JE, Topley N, Labeta MO (2013) Targeting the TLR co-receptor CD14 with TLR2-derived peptides modulates immune responses to pathogens. Sci Transl Med 5:185ra164
19. Raby AC, Colmont CS, Kift-Morgan A, Kohl J, Eberl M, Fraser D, Topley N, Labeta MO (2017) Toll-Like Receptors 2 and 4 Are Potential Therapeutic Targets in Peritoneal Dialysis-Associated Fibrosis. J Am Soc Nephrol 28:461–478
20. Morgan AH, Dioszeghy V, Maskrey BH, Thomas CP, Clark SR, Mathie SA, Lloyd CM, Kuhn H, Topley N, Coles BC, Taylor PR, Jones SA, O'Donnell VB (2009) Phosphatidylethanolamine-esterified eicosanoids in the mouse: tissue localization and inflammation-dependent formation in Th-2 disease. J Biol Chem 284:21185–21191

Chapter 7

Citrobacter rodentium Infection Model for the Analysis of Bacterial Pathogenesis and Mucosal Immunology

Catherine L. Kennedy and Elizabeth L. Hartland

Abstract

Citrobacter rodentium is a mouse restricted pathogen that was originally isolated from laboratory mouse colonies and causes transmissible colonic hyperplasia, characterized by thickening of the colon and inflammation. As a natural pathogen of mice, the infection model has proven critical to the development of our understanding of the pathogenesis of enteric disease and the mucosal immune response. In addition to this, some features of disease such as dysbiosis, inflammation, and wound healing replicate features of human inflammatory bowel diseases. As such, the *C. rodentium* infection model has become a key tool in investigations of many aspects of mucosal immunology.

Key words Colitis, Mucosal immunity, *Citrobacter rodentium*, Bacterial infection, Immune cell analysis, Bacterial culture

1 Introduction

Citrobacter rodentium is a mouse restricted pathogen that was originally isolated from laboratory mouse colonies and which causes transmissible murine colonic hyperplasia (TMCH). TMCH is characterized by thickening of the colon (hyperplasia), some loss of crypt architecture and increased inflammation [1]. *C. rodentium* carries the same virulence factors as the clinically relevant human diarrheagenic pathogens, enteropathogenic *Escherichia coli* (EPEC), and enterohemorrhagic *E. coli* (EHEC) [2]. All three are attaching and effacing (A/E) pathogens that induce histopathological lesions, termed A/E lesions, on the apical surface of host enterocytes [3]. A/E pathogens carry a pathogenicity island, the locus of enterocyte effacement (LEE), that encodes the components of a type 3 secretion system (T3SS), which comprises a needle-like structure that allows the pathogen to directly translocate effector proteins into the host cell. Several of these effector proteins are encoded within the LEE including the translocated intimin receptor, Tir, while many others are encoded in other parts

Brendan J. Jenkins (ed.), *Inflammation and Cancer: Methods and Protocols*, Methods in Molecular Biology, vol. 1725,
https://doi.org/10.1007/978-1-4939-7568-6_7, © Springer Science+Business Media, LLC 2018

of the genome [2]. A group of 21 core effectors, including all those encoded within the LEE and a number of non-LEE encoded (Nle) effectors, is shared by all A/E pathogens [4]. These effectors subvert various host cell processes, including actin filament formation, Rho GTPase function, host protein ubiquitination pathways, phagocytosis, apoptosis, and inflammatory signaling, all of which enables the bacteria to colonize the host intestinal tract, multiply and cause disease [3, 5]. EPEC and EHEC colonize mice poorly, so *C. rodentium* has become an invaluable tool for understanding the role of effector proteins in virulence [1, 6–11].

In addition to its role as a surrogate pathogen for EPEC and EHEC, *C. rodentium* is an important tool for studying the enteric mucosal immune response due to its ability to cause colitis without significant invasion or systemic inflammation. Although early reports highlighted a role for Th1 cells [12], more recent studies have defined a key role for type 3 innate lymphoid cells (ILC3s) in the innate stages of infection working with epithelial cells via lymphotoxin β and IL-22 to maintain epithelial integrity and prevent systemic infection [13–16], although ILC3s as the key source of IL-22 is questionable [17]. Neutrophils [18, 19], CD4+ T helper 17 (Th17) [20–22], Th22 [22, 23], and B cells (particularly serum IgG) [24] are also important in the resolution of infection.

Finally, *C. rodentium* infection models have been used to probe the role of the microbiota in containing enteric infection, an emergent and rapidly expanding field [25, 26]. Herein we describe the establishment and monitoring of the *C. rodentium* mouse infection model, analysis of infection parameters using gross and histopathological measures and the preparation of colonic tissue for flow cytometric analysis.

2 Materials

2.1 Citrobacter rodentium Infection Model

1. Mice aged 6–8 weeks, male or female.
2. *Citrobacter rodentium* isolate ICC169 (*see* **Note 1**).
3. Luria agar (LA) and Luria broth (LB) supplemented with relevant antibiotics.
4. Steel gavage needles, 20 gauge, 38 mm length; and 1 mL syringes.

2.2 Preparation of Colon for FACS

1. Petri dishes.
2. Small dissection kit.
3. 50 and 15 mL conical tubes.
4. 70 μm cell strainers.
5. No. 10 or 11 scalpel blades.

6. Plastic Pasteur pipettes.
7. Ca^{2+}/Mg^{2+}-free Hanks balanced salt solution (fHBSS).
8. Collection buffer (5 mL per sample): RPMI containing 1 mM dithiothreitol (DTT).
9. Dissociation buffer (20 mL per sample): fHBSS containing 3 mM ethylenediaminetetraacetic acid (EDTA) and 0.5 mM DTT.
10. Wash buffer A: Phosphate buffered saline (PBS) containing 1 mM EDTA, 3% fetal calf serum (FCS).
11. Digestion cocktail (10 mL per sample): Ca^{2+}/Mg^{2+}-replete HBSS (cHBSS), 0.5% bovine serum albumin (BSA), 0.5 mg/mL Collagenase (*see* **Note 2**), 5 U/mL Dispase II, 0.1 mg/mL DNAse I (*see* **Note 3**).
12. Wash buffer B: PBS, 3% FCS
13. Percoll solutions: Make up a 90% Percoll solution by adding 9 parts Percoll to one part 10× PBS. Then dilute the 90% solution using 1× PBS, 1 mM EDTA to desired concentrations (*see* **Note 4**).

3 Methods

The following description of infection of mice with *C. rodentium* and subsequent monitoring has been approved by the University of Melbourne Animal Ethics Committee and is routinely used in the laboratory. However, all procedures must meet the requirements of a relevant institutional animal ethics committee.

3.1 C. rodentium Infection Model: Infection

1. Set up an overnight culture of *C. rodentium* ICC169 by inoculating a 10 mL LB broth, supplemented with 50 μg/mL nalidixic acid, with a single colony. Derivatives of *C. rodentium* that carry gene disruptions and/or plasmids may require additional antibiotic selection.
2. Incubate overnight (approximately 16 h) at 37 °C with shaking so that the culture reaches stationary phase.
3. Centrifuge the culture at 1520 × *g* for 10 min at room temperature to pellet the cells.
4. Pour off supernatant and resuspend the pellet in 1 mL PBS (i.e., 0.1 times the volume of the overnight culture).
5. Determine the optical density at 600 nm (OD_{600}) of the resuspended pellet by taking a 10 μL sample and diluting it in 990 μL PBS. For *C. rodentium* cultures, an OD_{600} of 1.0 equates to approximately 1×10^9 colony forming units (cfu)/mL (*see* **Note 5**).

6. Calculate the volume of inoculum required and the dilution required to give a final OD_{600} of 5.0 such that each mouse receives 1×10^9 cfu in 200 μL of inoculum (*see* **Notes 6** and 7).
7. The accuracy of the inoculum preparation should be checked in two ways:
   (a) Check the OD_{600} of the inoculum by diluting it 1/20 to ensure that the correct concentration has been attained prior to gavage.
   (b) Serially dilute 100 μL of the inoculum tenfold until dilutions of 10^{-6}, 10^{-7}, and 10^{-8} have been reached and plate 100 μL of each in duplicate onto LA supplemented with the relevant antibiotics. Culture overnight at 37 °C and the following day count the number of colonies on the 10^{-7} plates and calculate the cfu/mL.
   Both techniques are important as the OD_{600} ensures that the dilutions have been performed correctly and the colony count shows that viability correlates with the OD_{600} reading.
8. Using a straight, 20 gauge, 38 mm steel gavage needle attached to a 1 mL syringe, draw 200 μL of inoculum into the syringe (*see* **Note 8**).
9. Weigh the mouse then restrain by scruffing high around the shoulders and neck to restrict excessive movement of the head and secure tail against the palm so that the body of the mouse is straight.
10. Insert the gavage needle into the mouth of the mouse, guiding it to the back of the throat. Tip the head of the mouse back using the gavage needle such that the needle is in line with the line of the mouse's body. The gavage needle should slide easily down the throat and esophagus of the mouse and the inoculum should be able to be expelled without any resistance. If force is required at any stage of gavage, the gavage has not been executed properly and the needle should be removed and the mouse allowed to rest before reattempting (*see* **Note 9**).
11. Check the nares of the mouse to ensure the inoculum has not flowed into the lung or nasopharynx (as evidenced by bubbles around the nostrils) and then release the mouse into its cage.
12. Observe the mouse for 5 min to ensure it is breathing and behaving normally.

3.2 C. rodentium *Infection Model: Monitoring*

1. Weigh mice daily as measure of overall health. C57BL/6 mice generally tolerate *C. rodentium* infection well and will not lose weight over the course of infection. Other mouse strains (e.g., C3H/HeJ) or mice carrying genetic mutations such may lose significant amounts of weight. Weight loss of 10% or greater in

1 day or greater than 15% compared to the starting weight indicates the mouse should be killed for ethical reasons.

2. Collect fecal pellets from the mice at regular intervals to monitor *C. rodentium* colonization levels. Every 2 days will give a good picture of colonization kinetics.
   (a) Mice should be distributed into individual clean boxes and allowed to defecate.
   (b) The pellets should be collected into preweighed 1.5 mL tubes using forceps. Forceps must be soaked in 70% ethanol between uses.
   (c) Note the consistency of the fecal pellet and determine if there is any evidence of diarrhea (*see* **Note 10**).
   (d) Weigh the pellets and resuspend in PBS to a final concentration of 100 mg feces/mL. The pellets can be emulsified in the PBS using plastic pestles designed to fit in 1.5 mL tubes, or on a vortex with an attachment to hold 1.5 mL tubes.
   (e) Serially dilute the fecal emulsion tenfold in PBS. Wide bore pipette tips are necessary when pipetting the neat and 10^{-1} dilutions, but it is preferable to change to normal size pipette tips for the remaining dilutions. Plate 100 μL of three consecutive dilutions onto LA supplemented appropriate antibiotics and culture overnight at 37 °C. Count colonies on plates where between 30 and 300 colonies have grown and determine cfu/g feces (*see* **Note 11**).
3. Monitor for other qualitative signs of infection including;
   (a) Appearance (scruffy, unkempt, or skin tenting as evidence of dehydration).
   (b) Behavior and activity levels (reduced activity, hunched, not stretching to get to food source). Hunching is a clear sign of fulminant infection and mice showing signs of hunching should be closely monitored and carefully handled to minimize stress.
4. Follow the course of infection as long as required. Mice can be killed at desired time points depending on which phase of infection is of interest. Various measures of disease can be analyzed at the time of killing, including:
   (a) Colon and cecum weight and length: Fulminant infection frequently results in shortening and thickening of the colon and shrinkage of the cecum.
   (b) Histopathology: Hematoxylin and eosin staining to show colonic hyperplasia, inflammatory infiltrate, and changes to crypt and epithelial layer architecture (Fig. 1).

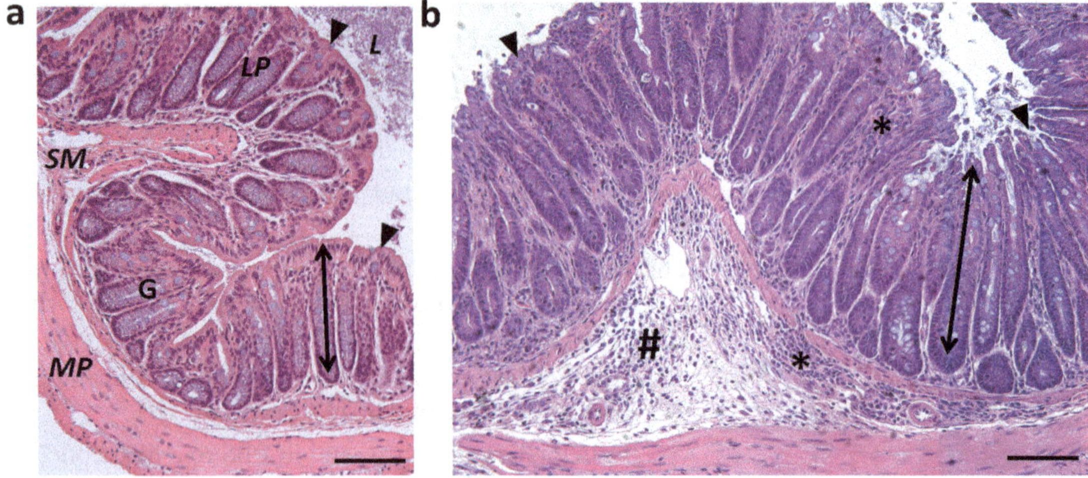

Fig. 1 Representative micrographs of H&E stained transverse sections of distal colon. (**a**) Uninfected tissue. *L* denotes lumen; *LP* denotes lamina propria; *SM* denotes submucosa; *MP* denotes muscularis propria. Crypt height, indicated by *double-headed arrow*, is approximately 150 μm and crypts are lined with goblet cells, G. Arrowheads indicate neatly arranged epithelial cells. (**b**) Infected tissue. Inflammatory infiltrate (*) evident in the lamina propria and submucosal space. Extensive edema in submcosa (#). Crypt hyperplasia (*double-headed arrow*) evident with crypt height approximately 250 μm. Arrowheads indicate disruption of the epithelial layer. Note also the absence of goblet cells in the crypts. Scale bar, 100 μm

(c) Immunohistochemistry—Frozen: To spatially identify molecules or cells of interest and show *C. rodentium* colonization.

(d) Flow cytometry analysis: To identify rare cell types and quantify cellular infiltrates. The preparation of a single cell suspension from colonic tissue is described below.

3.3 Tissue Dissociation for FACS Analysis

1. Kill mouse according to relevant ethical guidelines.
2. Excise colon and/or cecum, clean away any mesentery, cut longitudinally and rinse in ice cold HBSS to remove feces.
3. Transfer tissue to a 10 mL conical tube containing 5 mL collection buffer and store on ice.
4. Shake tube containing colon to remove any remaining feces and mucus and empty into petri dish.
5. Cut up colon and/or cecum into 10–15 pieces and transfer to 50 mL tube containing 10 mL Dissociation buffer (*see* **Note 12**).
6. Incubate with movement (orbital shaker or rocker), for 15 min at 37 °C (*see* **Note 13**).
7. Vortex tube to dissociate epithelial layer from lamina propria.

8. Pour supernatant through 70 μm cell strainer into 50 mL Falcon containing 25 mL Wash buffer A. Store Falcon tube on ice.
9. Transfer intact tissue from strainer into 10 mL fresh Dissociation buffer and incubate as for **step 6**.
10. Vortex again and strain into the same 50 mL Falcon tube. Strained portion contains epithelial cell and intraepithelial lymphocyte (IEL) fraction. IELs can be further purified using Percoll density gradient centrifugation (*see* **steps 19–25**).
11. Collect remaining lamina propria (LP) tissue into a petri dish and wash once in 15 mL cHBSS by adding the cHBSS directly to the plate and then aspirating off again (*see* **Note 14**).
12. Mince tissue to a fine paste using scalpel blade (*see* **Note 15**).
13. Transfer minced tissue into 5 mL Digestion cocktail in a 15 mL Falcon tube and incubate at 37 °C for 15 min with movement (orbital shaker or rocker).
14. Add 5 mL Wash buffer B and pipette ~15 times using plastic Pasteur pipette.
15. Stand for 5 min to let large pieces settle and strain supernatant though fresh 70 μm cell strainer into a 50 mL Falcon containing 25 mL Wash buffer A and store filtrate on ice.
16. Repeat **steps 13–15**; however, the sample can be strained without allowing larger pieces to settle as they will be collected by the filter. Discard strainer and remaining tissue (*see* **Note 16**).
17. Strained portion contains mesenchymal/muscle cells and lamina propria lymphocytes (LPLs). LPLs can be further purified using Percoll density gradient centrifugation (*see* **steps 19–25**).
18. Centrifuge 50 mL falcon tubes containing the EpC/IEL or LP/LPL fractions at 400 × *g* for 20 min at 4 °C. Wash pellet in 10 mL Wash buffer A.
19. The remaining cell pellets can be used for FACS analysis (*see* **Note 17**) or can be further purified using Percoll density gradient centrifugation to isolate lymphocytes.
20. To further isolate lymphocytes, cells in cold Wash buffer A and remove as much supernatant as possible.
21. Resuspend in 8 mL 40% Percoll, 1 mM EDTA in a 15 mL Falcon tube (*see* **Note 4**).
22. Underlay cell suspension with 4 mL 80% Percoll 1 mM EDTA using a thin 1 mL Pasteur pipette (*see* **Note 18**).
23. Spin at 663 × *g* for 20 min at room temperature and allow centrifuge to decelerate without the brake on.

24. Epithelial and other lamina propria cells will collect at the top of the tube, lymphocytes (IELs, LPLs, or total) will collect at the interphase of the two densities (*see* **Note 19**).
25. Collect the lymphocyte fraction and resuspend in Wash buffer A to a final volume of 20 mL. Spin at 400 × *g* for 10 min at room temperature to pellet the cells. Lymphocytes are ready for downstream analysis including stimulation for cytokine expression.

This technique has been successfully used by our laboratory to identify even rare cell types such as MAIT cells and regulatory T-cells.

4 Notes

1. There are two strains of *C. rodentium* commonly used for infection models; DSB100 and ICC168 (or the nalidixic resistant or bioluminescent derivatives of ICC168, which are ICC169 and ICC180, respectively [27, 28]). A third strain, EX-33, was isolated from a different outbreak; however, it appears to mediate the same disease pathology [29, 30].
2. The nomenclature of collagenase preparations is different across diverse companies. The key feature to look for is low tryptic activity. Collagenase Type IV from ThermoFisher Scientific, Type 4 from Worthington and Type D from Sigma Aldrich all have above average collagenase activity and low tryptic activity so are ideal. Collagenase Type 3 from Worthington has low secondary protease activity and normal collagenase activity and is also suitable.
3. To save time and enhance reproducibility, prepare a 10× concentrated stock of Collagenase/Dispase in cHBSS, 0.5% BSA and freeze in 1 mL aliquots for up to 6 months. Dilute in cHBSS, 0.5% BSA immediately before use. DNase should be aliquoted separately in dH_2O.
4. For clear demarcation of the Percoll layers, PBS containing phenol red indicator or RPMI, supplemented with 1 mM EDTA, can be used to make up the 40% solution. This way, the interphase is clearly identified at the color change.
5. The concentrated preparation from a healthy overnight culture should have an OD_{600} of around 14.0. Much greater than this (>17.0) could indicate a high number of dead or dying cells, resulting in the final dose containing a lower proportion of healthy, infective *C. rodentium* cells. Much lower than this (<11.0) indicates too short a culture time (so the bacteria may not have reached stationary phase), problems with the

culture conditions or a deficiency in the strain if a mutant is being used.

6. An example calculation is as follows:
   (a) Inoculum is required for infection of 10 mice at 200 μL per mouse. Therefore, a minimum of 2000 μL plus overage is required = 2500 μL.
   (b) The calculated OD_{600} of the concentrated culture is 15.4 and the final viable count required is 1.0×10^9 cfu/200 μL, or 5.0×10^9 cfu/mL which is equivalent to an OD_{600} of 5.0.

$$C1V1 = C2V2$$

$$15.4_{OD600} \times V1 = 5.0_{OD600} \times 2500\,\mu L$$

$$V1 = 12,500/15.4$$

$$V1 = 812\,\mu L$$

   Therefore, 812 μL of the concentrated culture must be diluted in 1688 μL PBS to give 2500 μL inoculum at a concentration of OD_{600} 5.0.

7. A reduced dose of $1.0\text{–}5.0 \times 10^8$ cfu can be used to establish infection in mice that may succumb to more severe disease. While the higher dose of 1.0×10^9 cfu/mouse more reproducibly establishes infection, it is often necessary to balance this with animal welfare and eliciting an infection that the mice can clear so that the full immune response can be studied.

8. Reusable steel gavage needles can be stored in 100% ethanol between uses to eliminate contamination. Before gavage, the needles are rinsed three times in 70% ethanol and three times in sterile PBS by drawing 1 mL into the syringe and expelling it. The gavage needle does not need to be cleaned between mice, but should be cleaned thoroughly between different *C. rodentium* strains.

9. There are two main issues with gavage which may require euthanasia of the mouse. Firstly, the needle may pass into the bronchus rather than the esophagus. This can be detected if the mouse starts to choke, show signs of difficulty in breathing, or fluid or bubbles are visible around the nares. Also, the gavage needle will not be able to be inserted very far as the lungs sit above the stomach. If it is suspected that the gavage needle has been inserted into the bronchus, immediately remove the needle and release the mouse and observe to ensure it is breathing normally before reattempting the gavage. The second issue with gavage is esophageal rupture. This is more likely to occur is the mouse is not scuffed securely with the body held

in a straight line and will *only* occur if force is used to insert the needle. It can be difficult to detect if esophageal rupture has occurred during gavage; however, if the mouse appears scruffy and is losing weight over the first 2 days of infection (when *C. rodentium* is only barely colonizing the gut) it is likely that rupture has occurred and the mouse should be euthanized.

10. C57BL/6 mice do not develop fulminant diarrhea during infection with *C. rodentium*, although loose stools are usually evident. Diarrhea is detectable in some mice carrying mutations in host defense genes and can be a helpful descriptor of susceptibility to disease. Diarrhea can be graded on a scale of 0–4 as follows [8]:

0—(no diarrhea)	Solid stool with no sign of soiling around the anus. The stool is very firm when subjected to pressure with tweezers
1—(very mild diarrhea)	Formed stools that appear moist on the outside. Stool is less firm when pressure applied with tweezers.
2—(mild diarrhea)	Formed stools that appear moist on the outside. Stools will easily submit to pressure applied with tweezers.
3—(diarrhea)	No formed stools with a mucous-like appearance. Mouse takes a long time to pass stool and soiling around the anus and tail may be evident.
4—(severe, watery diarrhea)	Mostly clear or mucous-like liquid stool with very minimal solid present and considerable soiling around anus. Mouse may not be able to pass stool at all. Occasionally, blood may be observed in the stool.

11. There will be some variability in colonization levels between mice; however, as a guide, it is best to start by plating an aliquot of neat, 10^{-1}, 10^{-2} at day 2 post infection. After overnight culture, count the plates that have between 30 and 300 colonies and use this as the basis for determining how far the sample must be diluted at later time points—i.e., if the optimal dilution for determining cfu/g at day 2 is 10^{-1}, at day 4 dilute out to 10^{-4} and plate 10^{-2}, 10^{-3}, and 10^{-4}. The colonization level will increase until day 10, then plateau until around day 14, then start to decrease until the infection is cleared at between days 18 and 24. The period of clearance can be quite variable between bacterial and mouse strains so more frequent monitoring is often required.

12. Cutting the tissue to smaller pieces helps with the movement of the tissue in the buffer and encourages the nonenzymatic dissociation.

13. Incubation in the Dissociation buffer can be done at room temperature as well.
14. EDTA inhibits collagenase activity, so washing the tissue in cHBSS is important for the efficient digestion of the lamina propria tissue in the next steps.
15. Tissue should be minced so the fragments are of a size that can be easily aspirated in a plastic Pasteur pipette. This creates a greater surface area for the enzymes to act on and also facilitates mechanical dissociation by pipetting.
16. It is likely that some larger pieces of tissue will remain after only two enzymatic dissociation steps; however, this is preferable to complete breakdown which may result in overdigestion of the sample and loss of cell surface receptors.
17. If the single cell suspension is to be run without further purification, it is essential to include 1 mM EDTA in the buffers to prevent clumping of the epithelial cells and to re-strain the cells immediately before running if the cells have been stored before analysis.
18. To underlay the 80% Percoll solution, use a fine Pasteur pipette which can reach to the base of the 15 mL Falcon tube. Very slowly expel the 80% Percoll solution into the bottom of the tube. The higher density 80% Percoll solution will remain in the bottom of the tube without mixing into the 40% solution. The efficacy of this will be very obvious if the 40% solution is made up using PBS containing phenol red or RPMI and the 80% solution is made up using normal PBS.
19. It can be helpful to remove the top layer of epithelial cells and much of the 40% Percoll before collecting the cells at the interphase to prevent contamination of the pipette and sample due to passing through the epithelial cells.

References

1. Mundy R, MacDonald TT, Dougan G, Frankel G, Wiles S (2005) *Citrobacter rodentium* of mice and man. Cell Microbiol 7:1697–1706
2. Petty NK, Bulgin R, Crepin VF, Cerdeno-Tarraga AM, Schroeder GN, Quail MA et al (2010) The *Citrobacter rodentium* genome sequence reveals convergent evolution with human pathogenic *Escherichia coli*. J Bacteriol 192:525–538
3. Wong AR, Pearson JS, Bright MD, Munera D, Robinson KS, Lee SF et al (2011) Enteropathogenic and enterohaemorrhagic *Escherichia coli:* even more subversive elements. Mol Microbiol 80:1420–1438
4. Iguchi A, Thomson NR, Ogura Y, Saunders D, Ooka T, Henderson IR et al (2009) Complete genome sequence and comparative genome analysis of enteropathogenic *Escherichia coli* O127:H6 strain E2348/69. J Bacteriol 191:347–354
5. Santos AS, Finlay BB (2015) Bringing down the host: enteropathogenic and enterohaemorrhagic *Escherichia coli* effector-mediated subversion of host innate immune pathways. Cell Microbiol 17:318–332
6. Feuerbacher LA, Hardwidge PR (2014) Influence of NleH effector expression, host genetics, and inflammation on *Citrobacter rodentium* colonization of mice. Microbes Infect 16:429–433

7. Pearson JS, Giogha C, Muhlen S, Nachbur U, Pham CL, Zhang Y et al (2017) EspL is a bacterial cysteine protease effector that cleaves RHIM proteins to block necroptosis and inflammation. Nat Microbiol 2:16258
8. Pearson JS, Giogha C, Ong SY, Kennedy CL, Kelly M, Robinson KS et al (2013) A type III effector antagonizes death receptor signalling during bacterial gut infection. Nature 501:247–251
9. Sham HP, Shames SR, Croxen MA, Ma C, Chan JM, Khan MA et al (2011) Attaching and effacing bacterial effector NleC suppresses epithelial inflammatory responses by inhibiting NF-kappaB and p38 mitogen-activated protein kinase activation. Infect Immun 79:3552–3562
10. Wickham ME, Lupp C, Vazquez A, Mascarenhas M, Coburn B, Coombes BK et al (2007) *Citrobacter rodentium* virulence in mice associates with bacterial load and the type III effector NleE. Microbes Infect 9:400–407
11. Ma C, Wickham ME, Guttman JA, Deng W, Walker J, Madsen KL et al (2006) *Citrobacter rodentium* infection causes both mitochondrial dysfunction and intestinal epithelial barrier disruption *in vivo*: role of mitochondrial associated protein (Map). Cell Microbiol 8:1669–1686
12. Simmons CP, Goncalves NS, Ghaem-Maghami M, Bajaj-Elliott M, Clare S, Neves B et al (2002) Impaired resistance and enhanced pathology during infection with a noninvasive, attaching-effacing enteric bacterial pathogen, *Citrobacter rodentium,* in mice lacking IL-12 or IFN-gamma. J Immunol 168:1804–1812
13. Cella M, Fuchs A, Vermi W, Facchetti F, Otero K, Lennerz JK et al (2009) A human natural killer cell subset provides an innate source of IL-22 for mucosal immunity. Nature 457:722–725
14. Macho-Fernandez E, Koroleva EP, Spencer CM, Tighe M, Torrado E, Cooper AM et al (2015) Lymphotoxin beta receptor signaling limits mucosal damage through driving IL-23 production by epithelial cells. Mucosal Immunol 8:403–413
15. Tumanov AV, Koroleva EP, Guo X, Wang Y, Kruglov A, Nedospasov S et al (2011) Lymphotoxin controls the IL-22 protection pathway in gut innate lymphoid cells during mucosal pathogen challenge. Cell Host Microbe 10:44–53
16. Zheng Y, Valdez PA, Danilenko DM, Hu Y, Sa SM, Gong Q et al (2008) Interleukin-22 mediates early host defense against attaching and effacing bacterial pathogens. Nat Med 14:282–289
17. Rankin LC, Girard-Madoux MJ, Seillet C, Mielke LA, Kerdiles Y, Fenis A et al (2016) Complementarity and redundancy of IL-22-producing innate lymphoid cells. Nat Immunol 17:179–186
18. Spehlmann ME, Dann SM, Hruz P, Hanson E, McCole DF, Eckmann L (2009) CXCR2-dependent mucosal neutrophil influx protects against colitis-associated diarrhea caused by an attaching/effacing lesion-forming bacterial pathogen. J Immunol 183:3332–3343
19. Wang Y, Koroleva EP, Kruglov AA, Kuprash DV, Nedospasov SA, YX F et al (2010) Lymphotoxin beta receptor signaling in intestinal epithelial cells orchestrates innate immune responses against mucosal bacterial infection. Immunity 32:403–413
20. Geddes K, Rubino SJ, Magalhaes JG, Streutker C, Le Bourhis L, Cho JH et al (2011) Identification of an innate T helper type 17 response to intestinal bacterial pathogens. Nat Med 17:837–844
21. Ishigame H, Kakuta S, Nagai T, Kadoki M, Nambu A, Komiyama Y et al (2009) Differential roles of interleukin-17A and -17F in host defense against mucoepithelial bacterial infection and allergic responses. Immunity 30:108–119
22. Backert I, Koralov SB, Wirtz S, Kitowski V, Billmeier U, Martini E et al (2014) STAT3 activation in Th17 and Th22 cells controls IL-22-mediated epithelial host defense during infectious colitis. J Immunol 193:3779–3791
23. Basu R, O'Quinn DB, Silberger DJ, Schoeb TR, Fouser L, Ouyang W et al (2012) Th22 cells are an important source of IL-22 for host protection against enteropathogenic bacteria. Immunity 37:1061–1075
24. Simmons CP, Clare S, Ghaem-Maghami M, Uren TK, Rankin J, Huett A et al (2003) Central role for B lymphocytes and CD4+ T cells in immunity to infection by the attaching and effacing pathogen *Citrobacter rodentium.* Infect Immun 71:5077–5086
25. Keeney KM, Yurist-Doutsch S, Arrieta MC, Finlay BB (2014) Effects of antibiotics on human microbiota and subsequent disease. Annu Rev Microbiol 68:217–235
26. Collins JW, Keeney KM, Crepin VF, Rathinam VA, Fitzgerald KA, Finlay BB et al (2014) *Citrobacter rodentium*: infection, inflammation and the microbiota. Nat Rev Microbiol 12:612–623
27. Ghaem-Maghami M, Simmons CP, Daniell S, Pizza M, Lewis D, Frankel G et al (2001) Intimin-specific immune responses prevent

bacterial colonization by the attaching-effacing pathogen *Citrobacter rodentium*. Infect Immun 69:5597–5605

28. Wiles S, Clare S, Harker J, Huett A, Young D, Dougan G et al (2004) Organ specificity, colonization and clearance dynamics in vivo following oral challenges with the murine pathogen *Citrobacter rodentium*. Cell Microbiol 6:963–972

29. Luperchio SA, Newman JV, Dangler CA, Schrenzel MD, Brenner DJ, Steigerwalt AG et al (2000) *Citrobacter rodentium*, the causative agent of transmissible murine colonic hyperplasia, exhibits clonality: synonymy of *C. rodentium* and mouse-pathogenic *Escherichia coli*. J Clin Microbiol 38:4343–4350

30. Nakagawa M, Sakazaki R, Muto T, Saito M, Hagiwara T (1969) Infectious megaenteron of mice. II Detection of coliform organisms of an unusual biotype as the primary cause. Jpn J Med Sci Biol 22:375–382

Chapter 8

In Vivo Infection Model of Severe Influenza A Virus

Ashley Mansell and Michelle D. Tate

Abstract

The lung is constantly exposed to both environmental and microbial challenge. As a "contained" organ, it also constitutes an excellent "self-contained" tissue to examine inflammatory responses and cellular infiltration into a diseased organ. Influenza A virus (IAV) causes both mild and severe inflammation that is strain specific following infection of the lung epithelium that spreads to other cells of the lung environment. Here, we describe a method of intranasal inoculation of the lung with IAV that can be used as a preclinical model of infection. Mice can be monitored for clinical signs of infection and tissue and lung fluid collected for further analysis to dissect the immunological consequences of IAV infection. Importantly, this method can be modified to introduce other pathogens, therapies and environmental stimuli to examine immune responses in the lung.

Key words Intranasal, Influenza A virus, Anesthetic, Clinical signs of disease, PR8, HKx31, Bronchoalveolar lavage (BAL)

1 Introduction

Influenza A viruses (IAV) are a major cause of morbidity and severe illness globally. The emergence of highly pathogenic H5N1 and H7N9 avian IAV strains predominately across Asia has caused sporadic infections in humans with high mortality. The mouse model of IAV infection provides a convenient system to examine virus replication, disease pathogenesis and the inflammatory response elicited following intranasal infection of mice with IAV. Mice are not naturally infected with IAV, and intranasal inoculation with human seasonal strains leads to replication of the virus in the upper and lower respiratory tract but it generally does not result in severe disease [1, 2]. Highly Pathogenic Avian Influenza (HPAI) H5N1, H7N9, H9N2, and H4N8 viruses, and the 1918 H1N1 pandemic virus are capable of inducing disease in mice without the requirement of prior adaptation [3, 4].

The sequential passage of human isolates through mouse lung allows for the selection of virus mutants that show increased replication efficiency in vivo resulting in the induction of disease similar

Brendan J. Jenkins (ed.), *Inflammation and Cancer: Methods and Protocols*, Methods in Molecular Biology, vol. 1725, https://doi.org/10.1007/978-1-4939-7568-6_8,

to that observed in humans [5, 6]. The mouse adapted A/PR/8/34 (PR8) strain has been widely used in studies examining disease pathogenesis and the immune responses elicited following IAV infection of mice. PR8 was adapted to mice by >300 sequential passages in mouse lung [7] and is therefore highly virulent for mice, resulting in rapid weight loss and high mortality follow inoculation with as low as 50 plaque-forming units (PFU) [1, 5]. During the process of adaption, it was likely that PR8 acquired mutations associated with increased replication efficiency in the respiratory tract of mice and/or evasion of innate host responses. For example, PR8 is largely poor in its ability to infect macrophages, which are permissive to viral replication [1, 8]. HKx31 (H3N2) is a high-yielding reassortant of PR8 that expresses the hemagglutinin (HA) and neuraminidase (NA) of A/Aichi/2/68 (H3N2) from the Hong Kong pandemic of 1968. Unlike the mouse-adapted PR8 strain, HKx31 is similar to many pathogenic IAV strains such as H5N1 and H7N9 in its ability to infect macrophages [9, 10].

IAV of mice is characterized by the early production of proinflammatory cytokines (e.g., IL-6, MCP-1, TNFα, KC, and IL-1β), as well accumulation of inflammatory cells in the alveoli, including neutrophils, macrophages and lymphocytes, with subsequent recruitment of T cells and the development of humoral responses [2, 5]. Viral clearance is generally achieved 7–10 days after sublethal infection. Severe IAV infections of mice (i.e., following inoculation with mouse-adapted or HPAI viruses) are associated with a number of pathological features such as high viral loads, greater numbers of inflammatory infiltrate and elevated levels of inflammatory mediators [1, 2]. Vascular leak and pulmonary edema are hallmark pathological features of acute respiratory Distress Syndrome (ARDS) and have been observed during severe IAV infection of mice and humans [1, 11].

While the adaptive immune response plays an important role in the clearance of IAV and eventual resolution of infection, increasing evidence demonstrates the innate immune response to IAV infection plays a crucial role in the pathophysiology of disease. Innate immune recognition receptor such as Toll-like receptor (TLR)-2, TLR3, TLR4, and TLR7 [12, 13], have all been shown to play important roles in recognizing IAV infection and initiating inflammation as a response to infection. Increasing evidence from our and other laboratories also identifies a critical role for the nucleotide-binding domain and leucine-rich-repeat-containing (NLR) family of pattern-recognition molecules in inducing inflammation and contributing the pathophysiology and disease outcome during IAV challenge.

The NLRP3 inflammasome is an oligomeric innate immune intracellular signaling complex that senses many pathogen-, host-, and environmental-derived factors [14]. Inflammasome-induced cytokine release requires two signals: (1) upregulation of components of the NLRP3 inflammasome and synthesis of pro-IL-1β through activation of the prototypic inflammatory transcription factor NF-κB; and (2) inflammasome formation that results in IL-1β maturation and secretion. Following activation, NLRP3 binds to the adaptor protein, apoptosis-associated speck-like protein containing a CARD (ASC). ASC further recruits the enzyme caspase-1 to form the inflammasome complex initiating autocatalytic cleavage of caspase-1. The NLRP3 inflammasome is now recognized as a major route by which the innate immune system recognizes and responds during IAV infection [14]. To date, IAV single-stranded RNA (ssRNA) and proton flux via the IAV-encoded matrix-2 (M2) ion channel have been shown to activate the NLRP3 inflammasome [15, 16], which is important in the development of adaptive immune responses to IAV. Studies utilizing mice lacking components of the NLRP3 inflammasome have demonstrated its importance in eliciting rapid protective responses following infection with PR8 [15, 17]. Recently, we identified that the PB1-F2 protein from the PR8 and H7N9 strains of IAV induced NLRP3 inflammasome activation in mice via intranasal inoculation, contributing to severe disease pathophysiology [18, 19]. Importantly, intranasal delivery of a small molecule inhibitor of NLRP3 provided protection from PR8- and HKx31-induced lethality, commensurate with reduced lung inflammatory cytokine expression such as IL-6, MCP-1, TNFα, and IL-1β reduced inflammatory cellular infiltrates [5].

The intranasal inoculation method therefore provides an excellent animal model to (1) challenge mice with pulmonary focused pathogen models such as IAV, and (2) a means to therapeutically deliver intervention strategies that may mimic intranasal drug delivery similar to that possible for humans.

2 Materials

2.1 Intranasal Inoculation of Mice with Influenza Virus

1. Biological safety cabinet.
2. Influenza virus stock: In a BSL2 facility, influenza viruses are routinely grown in 10-day old embryonated hen's eggs and allanotic fluid aliquots and stored at −80 °C for several years (*see* **Note 1**).
3. Preparation of influenza virus inoculum: Remove aliquot of influenza virus from −80 °C. Thaw at room temperature and perform the following in a biological safety cabinet. Dilute influenza stock in sterile phosphate buffered saline (PBS) to desired plaque-forming units (PFU) in 50 μL, e.g., 50 PFU in 50 μL or 1000 PFU per mL (*see* **Note 2**).
4. Isoflurane.

5. Anesthetic machine or glass jar with screw lid containing cotton wool or tissues.
6. Steel mesh/grid that can be placed inside the glass jar on top of the tissues/tissues, so that mice cannot come into direct contact with the anesthetic.
7. P200 pipette and P200 pipette tips.
8. Male or female C57Bl/6 mice at 6–8 weeks of age.

2.2 Monitoring of Mice Following Influenza Infection

1. Monitoring sheet (*see* **Note 3**).
2. Weigh scale.
3. Small open lid container to place on weigh scale.

2.3 Euthanasia of Mice with Pentobarbitone

1. Pentobarbitone.
2. 1 mL syringe.
3. 29-gauge needle.
4. Dissection scissors and tweezers.

2.4 Collection of Bronchoalveolar Lavage (BAL)

1. 80% w/v ethanol.
2. Sterile phosphate-buffered saline (PBS).
3. 3 mL syringe.
4. 18-gauge needle.
5. 23-gauge needle that has been blunted by removing the bevel/tip with scissors.
6. 10 or 15 mL tubes.

2.5 Harvesting of Lung Tissue and Sera

1. 1.5 mL Eppendorf tubes.
2. Box containing wet ice.
3. Container containing liquid nitrogen.
4. 1 mL syringe.
5. 29-gauge needle.
6. Heparin-coated Eppendorf tube or commercial serum collection tube.

3 Methods

3.1 Intranasal Inoculation of Mice with Influenza Virus

1. Place the mouse cage into a biological safety cabinet.
2. Place a glass jar containing a screw lid into the biological safety cabinet.
3. Insert cotton wool or tissues into the bottom of the jar (*see* **Note 4**).

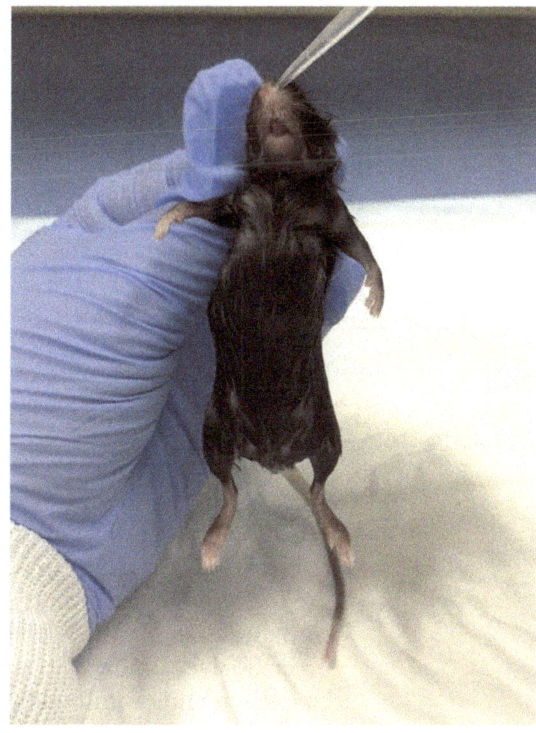

Fig. 1 Intranasal inoculation of mice with influenza virus. Holding the anesthetized mouse upright and pipetting the virus inoculum onto the nares

4. Place 100 μL of isoflurane onto the cotton wool or tissues and cover with a steel mesh/grid.
5. Place the mouse into jar containing the isoflurane.
6. Monitor the mouse carefully until it is anaesthetized and ensure that breathing is no longer rapid, nor there is any movement (*see* **Note 5**).
7. Remove the mouse from the jar or anesthetic machine and hold it upright (Fig. 1).
8. Slowly place 50 μL of the virus inoculum evenly over the two nares using a pipette.
9. Keep the mouse upright until the inoculum is completely inhaled.
10. Return the mouse to a cage and monitor until it regains consciousness and appears fully recovered from the effects of the anesthesia, i.e., alert and moving around freely.

3.2 Monitoring of Mice Following Influenza Infection

1. Following influenza virus infection, mice should be euthanized as per below and monitored in accordance with ethical approval.

2. For monitoring, each mouse needs to be easily identified, i.e., ear clipping, tattoos, or marking the tail.
3. Mice should be weighed daily by placing the mouse in an open lid container that is on top of a weighing scale.
4. Record the mouse weights on a monitoring sheet.
5. Score the mice daily for physical signs of disease. 0 = no visible signs of disease; 1 = slight ruffling of fur; 2 = ruffled fur, reduced mobility and 3 = ruffled fur, reduced mobility, rapid breathing (*see* **Note 6**).

3.3 Euthanasia of Mice with Pentobarbitone

1. Remove mouse from its cage.
2. Restrain the mouse by the scruff.
3. Inject >10 mg/kg of pentobarbitone into the peritoneal cavity (*see* **Note 7**).
4. Monitor the mouse and ensure euthanasia by measuring reflexes, i.e., pinching of the foot. Once mouse is euthanized, the contents of the lung can be examined for cellular infiltrates, cytokines, chemokines, and other cellular factors by extracting bronchoalveolar lavage as described below, or, the organ can be excised and examined by histological sectioning as described below.

3.4 Collection of BAL

1. Euthanize the mouse as per above.
2. Spray the mouse's coat with 80% ethanol ensuring the coat is wet to confidently "sterilize" the area.
3. If blood is required to be collected, this can be done prior to BAL (see below).
4. Using dissection scissors, expose the trachea of the mouse.
5. Carefully cut away the tissue that sounds the trachea (Fig. 2a).
6. Hold the mouse upright and carefully make a small incision in the trachea by inserting a 18-gauge needle into the trachea.
7. Fill a 3 mL syringe containing a blunted 23-gauge needle, with 1 mL of PBS.
8. While holding the mouse upright, carefully place the trip of the blunted needle into the trachea of the mouse (Fig. 2b).
9. Inject the 1 mL of PBS into the lung and immediately draw back on the syringe to recover the PBS (approx. 60–80% recovery).
10. Place the BAL into a 10 or 15 mL tube on ice.
11. Repeat **steps 6–9** twice to flush the lung a total of three times.
12. Store the tube containing the BAL on ice.
13. Spin the tubes containing BAL at 500 × *g*, 4 °C for 5 min.

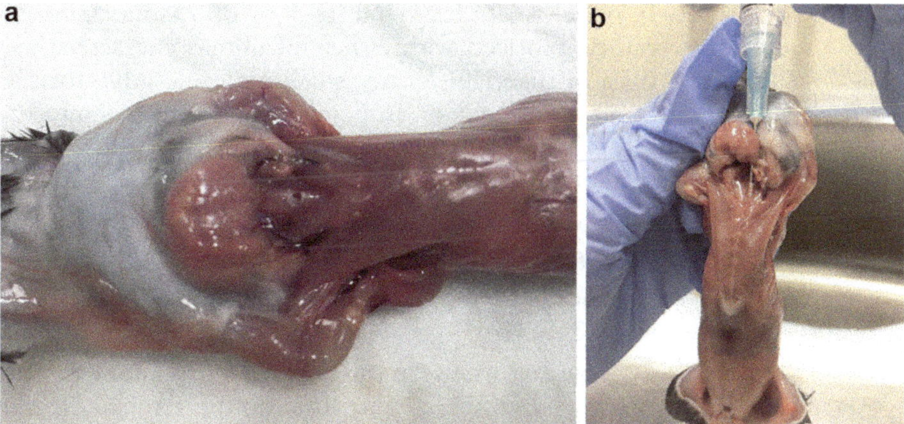

Fig. 2 Collection of BAL from mice. (**a**) Exposing and creating small incision in the trachea. (**b**) Inserting the blunted needle into the trachea and flushing the lungs with 1 mL of PBS

14. Remove the supernatant, aliquot in Eppendorf tubes and store at −80 °C for analysis, e.g., levels of proinflammatory cytokines via ELISA or cytokine bead array according to manufacturer's instructions. BAL can also be assayed for inflammasome activation by examining ASC speck formation by flow cytometry [20] (*see* accompanying Chapter 14).
15. The cell pellet can then be immediately utilized for flow cytometry analysis of cellular infiltrate (e.g., neutrophils, macrophages, T cells [1, 5]).

3.5 Harvesting of Lung Tissue and Sera

1. Euthanize the mouse as per above.
2. For collection of sera, harvest the blood directly from the heart by performing a cardiac puncture using a 1 mL syringe and 29-gauge needle. Place the blood in a heparin-coated Eppendorf tube or a commercial serum collection tube. Approximately 500 μL can be collected on average.
3. BAL can then be performed as per above without significantly impacting analysis of viral loads in the lung tissue.
4. Remove the lung tissue from the mouse.
5. Place the lung tissue in an Eppendorf tube.
6. Snap freeze the Eppendorf in liquid nitrogen.
7. Store sera and lung tissues at −80 °C for analysis, e.g., analysis of viral loads, cytokine levels, mRNA or protein expression.

4 Notes

1. The titer of the influenza stock should be determined by standard plaque assay on MDCK cells as previously described [21].

2. In place of 50 μL of viral stock or PBS as mock infection, this can be replaced with either inflammasome activators such as silica or nigericin, drugs, small molecule inhibitors, and antibodies dissolved or suspended in a total volume of 50 μL. Other pathogens such as viruses or bacteria can also be substituted in place of IAV at this step also.
3. Monitoring sheet should describe the ethical requirements for scoring of clinical signs of disease and weight loss.
4. An anesthetic machine if available can be used in replace of **steps 3–5**.
5. Do not leave mouse in the exposed to isoflurane for too long as this may result in lethality. If in doubt, remove the mouse and check if it is anaesthetized. If it is still breathing rapidly or shows signs of movement, reexpose to isoflurane in the jar. If the mouse is not anaesthetized enough or too deeply, the mouse will not inhale the virus inoculum or PBS through its nostrils.
6. Monitoring signs of clinical disease is a crucial ethical aspect of responsible monitoring of mice and animal welfare. All animal experimentation should be conducted in accordance with local ethics committee requirements which may vary. Always check with your institutional ethics and biosafety committee to obtain the relevant documentation and information relating to ethical handling and experimentation on animals and their scoring matrix and level of clinical signs of disease before ethical euthanasia of animals is required.
7. As an alternative to >10 mg/kg injection of pentobarbitone, mice can be euthanized by CO_2 asphyxiation. Cervical dislocation as a method of euthanasia is not recommended, however, as it can cause bleeding around the lung.

Acknowledgment

This work was supported by the Victorian State Government Operational Infrastructure Scheme, the National Health and Medical Research Council of Australian Project and Fellowship Grants 1079924, 1098298, and 1123319.

References

1. Tate MD, Pickett DL, van Rooijen N, Brooks AG, Reading PC (2010) Critical role of airway macrophages in modulating disease severity during influenza virus infection of mice. J Virol 84:7569–7580
2. Tate MD, Schilter HC, Brooks AG, Reading PC (2011) Responses of mouse airway epithelial cells and alveolar macrophages to virulent and avirulent strains of influenza A virus. Viral Immunol 24:77–88

3. Lai C, Wang K, Zhao Z, Zhang L, Gu H, Yang P et al (2017) C-C motif chemokine ligand 2 (CCL2) mediates acute lung injury induced by lethal influenza H7N9 virus. Front Microbiol 8:587
4. Perrone LA, Plowden JK, Garcia-Sastre A, Katz JM, Tumpey TM (2008) H5N1 and 1918 pandemic influenza virus infection results in early and excessive infiltration of macrophages and neutrophils in the lungs of mice. PLoS Pathog 4:e1000115
5. Tate MD, Ong JD, Dowling JK, McAuley JL, Robertson AB, Latz E et al (2016) Reassessing the role of the NLRP3 inflammasome during pathogenic influenza A virus infection via temporal inhibition. Sci Rep 6:27912
6. Sweet C, Smith H (1980) Pathogenicity of influenza virus. Microbiol Rev 44:303–330
7. Taylor RM (1941) Experimental infection with influenza a virus in mice: the increase in intrapulmonary virus after inoculation and the influence of various factors thereon. J Exp Med 73:43–55
8. Londrigan SL, Tate MD, Brooks AG, Reading PC (2012) Cell-surface receptors on macrophages and dendritic cells for attachment and entry of influenza virus. J Leukoc Biol 92:97–106
9. Gu J, Xie Z, Gao Z, Liu J, Korteweg C, Ye J et al (2007) H5N1 infection of the respiratory tract and beyond: a molecular pathology study. Lancet 370:1137–1145
10. Nicholls JM, Chan MC, Chan WY, Wong HK, Cheung CY, Kwong DL et al (2007) Tropism of avian influenza A (H5N1) in the upper and lower respiratory tract. Nat Med 13:147–149
11. Short KR, Kroeze EJ, Fouchier RA, Kuiken T (2014) Pathogenesis of influenza-induced acute respiratory distress syndrome. Lancet Infect Dis 14:57–69
12. Shirey KA, Lai W, Scott AJ, Lipsky M, Mistry P, Pletneva LM et al (2013) The TLR4 antagonist Eritoran protects mice from lethal influenza infection. Nature 497:498–502
13. Ichinohe T (2010) Respective roles of TLR, RIG-I and NLRP3 in influenza virus infection and immunity: impact on vaccine design. Expert Rev Vaccines 9:1315–1324
14. Iwasaki A, Pillai PS (2014) Innate immunity to influenza virus infection. Nat Rev Immunol 14:315–328
15. Thomas PG, Dash P, Aldridge JR Jr, Ellebedy AH, Reynolds C, Funk AJ et al (2009) The intracellular sensor NLRP3 mediates key innate and healing responses to influenza A virus via the regulation of caspase-1. Immunity 30:566–575
16. Ichinohe T, Pang IK, Iwasaki A (2010) Influenza virus activates inflammasomes via its intracellular M2 ion channel. Nat Immunol 11:404–410
17. Allen IC, Scull MA, Moore CB, Holl EK, McElvania-TeKippe E, Taxman DJ et al (2009) The NLRP3 inflammasome mediates in vivo innate immunity to influenza A virus through recognition of viral RNA. Immunity 30:556–565
18. McAuley JL, Tate MD, MacKenzie-Kludas CJ, Pinar A, Zeng W, Stutz A et al (2013) Activation of the NLRP3 inflammasome by IAV virulence protein PB1-F2 contributes to severe pathophysiology and disease. PLoS Pathog 9: e1003392
19. Pinar A, Dowling JK, Bitto NJ, Robertson AA, Latz E, Stewart CR et al (2017) PB1-F2 peptide derived from avian influenza A virus H7N9 induces inflammation via activation of the NLRP3 inflammasome. J Biol Chem 292:826–836
20. Sester DP, Zamoshnikova A, Thygesen SJ, Vajjhala PR, Cridland SO, Schroder K et al (2016) Assessment of inflammasome formation by flow cytometry. Curr Protoc Immunol 114:14.40.11–14.40.29
21. Anders EM, Hartley CA, Reading PC, Ezekowitz RA (1994) Complement-dependent neutralization of influenza virus by a serum mannose-binding lectin. J Gen Virol 75:615–622

Chapter 9

In Vivo Models for Inflammatory Arthritis

Gareth W. Jones, David G. Hill, Katie Sime, and Anwen S. Williams

Abstract

In vivo mouse models of inflammatory arthritis are extensively used to investigate pathogenic mechanisms governing inflammation-driven joint damage. Two commonly utilized models include collagen-induced arthritis (CIA) and methylated bovine serum albumin (mBSA) antigen-induced arthritis (AIA). These offer unique advantages for modeling different aspects of human disease. CIA involves breach of immunological tolerance resulting in systemic autoantibody-driven arthritis, while AIA results in local resolving inflammatory flares and articular T cell-mediated damage. Despite limitations that apply to all animal models of human disease, CIA and AIA have been instrumental in identifying pathogenic mediators, immune cell subsets and stromal cell responses that determine disease onset, progression, and severity. Moreover, these models have enabled investigation of disease phases not easily studied in patients and have served as testing beds for novel biological therapies, including cytokine blockers and small molecule inhibitors of intracellular signaling that have revolutionized rheumatoid arthritis treatment.

Key words Inflammatory arthritis, Rheumatoid arthritis, Collagen-induced arthritis, Antigen-induced arthritis, Histopathology

1 Introduction

Rheumatoid arthritis (RA) is an autoimmune, chronic inflammatory disease of the joints that results in articular degradation, and is associated with pain, stiffness, loss-of-function and systemic comorbidities [1]. Models of inflammatory arthritis have provided insight into the mechanisms that underpin the pathogenesis of RA and other inflammatory arthritides [2, 3]. These include spontaneous mouse models (e.g., $TNF\Delta^{ARE}$ mouse), models that require passive immunization strategies (e.g., collagen antibody-induced arthritis and K/BxN serum-transfer arthritis), and arthritis that is induced by adjuvants with or without antigenic stimulation (Table 1). This chapter focuses upon the collagen-induced arthritis (CIA) and methylated bovine serum albumin (mBSA) antigen-induced arthritis (AIA) models in mice.

CIA has long been considered the gold standard model for preclinical RA studies and involves the administration of

Brendan J. Jenkins (ed.), *Inflammation and Cancer: Methods and Protocols*, Methods in Molecular Biology, vol. 1725,
https://doi.org/10.1007/978-1-4939-7568-6_9,

Table 1
Conventional arthritis models induced in rats and mice by adjuvants and/or antigens

Model	Rat or mouse	Phenotype	Adjuvant	Antigen	Strain	Citation
Pristane induced arthritis	Rat	Polyarticular	2,6,10,14-Tetramethyl-pentadecane	None	Lewis (LEW), Dark Agouti (DA), DxEA	[27]
Oil-induced arthritis	Rat	Polyarticular	Avridine, Freund's incomplete adjuvant (FIA)	None	LEW, DA	[28]
Adjuvant-induced arthritis	Rat	Polyarticular	Mycobacterial components	None	Holtzman, Charles River (CD) strain, albino rats (CFN strain), LEW	[29, 30]
Streptococcal cell-wall	Rat	Polyarticular	Streptococcal cell-wall fragments	None	Sprague-Dawley (S-D)	[31]
Cartilage protein-induced arthritis	Rat	Polyarticular	FIA	Cartilage oligomeric matrix protein (COMP)	DA, DxEA	[32]
	Mouse	Polyarticular	Dodecyl dioctadecyl ammonium bromide	Proteoglycan	BALB/c, C3H	[33]
	Mouse	Polyarticular	FCA	COMP	C3H	[34]
Collagen-induced arthritis	Rat	Polyarticular	FIA or Freund's complete adjuvant (FCA)	Type II collagen (CII), Type XI collagen (CXI)	LEW, DA, Wistar, S-D	[35, 36]
	Mouse	Polyarticular	FCA	Type II collagen (CII)	DBA/1, B10.M-DR1, B10.M-DR4a, B10.RIII, B10.Q I, DBA-TCR Tg, C57BL/6	[4, 8]
Antigen-induced arthritis	Rat	Monoarticular	FCA	Methylated bovine serum albumin (mBSA)	LEW	[37]
	Mouse	Monoarticular	FCA	mBSA (±Bordetella pertussis)	C57BL/6, BALB/c	[12, 13]

heterologous type II collagen (CII) in complete Freund's adjuvant (CFA) to susceptible mouse strains [4]. Disease pathogenesis parallels characteristics of RA including a prearthritic phase, where loss of peripheral immune tolerance results in the generation of self- and CII-specific autoantibodies that trigger synovitis (inflammation of the synovial membrane). Susceptibility to CIA strongly associates with mouse strains expressing the major histocompatibility complex (MHC) class II I-A^q molecule, which interestingly mirrors the presence of risk alleles for human RA in MHC class II genes (HLA-DR1 and HLA-DR4) [5]. Consequently, DBA/1 is the most frequently used strain for CIA. Nevertheless, the "classical" CIA protocol has been adapted for use in C57BL/6 mice, facilitating studies in the large number of genetically altered strains available on this genetic background [6, 7]. However, it is important to recognize that despite the establishment of sustained CII-specific T- and B-cell responses in C57BL/6 mice, the clinical onset of inflammatory arthritis is delayed and the severity milder than observed in DBA/1 mice. Following the initial CII/CFA immunization in DBA/1 mice, clinical symptoms typically develop 20–25 days later as a polyarthritis primarily affecting the limbs. Disease peaks at approximately day 35, and is histopathologically characterized by synovial leukocyte infiltration, hyperplasia of the synovial lining, and cartilage and bone erosion [8] (Fig. 1). After this period, DBA/1 mice enter remission, but alternative immunization protocols utilizing homologous CII have resulted in a model featuring a chronic relapsing form of CIA that mimics the recurrent flares of synovitis seen in clinical RA [9–11].

The AIA model involves a local mBSA challenge, delivered into the knee joint of mice previously immunized with the same antigen (Fig. 2a) [12, 13]. Consequently, the model does not feature the breach of immune tolerance that results in systemic polyarticular disease as seen in RA, and recapitulated in CIA. Rather, following intra-articular (i.a.) delivery of mBSA, onset of joint inflammation is immediate and confined to the challenged joint. Development of AIA is dependent on $CD4^+$ T-lymphocytes, and the kinetics of synovial leukocyte infiltration that leads to cartilage and bone erosion is highly reproducible [14]. Synovitis is characterized by early neutrophil and macrophage recruitment, and a chronic phase of AIA features a prominence of synovial T cell infiltrates. Chronicity is observed provided an efficient retention of antigen within the joint is achieved [15, 16]. The C57BL/6 strain of mice is highly susceptible to mBSA AIA, which has facilitated the study of individual immune pathways and functions (e.g., cytokines, cytokine receptors, downstream signaling pathways, transcriptional regulators, and immune cells) using transgenic and gene deficient mice. Modification of the "classical" AIA protocol has yielded models with altered clinical characteristics. Through the adoptive transfer of ovalbumin (OVA)-specific T cells and the use of OVA as the

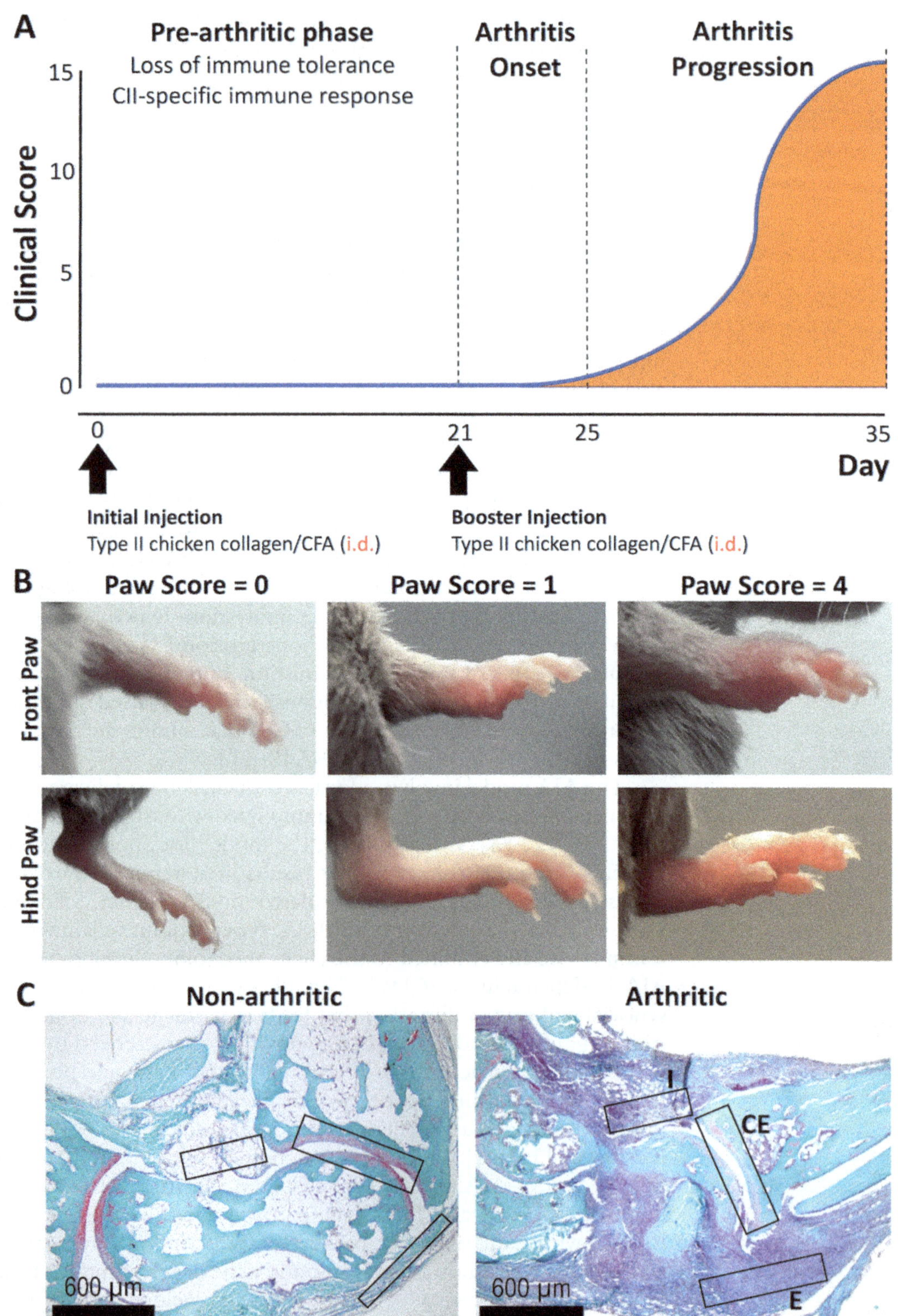

Fig. 1 Collagen-induced arthritis. (**a**) Timeline of the CIA model demonstrating the progression of clinical score. During the prearthritic phase, CII-specific immune responses are established associated with breach of

priming antigen, mice develop an AIA-like pathology accompanied by autoimmunity including the generation of self-reactive collagen-specific T- and B-cells and rheumatoid factor autoantibodies [17, 18]. Through repeated intra-articular administration of antigen, AIA has also been refined to study recurrent flares of disease, which models disease relapses as is seen in clinical RA [19, 20]. Approaches that allow for the development of a more chronic form of AIA have also facilitated the investigation of discrete synovial pathotypes. For example, repeated flares of AIA or the use of gene deficient mice that lack regulatory cytokines results in synovitis featuring ectopic lymphoid-like follicles, a histopathological characteristic seen in RA patients with severe synovitis and inferior responses to biological treatment (e.g., anti-TNF) [20, 21].

Here, we outline protocols for the induction and histopathological evaluation of disease in CIA and AIA. These models serve well to investigate molecular mechanisms underpinning arthritis progression and systemic comorbidities linked with RA, and provide a preclinical testing ground for novel therapeutics.

2 Materials

Unless otherwise stated, all solutions and buffers should be prepared in distilled water.

2.1 Animal Ethics

Animal experiments should be approved and performed with ethical consent from relevant local and national authorities. In the UK, animal experiments comply with the Animals (Scientific Procedures) Act 1986, and are performed under the authority of a Home Office Project License. Experiments should be designed and performed with good practice and incorporate refinements that improve animal welfare (*see* **Note 1**), using the minimum number of mice necessary to achieve scientifically valid data (*see* **Note 2**).

2.2 Collagen-Induced Arthritis

1. Inbred DBA/1 mice (MHC class II haplotype I-A^q), normally male, at 8–10 weeks of age and sourced from an approved supplier for scientific research (*see* **Note 3**).

Fig. 1 (continued) immunological tolerance. Onset of inflammatory arthritis occurs at day 21–25 and peaks at approximately day 35. Arrows indicate the days of the initial and booster immunizations. Routes of administration are shown in red. (**b**) Representative images for daily paw scoring: front and hind paws with a clinical score of 0 (left), 1 (middle), and 4 (right). (**c**) Histopathological assessment of ankle joints in CIA as determined by hematoxylin, fast green, and safranin O staining at day 35. Boxes highlight areas of inflammatory infiltrate (I), cartilage erosion (CE), and exudate (E)

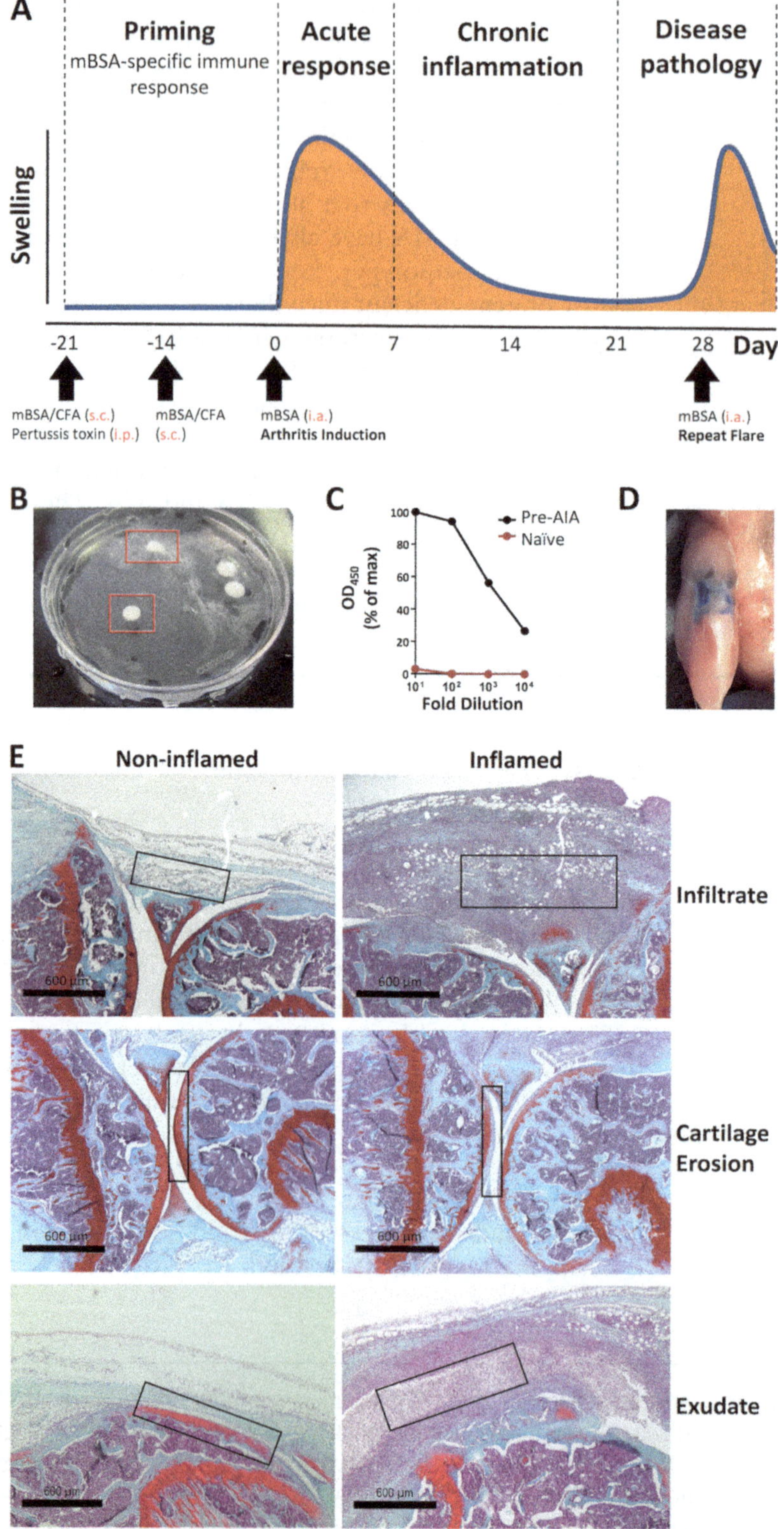

Fig. 2 mBSA antigen induced arthritis. (**a**) Schematic representation of the kinetics of joint swelling in AIA. During the priming phase from day −21 to day 0, an antigen-specific response to mBSA is established. *Arrows*

2. Heat-killed *Mycobacterium tuberculosis* strain H37Ra, desiccated, 100 mg vials (Difco™ brand from BD Biosciences).
3. Incomplete Freund's adjuvant (IFA; Sigma-Aldrich).
4. Type II collagen from chick.
5. 10 mM acetic acid.
6. Sterile water for injection.
7. Pestle and mortar.
8. A 10 mL glass syringe with metal luer lock for preparing the CII/CFA emulsion.
9. Blunt 18 gauge (G) needles for preparing the CII/CFA emulsion.
10. Disposable 1 mL syringes and needles (27 G × $^1/_2''$) for injecting CII/CFA emulsion.
11. Micrometer (e.g., POCO 2T, 0–10 mm range, 0.1 mm increments from Kroeplin Längenmesstechnik).

2.3 mBSA Antigen-Induced Arthritis

1. Inbred C57BL/6 mice, normally male, at 8–10 weeks of age and sourced from an approved supplier for scientific research (*see* **Note 4**).
2. Complete Freund's adjuvant (CFA).
3. Methylated bovine serum albumin (mBSA; *see* **Note 5**).
4. Sterile water for injection.
5. Pertussis toxin from *Bordetella pertussis* (Sigma-Aldrich).
6. Sterile Dulbecco's phosphate buffered saline (PBS).
7. A 10 mL glass syringe with metal luer lock for preparing the mBSA/CFA emulsion.
8. Blunt 18 G needles for preparing the mBSA/CFA emulsion.

Fig. 2 (continued) indicate days of antigen or adjuvant challenge and routes of administration (shown in *red*). (**b**) A stable mBSA/CFA emulsion can be tested by placing droplets onto a petri dish of cold water. An emulsion suitable for injection will result in a droplet that remains intact and immiscible in water (bottom box), while an unstable emulsion will disperse (top box). (**c**) The establishment of an antigen-specific mBSA response, prior to induction of AIA by i.a. mBSA challenge, can be determined by measuring serum mBSA-specific antibody (IgG) titers. Here, serum was taken prearthritis induction (day −1) and anti-mBSA antibody titers were determined by ELISA. Serum from nonchallenged mice was used as control. (**d**) Intra-articular injections can be practiced on dead mice using dye or ink. Successful injections can be confirmed by removing the skin over the joint to visualize dispersion of the injected dye. (**e**) Histological assessment of AIA as determined by hematoxylin, fast green, and safranin O staining of knee joints at day 10. Boxes highlight areas of inflammatory infiltrate (top), cartilage erosion detected by loss of red safranin O staining of the articular cartilage (middle), and synovial exudate (bottom). The inflamed knee from an AIA-challenged mouse (right) is compared with the contralateral nonchallenged control knee of the same mouse (left)

9. Disposable 1 mL and 10 mL syringes, 26 G × $^5/_8''$ and 21 G × $1^1/_2''$ needles.
10. 0.5 mL insulin syringes, 29 G with 10 μL volume markings.
11. 70% (v/v) ethanol.
12. Micrometer.

2.4 Histological Assessment of Inflammatory Arthritis

1. 10% (v/v) formalin solution, neutral buffered.
2. Formic acid decalcification solution: 10% (v/v) formic acid, 2% (w/v) formaldehyde. Dilute 100 mL of ≥ 95% formic acid and 50 mL of 37–41% (w/v) formaldehyde solution in distilled water to a final volume of 1 L.
3. Harris Hematoxylin.
4. 1% (v/v) acetic acid.
5. 0.2% (w/v) safranin O solution (*see* **Note 6**).
6. 0.01% (w/v) fast green solution (*see* **Note 6**).
7. Xylene, and 70%, 90%, and 100% ethanol for histology.
8. DPX mounting medium.

3 Methods

3.1 Preparation of a Collagen in Complete Freund's Adjuvant Emulsion for CIA

1. To prepare the complete Freund's adjuvant (CFA), grind one 100 mg vial of *Mycobacterium tuberculosis* into a fine powder using a pestle and mortar. Add 20 mL of incomplete Freund's adjuvant (IFA) to make a 5 mg/mL solution of *M. tuberculosis* in IFA. Vortex the resulting CFA before use to thoroughly suspend the *M. tuberculosis* (*see* **Note 7**).
2. Dissolve the type II collagen (CII) to the desired concentration of 4 mg/mL by adding 2.5 mL of 10 mM acetic acid to 10 mg of CII. Stir gently for several hours or overnight at 4 °C (*see* **Note 8**).
3. To 2.5 mL of the prepared CII solution, add an equal volume of CFA. Using the glass syringe and a 18 G blunt fill needle, prepare a white CII/CFA emulsion by repeated passing (i.e., uptake and removal of the liquid from the syringe) through the needle. Keep all reagents on ice as much as possible during emulsification, to help prevent denaturing of CII (*see* **Note 9**).
4. Test the emulsion by placing droplets onto a petri dish (or other suitable receptacle) containing water. A droplet of stable emulsion will initially sink below the water surface on impact then float back to the surface, remaining intact (as shown in Fig. 2b for preparation of mBSA/CFA emulsion). An unstable emulsion will disperse.
5. Keep the CII/CFA emulsion on ice.

3.2 Immunization of Mice for CIA

1. Using a 18 G blunt fill needle, carefully transfer emulsion into the immunization syringe by slowly drawing on the plunger. Avoid introducing air into the injecting syringe to maintain accurate, reproducible injection volumes. Attach a 27 G × $^{1}/_{2}''$ needle to the immunization syringe and place on ice (*see* **Note 10**).
2. Anaesthetize mice using isoflurane, or an anesthetic of choice (see **Note 11**).
3. Choose an injection site on the dorsal side of the mouse that is as close as possible to the base of the tail. A second injection will be given 21 days after this initial immunization, therefore be sure to leave sufficient space above the immunization site for the booster injection. 100 μL of CII/CFA emulsion must be slowly injected intradermally (i.d.), split over two 50 μL injections (*see* **Note 12**).
4. To ensure CIA induction of a high incidence, a booster or secondary immunization is given 21 days after the primary immunization (Fig. 1a). Prepare an identical formulation of CII/CFA as used as for the primary immunization.
5. The first signs of arthritis development are visible between days 20 and 25 after the initial immunization (Fig. 1a). Animals should be examined daily for arthritis incidence (*see* **Notes 13** and **14**).

3.3 Clinical Assessment of Inflammatory Arthritis in CIA

1. CIA incidence and progression is monitored by assigning an arthritis severity score to each paw. This is a subjective scoring system that considers the level of inflammation and the number of joints affected. Each paw should be scored individually on a scale of 0–5, with 5 indicating the most severe inflammation and ankyloses of the limb (Fig. 1b and Table 2).

Table 2
Clinical scoring of peripheral joint swelling in CIA

Paw score	Description
0	Normal
1	Erythema and mild swelling confined to the tarsals or ankle joint
2	Erythema and mild swelling extending from the ankle to the tarsals
3	Erythema and moderate swelling extending from the ankle to metatarsal joints
4	Erythema and severe swelling encompassing the ankle, foot, and digits
5	Deformed paw or joint with ankylosis

The graded scoring system above provides a macroscopic measure of joint swelling. Each paw is assigned a score, according to the table. The sum of scores in all four paws results in a clinical score for each animal

2. Arthritic joints are easily distinguished from normal nonarthritic joints. However, the subjectivity of quantifying the severity and progression of the arthritis in each limb by this method alone can be problematic for new users. A micrometer measurement across the mid-foot provides a quantitative measure of hind paw thickness (swelling). This measurement relies heavily on precision and reproducibility of micrometer placement from mouse to mouse.
3. Three approaches are used to clinically evaluate arthritis progression and severity. These include score per limb (paw score), sum of the scores per mouse (clinical score), and hind paw diameter measurement per mouse or per experimental group. The severity of CIA is further evaluated by histopathology (*see* Subheading 3.8 and Fig. 1c).

3.4 Preparation of a mBSA in Complete Freund's Adjuvant Emulsion for AIA

1. Dissolve 10 mg of mBSA antigen in 5 mL of injection water in a sterile universal cylinder, to yield a 2 mg/mL mBSA solution. Once dissolved, keep on ice.
2. Vortex a 10 mL vial of CFA to ensure that *M. tuberculosis* sediment is fully suspended. Remove 5 mL CFA from the vial using a 10 mL syringe and 21 G needle. The remaining 5 mL of CFA can be stored in the fridge until the booster injection is prepared 7 days later.
3. Change the needle on the syringe to an 18 G blunt fill needle. With force, inject the CFA into the mBSA solution. Using the glass syringe and a 18 G blunt fill needle, make a white emulsion by repeated uptake and flushing of the mBSA/CFA mixture (*see* **Note 9**).
4. Test the emulsion by placing droplets onto a petri dish (or other suitable receptacle) containing water. A droplet of stable emulsion will initially sink below the water surface on impact then float back to the surface, remaining intact (Fig. 2b). An unstable emulsion will disperse.
5. Keep the mBSA/CFA emulsion on ice.

3.5 Immunization of Mice to Induce an mBSA-Specific Immune Response for AIA

1. Check the supplied concentration of Pertussis toxin, which may vary according to batch and source, and dilute in PBS to 1.6 μg/mL.
2. Using 1 mL syringes and 26 G needles, immunize 8–10-week-old C57BL/6 mice with 100 μL (equivalent to 100 μg) of the prepared mBSA/CFA emulsion subcutaneously (s.c.) on the right hind flank (*see* **Note 15**).
3. Using 1 mL syringes and 26 G needles, administer 100 μL (equivalent to 160 ng) of the prepared Pertussis toxin intraperitoneally (*see* **Note 16**). The immunizations outlined in **steps 2** and **3** systemically prime the mice for an antigen-specific

response to mBSA. These are performed 21 days prior to the induction of joint inflammation, and is thus referred to as day −21 of AIA (Fig. 2a).

4. Prepare a second identical emulsion 7 days later (i.e., at day −14), and as before immunize mice subcutaneously with 100 μL of mBSA/CFA, this time on the left hind flank (*see* **Note 17**).

3.6 Induction of AIA by Intra-articular Injection of mBSA

1. 21 days after the initial immunization (i.e., on day 0), mice are administered 10 μL of a 10 mg/mL mBSA solution intra-articularly to induce inflammatory arthritis. For this, dissolve 10 mg of mBSA in 1 mL sterile injection water. Once dissolved, keep on ice. The right knee is injected to induce a unilateral, local form of inflammatory arthritis. The left control knee is injected with sterile water (*see* **Note 18**).
2. Anaesthetize mice using isoflurane, or an anesthetic of choice.
3. Using a 29 G insulin syringe, draw up approximately 100 μL of the mBSA solution. By inverting the tube, and while removing any air bubbles, adjust the volume in the syringe to 10 μL.
4. Using your fingers wetted in 70% ethanol, part the hair over the knee joint along the patellar ligament. This will allow visualization of the patellar ligament which will be used as a guide for intra-articular injection (*see* **Note 19**).
5. Using the insulin syringe insert the needle tip into the space underneath the patellar ligament (the infrapatellar fat pad region) and administer 10 μL of mBSA solution. This will result in a symmetrical distribution around the patellar ligament (Fig. 2d). Leave the needle tip inserted for a few seconds to avoid leakage, and then withdraw (*see* **Note 20**).
6. Administer an identical 10 μL dose of sterile water into the control left knee, and allow mice to recover from anesthesia.

3.7 Clinical Assessment of Inflammatory Arthritis in AIA

For clinical evaluation of arthritis development, joint swelling can be quantified using a micrometer. For this, mice can be anaesthetized briefly using an appropriate general anesthetic. To quantify knee joint swelling (in mm), subtract the joint diameter of the control left knee from the diameter of the arthritic right knee and graph throughout the time course of AIA (*see* **Note 21**).

3.8 Histopathological Evaluation of Inflammatory Arthritis in CIA and AIA

1. Kill mice using an appropriate humane method at desired time points of CIA or AIA, and remove whole joints by cutting through the bones distal and proximal to the joint of interest without damaging the joint. For example, for the knee joint in AIA cut through the proximal femur and the distal tibia and fibula bones.

2. Remove skin and place samples in 10% neutral buffered formalin solution for 4 days.
3. Transfer samples to formic acid decalcification solution (*see* **Note 22**) until decalcification is complete as confirmed by X-ray (typically 3–4 days).
4. Process samples into paraffin blocks, embedding the tissue in the orientation of interest for downstream sectioning.
5. Prepare parasagittal sections of 6–7 μm. For knee joints, adjust the plane of sectioning to ensure the patella, the whole patellar ligament, the femoral and tibial head growth plates, and the menisci are all visible within each section. Avoid midsagittal sections, as the presence of the cruciate ligaments will prevent detection of articular cartilage erosion by histological staining.
6. Dewax tissue sections in Xylene and rehydrate through decreasing concentrations of 100%, 90% and 70% ethanol, and distilled water following standard histological practice.
7. Stain in Harris hematoxylin for 2 min. Wash excess stain under running tap water.
8. Stain in fast green solution for 5 min.
9. Dip briefly (approx. 2 s) in 1% (v/v) acetic acid.
10. Stain in safranin O solution for 5 min.
11. Dip in distilled water (approx. 5 s) followed by 30 s in each of 70%, 90% and 100% ethanol (*see* **Note 23**). Dehydrate and clear in three changes of xylene following standard histological practice. Place coverslips on the slides using DPX mountant.
12. Histopathologically score inflammatory arthritis in consultation with rheumatologists and pathologists. Hematoxylin staining is used to detect synovial cellular infiltration, while proteoglycan detection by safranin O is used to track erosion of articular cartilage (Figs. 1c and 2e). Our in-house scoring of arthritic indices involves two independent observers blinded to the experimental groups scoring subsynovial inflammation (0 is normal; 5 is ablation of synovial adipose tissue by inflammatory infiltrate), synovial exudate (0 is normal; 3 is a substantial number of leukocytes with large fibrin deposits), synovial hyperplasia and pannus formation (0 is normal or up to three layers thick; 3 represents over three layers thick with overgrowth over joint surfaces and evidence of cartilage loss), and joint erosion (0 is normal; 3 is destruction of articular cartilage with significant erosion to underlying bone). The arthritic index, or disease score, is the aggregate score for all four parameters.

4 Notes

1. Approaches should be employed to improve mouse wellbeing during inflammatory arthritis experiments. For example, use of tangle-free bedding to minimize arthritic limbs being caught, the handling and restraining of mice on soft surfaces (e.g., Vetbed®), the proactive rather than reactive use of analgesia, and the use of general anesthetic. Temgesic (buprenorphine), which can be administered by subcutaneous injection or more conveniently in drinking water, can be used for analgesia. Inhalable isoflurane is a suitable anesthetic. Herein, we outline the techniques required for establishing CIA and AIA, but not the frequency and doses of analgesics and anesthetics used. Investigators should discuss the choice and use of analgesics and anesthetics with their animal welfare advisors. Further refinements should be adopted that can improve mouse well-being in inflammatory arthritis models, a comprehensive review of which can be found elsewhere [22].
2. The appropriate number of mice for experiments should be determined by statistical power analysis. For this, G*Power (http://www.gpower.hhu.de/en.html) is a useful tool for computing statistical power [23]. Where no preliminary data is available for power analysis, pilot experiments should be designed using small group sizes and the resource equation [24].
3. Female DBA/1 mice can also be used; however, differences in disease incidence and severity due to sex should be accounted for in the experimental design. Alternative CIA susceptible strains are available, but it should be appreciated that the kinetics of disease onset and severity will vary with genetic background [8]. For establishing CIA in C57BL/6 mice, refinements to the protocol provided herein are described elsewhere [6].
4. Female C57BL/6 mice may also be used. Other strains that demonstrate good severity and chronicity in AIA are described elsewhere [12]. The severity and kinetics of AIA varies with genetic background.
5. Efficient retention of antigen within the joint is required to establish chronicity. Bovine serum albumin has an isoelectric point (pI) of 4.5. Methylation of bovine serum albumin results in a pI $\geq$8.5, which allows the sustained retention of antigen within the joint via adherence to negatively charged noncartilaginous collagenous tissue and articular cartilage [15, 16].
6. In-house optimizations with different concentration of safranin O and fast green should be performed, using the provided concentrations as a starting point. Source and batch variations,

and the processing of tissue, can result in differences in the degree of tissue staining.

7. The CFA can be prepared in batches and stored at −20 °C in sealed glass vials for at least 12 months. When using previously frozen CFA, ensure that the adjuvant is thawed, and microbial particles thoroughly resuspended by vortex before use.
8. Collagen is not soluble in water or commonly used buffers. A concentration of 10 mM acetic acid will solubilize CII without causing adverse effects to the mouse. It is essential that the CII is dissolved before preparing the emulsion. Salts (e.g., NaCl and PBS) may precipitate CII from solution, thus glassware must be salt-free. We prefer to prepare the solution in the glass vial in which the collagen is supplied. CII solution is a clear, colorless liquid. It is advisable to freshly prepare the CII solution before each injection, and to begin the procedure at least 12 h in advance of when the CII solution is needed.
9. When preparing an emulsion of antigen solution and CFA, ensure to keep their ratios at 1:1. We find that repeated, forceful flushing of the antigen/CFA mixture through an 18 G blunt end needle is the best way of achieving a stable emulsion. This typically requires 10–20 passes through the needle and keeping solutions on ice prior to preparing the emulsion. Alternatively, emulsions can be made using a sonicator or tissue homogenizer, protocols for which can be found elsewhere. Due to viscosity, expect to lose emulsion during preparation and loading of immunization syringes. 5 mL of antigen/CFA emulsion is typically sufficient for 25–30 mice.
10. Operators are advised to work with small volumes and to prepare the immunization syringe just before injection. The acetic acid in the CII/CFA emulsion will slowly begin to dissolve the plastic in the syringe and will compromise the ability of the researcher to inject. Expected time for each injection is less than 2 min per mouse for an experienced researcher.
11. It is advised that animals are anesthetized for immunization. It is easier to inject the emulsion into the correct tissue layer while the mice are under anesthetic (e.g., isoflurane).
12. The operator will feel noticeable tissue resistance to the injection. A rapid and/or easy injection is indicative of a subcutaneous injection. Animals will not develop arthritis or arthritis incidence will be poor if the injection is administered by the wrong route. The first and booster injection sites should be spread out to avoid irritation. For example, the first injection administered on the right flank, and the booster immunization on the left.
13. The incidence of CIA in male DBA/1 mice is high (approximately 95–100%) if care is taken to prepare high-quality emulsions and the correct immunization technique is mastered. The

time course of CIA is very consistent from experiment to experiment.

14. It is advised that analgesia be administered in the drinking water (e.g., Buprenorphine hydrochloride at 400 μg/L) from day 20.
15. The mBSA/CFA emulsion is viscous. Draw up the emulsion into the syringe with a 18 G blunt fill needle attached. Turn the syringe upward and gently tap to remove air bubbles, which will rise slowly to the top. Air bubbles can be easily identified by holding the syringe up against a strong light. Attach the needle, and adjust the volume as desired, ensuring to remove the dead space volume within the needle.
16. Concurrent administration of *Bordetella pertussis* toxin as a further adjuvant bolsters antigen-specific T cell responses in autoimmune and chronic inflammatory disease models. In AIA, this supports establishing chronicity through promoting a more aggressive inflammatory response resulting in erosive pathology.
17. It is best to inject into different sites, not too close together to avoid irritation and coalescing of injection sites [22].
18. The establishment of an antigen-specific antibody response to mBSA can be confirmed prior to induction of joint inflammation by intra-articular injection of mBSA. For this, peripheral blood should be recovered by tail vain sampling, and serum antibody titers to mBSA (Fig. 2c) determined by enzyme-linked immunosorbent assay (ELISA) as described previously [19].
19. Successful intra-articular injection requires practice. In our experience, training is best achieved using dead mice and injecting dye or ink that will allow visualization of the injected area (Fig. 2d). Some prefer to perform the injection under a dissection microscope, which allows easier visualization of the patellar ligament. Alternatively, some groups make a small incision in the skin overlying the patellar ligament, which will heal without the need for stiches and again aid visualization [25].
20. To induce recurrent flares of AIA, and promote chronicity associated with a sustained response to mBSA within the joint, identical intra-articular administrations of mBSA can be performed at desired time points [19, 20]. Recurrent challenges with mBSA results in a strong T cell-dependent antigen-specific response and exacerbated joint erosion. Other groups have demonstrated that recurrent flares of disease can also be induced by intravenous injection of mBSA [26]. Here, despite the systemic administration of mBSA, the contralateral control joint is not affected, with arthritic flare only observed in a hyper-reactive, previously inflamed joint.

21. We suggest measuring knee-joint diameters at day 0 (preinduction of arthritis), day 1, day 2, and day 3 during the first week. Thereafter, measurement should be taken at day 7, day 10, day 14, day 21, day 28, and day 35. Typically, day 35 is considered the endpoint of the AIA model. For experiments where recurrent-flares of inflammation are induced by repeat intra-articular injection [19], knee joint diameters should again be measured daily for 3 days, before continuing with twice-weekly measurements. We find that these intervals will allow robust tracking of arthritis induction and resolution of joint inflammation (Fig. 2a).
22. Alternatively, ethylenediaminetetraacetic acid (EDTA) may be used to decalcify joint tissue, which may better preserve some antigens of interest for downstream immunohistochemical analysis. Decalcification in 200 mM EDTA, prepared in 10% neutral buffered formal saline, will require longer for complete decalcification, and the solution should be refreshed every 3–4 days to maximize efficiency.
23. It is important not to incubate the slides too long in ethanol, as safranin O is highly soluble in water and ethanol. Prolonged washing will remove the stain from the articular cartilage. Control nonarthritic joints should be stained alongside, as a positive control for safranin O staining of proteoglycans in the articular cartilage.

Acknowledgments

G.J. is supported by an Arthritis Research UK Career Development Fellowship (20305). D.H. is supported by a Medical Research Council PhD studentship and Life Science Research Network Wales, an initiative funded through the Welsh Government's Ser Cymru program. K.S. is supported by a PhD studentship funded through a generous donation from The Elizabeth Owens Bequest at Cardiff University.

References

1. Smolen JS, Aletaha D, McInnes IB (2016) Rheumatoid arthritis. Lancet S0140-6736:30173–30178
2. Asquith DL, Miller AM, McInnes IB, Liew FY (2009) Animal models of rheumatoid arthritis. Eur J Immunol 39:2040–2044
3. Brand DD (2005) Rodent models of rheumatoid arthritis. Comp Med 55:114–122
4. Courtenay JS, Dallman MJ, Dayan AD, Martin A, Mosedale B (1980) Immunisation against heterologous type II collagen induces arthritis in mice. Nature 283:666–668
5. Luross JA, Williams NA (2001) The genetic and immunopathological processes underlying collagen-induced arthritis. Immunology 103:407–416
6. Inglis JJ, Criado G, Medghalchi M, Andrews M, Sandison A, Feldmann M, Williams RO (2007) Collagen-induced arthritis in C57BL/6 mice is associated with a robust

and sustained T-cell response to type II collagen. Arthritis Res Ther 9:R113

7. Campbell IK, Hamilton JA, Wicks IP (2000) Collagen-induced arthritis in C57BL/6 (H-2b) mice: new insights into an important disease model of rheumatoid arthritis. Eur J Immunol 30:1568–1575
8. Brand DD, Latham KA, Rosloniec EF (2007) Collagen-induced arthritis. Nat Protoc 2:1269–1275
9. Boissier MC, Feng XZ, Carlioz A, Roudier R, Fournier C (1987) Experimental autoimmune arthritis in mice. I. Homologous type II collagen is responsible for self-perpetuating chronic polyarthritis. Ann Rheum Dis 46:691–700
10. Holmdahl R, Jansson L, Larsson E, Rubin K, Klareskog L (1986) Homologous type II collagen induces chronic and progressive arthritis in mice. Arthritis Rheum 29:106–113
11. Malfait AM, Williams RO, Malik AS, Maini RN, Feldmann M (2001) Chronic relapsing homologous collagen-induced arthritis in DBA/1 mice as a model for testing disease-modifying and remission-inducing therapies. Arthritis Rheum 44:1215–1224
12. Brackertz D, Mitchell GF, Mackay IR (1977) Antigen-induced arthritis in mice. I. Induction of arthritis in various strains of mice. Arthritis Rheum 20:841–850
13. Brackertz D, Mitchell GF, Vadas MA, Mackay IR, Miller JF (1977) Studies on antigen-induced arthritis in mice. II. Immunologic correlates of arthritis susceptibility in mice. J Immunol 118:1639–1644
14. Wong PK, Quinn JM, Sims NA, van Nieuwenhuijze A, Campbell IK, Wicks IP (2006) Interleukin-6 modulates production of T lymphocyte-derived cytokines in antigen-induced arthritis and drives inflammation-induced osteoclastogenesis. Arthritis Rheum 54:158–168
15. van den Berg WB, van de Putte LB (1985) Electrical charge of the antigen determines its localization in the mouse knee joint. Deep penetration of cationic BSA in hyaline articular cartilage. Am J Pathol 121:224–234
16. van den Berg WB, van de Putte LB, Zwarts WA, Joosten LA (1984) Electrical charge of the antigen determines intraarticular antigen handling and chronicity of arthritis in mice. J Clin Invest 74:1850–1859
17. Maffia P, Brewer JM, Gracie JA, Ianaro A, Leung BP, Mitchell PJ, Smith KM, McInnes IB, Garside P (2004) Inducing experimental arthritis and breaking self-tolerance to joint-specific antigens with trackable, ovalbumin-specific T cells. J Immunol 173:151–156
18. Nickdel MB, Conigliaro P, Valesini G, Hutchison S, Benson R, Bundick RV, Leishman AJ, McInnes IB, Brewer JM, Garside P (2009) Dissecting the contribution of innate and antigen-specific pathways to the breach of self-tolerance observed in a murine model of arthritis. Ann Rheum Dis 68:1059–1066
19. Nowell MA, Williams AS, Carty SA, Scheller J, Hayes AJ, Jones GW, Richards PJ, Slinn S, Ernst M, Jenkins BJ, Topley N, Rose-John S, Jones SA (2009) Therapeutic targeting of IL-6 trans signaling counteracts STAT3 control of experimental inflammatory arthritis. J Immunol 182:613–622
20. Wengner AM, Hopken UE, Petrow PK, Hartmann S, Schurigt U, Brauer R, Lipp M (2007) CXCR5- and CCR7-dependent lymphoid neogenesis in a murine model of chronic antigen-induced arthritis. Arthritis Rheum 56:3271–3283
21. Jones GW, Bombardieri M, Greenhill CJ, McLeod L, Nerviani A, Rocher-Ros V, Cardus A, Williams AS, Pitzalis C, Jenkins BJ, Jones SA (2015) Interleukin-27 inhibits ectopic lymphoid-like structure development in early inflammatory arthritis. J Exp Med 212:1793–1802
22. Hawkins P, Armstrong R, Boden T, Garside P, Knight K, Lilley E, Seed M, Wilkinson M, Williams RO (2015) Applying refinement to the use of mice and rats in rheumatoid arthritis research. Inflammopharmacology 23:131–150
23. Faul F, Erdfelder E, Lang AG, Buchner A (2007) G*Power 3: a flexible statistical power analysis program for the social, behavioral, and biomedical sciences. Behav Res Methods 39:175–191
24. Charan J, Kantharia ND (2013) How to calculate sample size in animal studies? J Pharmacol Pharmacother 4:303–306
25. van den Berg WB, Joosten LA, van Lent PL (2007) Murine antigen-induced arthritis. Methods Mol Med 136:243–253
26. Lens JW, van den Berg WB, van de Putte LB (1984) Flare-up of antigen-induced arthritis in mice after challenge with intravenous antigen: studies on the characteristics of and mechanisms involved in the reaction. Clin Exp Immunol 55:287–294
27. Vingsbo C, Sahlstrand P, Brun JG, Jonsson R, Saxne T, Holmdahl R (1996) Pristane-induced arthritis in rats: a new model for rheumatoid arthritis with a chronic disease course influenced by both major histocompatibility

complex and non-major histocompatibility complex genes. Am J Pathol 149:1675–1683

28. Holmdahl R, Goldschmidt TJ, Kleinau S, Kvick C, Jonsson R (1992) Arthritis induced in rats with adjuvant oil is a genetically restricted, alpha beta T-cell dependent autoimmune disease. Immunology 76:197–202
29. Katz L, Piliero SJ (1969) A study of adjuvant-induced polyarthritis in the rat with special reference to associated immunological phenomena. Ann N Y Acad Sci 147:517–536
30. Zidek Z, Perlik F (1971) Genetic control of adjuvant-induced arthritis in rats. J Pharm Pharmacol 23:389–390
31. Cromartie WJ, Craddock JG, Schwab JH, Anderle SK, Yang CH (1977) Arthritis in rats after systemic injection of streptococcal cells or cell walls. J Exp Med 146:1585–1602
32. Carlsen S, Hansson AS, Olsson H, Heinegard D, Holmdahl R (1998) Cartilage oligomeric matrix protein (COMP)-induced arthritis in rats. Clin Exp Immunol 114:477–484
33. Hanyecz A, Berlo SE, Szanto S, Broeren CP, Mikecz K, Glant TT (2004) Achievement of a synergistic adjuvant effect on arthritis induction by activation of innate immunity and forcing the immune response toward the Th1 phenotype. Arthritis Rheum 50:1665–1676
34. Carlsen S, Nandakumar KS, Backlund J, Holmberg J, Hultqvist M, Vestberg M, Holmdahl R (2008) Cartilage oligomeric matrix protein induction of chronic arthritis in mice. Arthritis Rheum 58:2000–2011
35. Lu S, Carlsen S, Hansson AS, Holmdahl R (2002) Immunization of rats with homologous type XI collagen leads to chronic and relapsing arthritis with different genetics and joint pathology than arthritis induced with homologous type II collagen. J Autoimmun 18:199–211
36. Trentham DE, Townes AS, Kang AH (1977) Autoimmunity to type II collagen an experimental model of arthritis. J Exp Med 146:857–868
37. Griffiths RJ (1992) Characterisation and pharmacological sensitivity of antigen arthritis induced by methylated bovine serum albumin in the rat. Agents Actions 35:88–95

Chapter 10

Isolation of Mouse Primary Gastric Epithelial Cells to Investigate the Mechanisms of *Helicobacter pylori* Associated Disease

Le Son Tran and Richard L. Ferrero

Abstract

The gastrointestinal epithelium provides the first line of defense against invading pathogens, among which *Helicobacter pylori* is linked to numerous gastric pathologies, including chronic gastritis and cancer. Primary gastric epithelial cells represent a useful model for the investigation of the underlying molecular and cellular mechanisms involved in these *H. pylori* associated diseases. In this chapter, we describe a method for the isolation of primary gastric epithelial cells from mice and detection of epithelial cell adhesion molecule (EpCAM) expression in the isolated cells.

Key words Primary culture, Gastric epithelial cells, EpCAM, *Helicobacter pylori*

1 Introduction

Gastric epithelial cells (GECs) lining the stomach form the first line of defense against *Helicobacter pylori* (*H. pylori*) infection [1]. It has been shown that *H. pylori* can penetrate the gastric mucous layer and attach to the apical surface of GECs where the bacterium can initiate gastric inflammation [2]. Although, human gastric epithelial cell lines, such as AGS, MKN28 and Kato III cells, have been used for modeling *H. pylori* infection in vitro, these transformed cell lines harbor oncogenic mutations and have altered protein expression profiles after many passages in vitro. Therefore, these cell lines do not always reflect the normal signal transduction pathways present in primary cells [3]. For these reasons, the isolation of mouse primary GECs is of interest to the field of *H. pylori* infection and gastric pathogenesis. However, there are at least two major challenges in obtaining these cells. Although epithelial cells represent the most abundant cell population in the gastric glands, the presence of other types of cells within these glands, particularly fibroblasts, makes it difficult to obtain highly pure GEC cultures

Brendan J. Jenkins (ed.), *Inflammation and Cancer: Methods and Protocols*, Methods in Molecular Biology, vol. 1725,
https://doi.org/10.1007/978-1-4939-7568-6_10, © Springer Science+Business Media, LLC 2018

[4–7]. Another important issue is the low density and viability of isolated GECs, resulting from inefficient tissue dissociation methods and the cytotoxic effects of enzymatic digestion [8, 9]. Here, we introduce a simple and optimized method to establish mouse primary GEC cultures that have minimal levels of fibroblast contamination and can be employed for studying the responses of host epithelial cells to *H. pylori* infection, as well as validating previous findings obtained with immortalized cell lines.

2 Materials

2.1 Reagents for GEC Isolation

1. Mice: specific pathogen-free male or female C57BL/6 mice, of 3–4 weeks age (*see* **Note 1**).
2. 1× Hanks Balanced Salt Solution Hank's (HBSS) balanced salt solution without Ca^{2+} and Mg^{2+}, containing 100 U/mL penicillin and streptomycin (pen/strep) (*see* **Note 2**).
3. Digestion solution: 1.25 mg/mL bovine serum albumin (BSA), 0.72 mg/mL dispase II (Thermo Fisher Scientific) and 1 mg/mL collagenase A (Roche) in HBSS (*see* **Notes 3** and **4**).
4. GEC medium: 20% fetal calf serum (FCS), 2 mM of L-glutamine, 100 U/mL of pen/strep, 2.5 mg/mL of fungizone antimycotic solution, 1× insulin/transferrin/selenite (ITS) and 10 ng/mL mouse epidermal growth factor (EGF) in DMEM/F12 basal medium (*see* **Note 5**).
5. Coating solution: 3 mg/mL rat tail collagen type I. Dilute the collagen to a working concentration of 50 μg/mL in 20 mM acetic acid and filter the solution using a 0.22 μm filter membrane.
6. C Tubes for dissociation of tissues to obtain single-cell suspensions using a gentleMACS™ Dissociator (Miltenyi Biotec).

2.2 Reagents for Immunofluorescence Staining

1. Fixation buffer: 4% (w/v) Paraformaldehyde (PFA) (*see* **Note 6**).
2. Blocking buffer: 3% (w/v) BSA, 0.1% (w/v) saponin in phosphate—buffered saline (PBS).
3. Primary antibodies: 1 mg/mL rabbit anti-mouse EpCAM; 1 mg/mL rabbit anti-mouse Vimentin. Dilute to a final concentration of 5 μg/mL in blocking buffer (*see* **Note 7**).
4. Secondary antibodies: 1 mg/mL anti-rabbit IgG-Alexa Fluor® 488. Dilute 1:1000 in blocking buffer (*see* **Note 7**).
5. Nuclear dye: 20 mM of Hoechst 33342. Dilute 1:1000 in PBS.
6. Dako fluorescence mounting medium.

3 Methods

3.1 Isolation of Mouse Primary Gastric Epithelial Cells

1. Euthanize 3–4 week old mice by either CO_2 asphyxiation or cervical dislocation, as per institutional guidelines.
2. Open the abdomen and excise stomachs with fine curved scissors.
3. Open the stomachs by cutting along the greater curvature, then wash with HBSS supplemented with pen/strep to remove residual digesta.
4. Place the stomach tissues immediately in collection tubes containing HBSS supplemented with pen/strep. Following this step, the remaining procedure is undertaken in a laminar flow hood using aseptic techniques.
5. Transfer the stomachs to a 10 cm^2 dish containing 5 mL of freshly prepared digestion solution (*see* **Note 8**).
6. Remove the forestomach and finely mince the gastric glandular tissues into 1–2 mm^3 pieces with a sharp scalpel (*see* **Note 9**).
7. Transfer the digestion solution containing gastric pieces into a T75 tissue culture flask.
8. Shake at 150 cycle/min for 1 h, at 37 °C, 5% CO_2 (*see* **Note 10**).
9. During the incubation time, place sterilized coverslips in several additional wells for immunofluorescence staining to check the purity of the GEC cultures. Coat all wells with rat tail collagen I by adding 300 μL of 50 μg/mL collagen solution to each well and incubating at room temperature for 1 h (*see* **Note 11**).
10. After aspirating the collagen solution, rinse the wells three times with 300 μL of sterile PBS to remove the acid in the collagen solution. Air-dry the plates inside a laminar flow hood.
11. Following tissue digestion, pipette up and down 20 times with a 5 mL serological pipette to further dissociate gastric tissues (*see* **Note 12**).
12. Shake the flask at 150 cycle/min for a further 15 min, at 37 °C, 5% CO_2 (*see* **Note 13**).
13. Transfer the digested tissues from T75 flasks into 15 mL falcon tubes and pellet by centrifugation at 4 °C, 300 × *g* for 5 min (*see* **Note 14**).
14. Discard the digestion solution and avoid disturbing the cell pellets, then resuspend pellets in 2 mL of GEC medium.
15. Transfer cell suspensions into purple C tubes and homogenize by using the gentleMACS™ Dissociator (*see* **Note 15**).
16. Spin down the C tubes at 300 × *g*, discard the supernatants and resuspend each cell pellet in 1 mL of GEC media.

17. Cells are then counted using a hemocytometer and plated at 10^5 cells/mL per well in collagen-coated wells.
18. Cells are grown at 37 °C with 5% of CO_2 in a humidified incubator.
19. Change the culture medium every 2 days to remove cellular debris (*see* **Note 16**).
20. Epithelial cells are grown for 5 days before performing downstream analysis (immunofluorescence staining for EpCAM/Vimentin, co-culturing with *H. pylori* or stimulation with agonists/cytokines) (*see* **Note 17**).

3.2 Immunofluorescence Staining to Confirm the Purity of GEC Preparations

Immunofluorescence staining is performed for adhesion molecule EpCAM and Vimentin as standard markers of epithelial cells and fibroblasts, respectively [10]. This assay allows us to detect fibroblast contamination, as well as assess the purity of our GEC cultures (Fig. 1).

1. Aspirate the culture medium and wash cells with warm PBS for 5 min and gently discard PBS.
2. Fix cells with 4% PFA for 15 min at room temperature, and discard PFA in a fume hood (*see* **Note 18**).
3. Wash cells three times with PBS, 5 min per wash.
4. Block and permeabilize fixed cells in blocking buffer for 60 min, at room temperature.
5. Add 100 μL aliquots of diluted 5 μg/mL primary rabbit anti-mouse EpCAM or 5 μg/mL rabbit anti-Vimentin to a parafilm sheet (*see* **Note 19**).
6. Remove coverslips from plates and place upside down on the aliquots (cells facing the aliquot), then incubate in a humid chamber, overnight at 4 °C (*see* **Note 20**).
7. Wash coverslips three times with blocking buffer.
8. Add 100 μL of 1:1000 diluted secondary antibody, anti-rabbit IgG-Alexa Fluor® 488 for 2 h, at room temperature as described in **step 5**. From this point onwards, coverslips should be protected from light using foil.
9. Wash coverslips three times with blocking buffer.
10. Stain nuclei with 1:1000 dilution Hoechst 33342 for 5 min at room temperature.
11. Wash coverslips once in PBS.
12. Touch the edge of the coverslips on a paper towel and then aspirate any residual drops of PBS (*see* **Note 21**).
13. Mount coverslips with a small drop of mounting medium onto microscope slides (*see* **Note 22**).

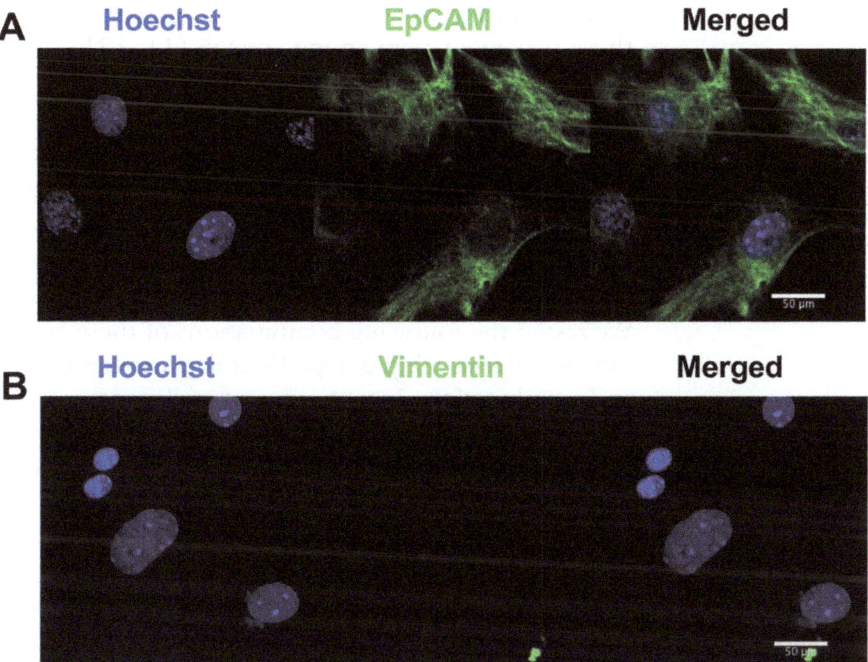

Fig. 1 Immunofluorescence staining of GECs for EpCAM and Vimentin, representing epithelial cell and fibroblast markers, respectively. Cells were isolated and cultured as described. At day 5 of culture, isolated cells appeared healthy and by indirect immunofluorescence reacted with an antibody specific for (**a**) EpCAM but not one specific for (**b**) Vimentin, confirming their epithelial origin. Cell nuclei were counterstained with Hoeschst 33342. In addition, cells obtained by this method can be employed for various in vitro assays (*e. g.* ELISA, Western blotting, TUNEL). We observed that these cells exhibited enhanced production of the neutrophil-chemoattractant chemokines, KC and MIP2, in response to stimulation with *H. pylori* bacteria (data not shown), consistent with previous findings using the mouse GSM06 gastric epithelial cell line [16]. Representative images were acquired using a Nikon confocal microscope, scale bar = 5 µm, 40× magnification

14. Seal the edges of the coverslips with nail polish and allow to air dry at room temperature. Slides can be stored at 4 °C until imaging.
15. Visualize EpCAM and vimentin staining on a confocal microscope (*see* **Note 23**).

4 Notes

1. The yield of isolated cells is approximately 1×10^5–5×10^5 cells per mouse stomach. The best GEC yields are obtained from mice no older than 3 weeks of age. In addition, there are fewer numbers of fibroblasts when using young compared with adult mice. It is likely that young mice have greater numbers of actively proliferating gastric epithelial stem cells than adult animals. Furthermore, epithelial cultures from adult rat and

rabbit stomachs were reported to contain more fibroblasts than those generated from young animals [11, 12].

2. Ca^{2+}- and $MgCl^{2+}$-free HBSS is used to facilitate tissue dissociation. Penicillin and streptomycin are added to HBSS to reduce bacterial and fungal contamination from the microbiota and/or the process of organ harvesting.
3. The enzymes used for the dissociation of gastric tissues and shown to be able to eliminate the fibroblast contamination for tissue digestion include collagenase, dispase and hyaluronidase. We tested the following combinations of these enzymes: combination 1 consisting of type IV collagenase and hyaluronidase, and combination 2 consisting of collagenase A and dispase [12, 13]. We found that the latter combination gave the best yield of GECs and the least degree of fibroblast contamination. This combination has therefore been used for the method described in this Chapter.
4. It is recommended to prepare 100× stock solutions of dispase II, collagenase A and BSA. Dry powdered forms of these proteins are dissolved in HBSS, filtered through 0.2 μm filter membranes and stored in single-use aliquots at −20 °C for long-term use.
5. The formulation of GEC medium described here has been adapted from that reported by Konda and Chiba [13].
6. Paraformaldehyde is a powder of polymerized formaldehyde that by itself cannot fix tissues. To be used as a fixative, paraformaldehyde has to be dissolved in warm PBS to become a formaldehyde solution. This step should be done in a fume hood as formaldehyde fumes are toxic.
7. The optimal working concentration of primary antibodies will vary depending on recommendations from the manufacturers.
8. To ensure maximal enzyme activity, the digestion solution should be made fresh by diluting enzyme stock solutions with HBSS to the appropriate final concentrations.
9. The forestomach in mice is predominantly lined with non-glandular stratified squamous epithelium [14].
10. Mechanical dissociation of gastric tissues by vigorous, side-to-side shaking of T75 flasks can remove intact gastric glands from the stomach tissues.
11. Rat tail collagen type I is used as a matrix for GECs to attach and proliferate.
12. This step will help to completely disperse the cells from partially digested tissues [4]. Furthermore, Moyer et al. reported that mechanic dissociation can reduce contamination by fibroblasts [15].

13. The digestion process should be no longer than the proposed times in this method as enzymatic digestion by collagenase and dispase can have damaging effects on cell surface membranes.
14. To prevent cell damage and therefore obtain higher yields, cells should be kept cold throughout all procedures except the digestion step.
15. The gentleMACs Dissociator is a benchtop instrument useful for generating single cell suspensions from tissues. We found that using this system (m_intestine_01 program) can increase GEC yields.
16. Although cellular clumps or debris can be removed by filtering cell suspensions through 70 μm cell strainers in **step 15** (Subheading 3.1), we found that this procedure significantly decreased the yield of GECs. Instead, we remove these clumps and debris by a change of medium on day 2 of the culture.
17. Primary GECs should not be grown for more than 5 days, as fibroblasts will overgrow the GECs.
18. Discard PFA as a hazardous waste.
19. If the anti-EpCAM and anti-Vimentin antibodies are of two different isotypes, dual staining for these markers can be performed simultaneously in one sample. Since our primary antibodies are from the same species (rabbit IgG), we stain them separately. In addition, an isotype antibody control or a secondary antibody control without the primary antibody should be used to confirm the specificity of primary antibodies.
20. To lift the coverslips, with one hand use a needle and the other hand hold a curved tweezer.
21. As much of the residual PBS as possible needs to be removed, so that the mounting medium spreads uniformly after mounting.
22. Warm the mounting medium to room temperature so that it is easier to pipette when mounting.
23. Glass coverslips can be replaced by Ibidi chambers(μ-Slide 8 Well, CAT: 80826), which are more convenient to handle than coverslips and are suitable for use in both upright micro scopes and live cell imaging.

Acknowledgments

This work was supported by funding from the National Health and Medical Research Council (NHMRC) to RLF (project APP1079930). Research at the Hudson Institute of Medical Research is supported by the Victorian Government's Operational Infrastructure Support Program. RLF holds an NHMRC Senior Research Fellowship (APP1079904).

References

1. Wadhwa R, Song S, Lee JS, Yao Y, Wei Q, Ajani JA (2013) Gastric cancer-molecular and clinical dimensions. Nat Rev Clin Oncol 10:643–655
2. Celli JP, Turner BS, Afdhal NH, Keates S, Ghiran I, Kelly CP, Ewoldt RH, McKinley GH, So P, Erramilli S, Bansil R (2009) Helicobacter pylori moves through mucus by reducing mucin viscoelasticity. Proc Natl Acad Sci U S A 106:14321–14326
3. Yokozaki H (2000) Molecular characteristics of eight gastric cancer cell lines established in Japan. Pathol Int 50:767–777
4. Terano A, Mach T, Stachura J, Sekhon S, Tarnawski A, Ivey KJ (1983) A monolayer culture of human gastric epithelial cells. Dig Dis Sci 28:595–603
5. Aziz F, Yang X, Wen Q, Yan Q (2015) A method for establishing human primary gastric epithelial cell culture from fresh surgical gastric tissues. Mol Med Rep 12:2939–2944
6. Viala J, Chaput C, Boneca IG, Cardona A, Girardin SE, Moran AP, Athman R, Memet S, Huerre MR, Coyle AJ, DiStefano PS, Sansonetti PJ, Labigne A, Bertin J, Philpott DJ, Ferrero RL (2004) Nod1 responds to peptidoglycan delivered by the *Helicobacter pylori* cag pathogenicity island. Nat Immunol 5:1166–1174
7. Wee JL, Chionh YT, Ng GZ, Harbour SN, Allison C, Pagel CN, Mackie EJ, Mitchell HM, Ferrero RL, Sutton P (2010) Protease-activated receptor-1 down-regulates the murine inflammatory and humoral response to *Helicobacter pylori*. Gastroenterol 138:573–582
8. Zavros Y, Van Antwerp M, Merchant JL (2000) Use of flow cytometry to quantify mouse gastric epithelial cell populations. Dig Dis Sci 45:1192–1199
9. Freshney RI (2010) Primary culture. Culture of animal cells: a manual of basic technique and specialized applications, 6th edn. John Wiley & Sons, Inc., Hoboken, NJ
10. Pollock K, Albares L, Wendt C, Hubel A (2013) Isolation of fibroblasts and epithelial cells in bronchoalveolar lavage (BAL). Exp Lung Res 39:146–154
11. Ota S, Razandi M, Sekhon S, Krause WJ, Terano A, Hiraishi H, Ivey KJ (1988) Salicylate effects on a monolayer culture of gastric mucous cells from adult rats. Gut 29:1705–1714
12. Matuoka K, Tanaka M, Mitsui Y, Murota SI (1983) Cultured rabbit gastric epithelial cells producing prostaglandin I2. Gastroenterol 84:498–505
13. Konda Y, Chiba T (2002) Rat gastric mucosal epithelial cell culture. Methods Mol Biol 188:17–25
14. Willet SG, Mills JC (2016) Stomach organ and cell lineage differentiation: from embryogenesis to adult homeostasis. Cell Mol Gastroenterol Hepatol 2:546–559
15. Moyer MP (1983) Culture of human gastrointestinal epithelial cells. Proc Soc Exp Biol Med 174:12–15
16. Ferrero RL, Ave P, Ndiaye D, Bambou JC, Huerre MR, Philpott DJ, Memet S (2008) NF-kappaB activation during acute Helicobacter pylori infection in mice. Infect Immun 76:551–561

Chapter 11

Dissecting Interleukin-6 Classic- and Trans-Signaling in Inflammation and Cancer

Christoph Garbers and Stefan Rose-John

Abstract

Interleukin-6 is a cytokine synthesized by many cells in the human body. IL-6 binds to a membrane bound IL-6R, which is only present on hepatocytes, some epithelial cells and some leukocytes. The complex of IL-6 and IL-6R binds to the ubiquitously expressed receptor subunit gp130, which forms a homodimer and thereby initiates intracellular signaling via the JAK/STAT and the MAPK pathways. IL-6R expressing cells can cleave the receptor protein to generate a soluble IL-6R (sIL-6R), which can still bind IL-6 and can associate with gp130 and induce signaling even on cells, which do not express IL-6R. This paradigm has been called IL-6 trans-signaling whereas signaling via the membrane bound IL-6R is referred to as classic signaling. We have generated several molecular tools to differentiate between IL-6 classic- and trans-signaling and to analyze the consequence of cellular IL-6 signaling in vivo.

Key words Interleukin-6, Interleukin-6 receptor, IL-6 trans-signaling, Soluble gp130, Inflammation, Cancer

1 Introduction

Interleukin-6 (IL-6) is a cytokine found drastically elevated in most situations in which the homeostasis of the body has been challenged. High IL-6 levels are found upon bacterial [1] and viral infection [2], in obesity [3], during sepsis [4, 5] and also in cancer [6]. In the past 10 years, the IL-6R neutralizing monoclonal antibody Tocilizumab has been tested in the clinic for the treatment of autoimmune diseases and the antibody is now approved in more than 100 countries. Recently, an IL-6 neutralizing antibody called Siltuximab has been approved for the treatment of patients with Castleman's disease [7].

IL-6 is a 184 amino acid long four-helical protein, which is structurally related to other cytokines such as IL-2, IL-7, IL-9, IL-15 and IL-21 but also to factors such as erythropoietin, growth hormone, prolactin and leptin [8, 9]. Binding of IL-6 to the IL-6R is not sufficient for signaling. Rather, the IL-6/IL-6R complex

Brendan J. Jenkins (ed.), *Inflammation and Cancer: Methods and Protocols*, Methods in Molecular Biology, vol. 1725, https://doi.org/10.1007/978-1-4939-7568-6_11,

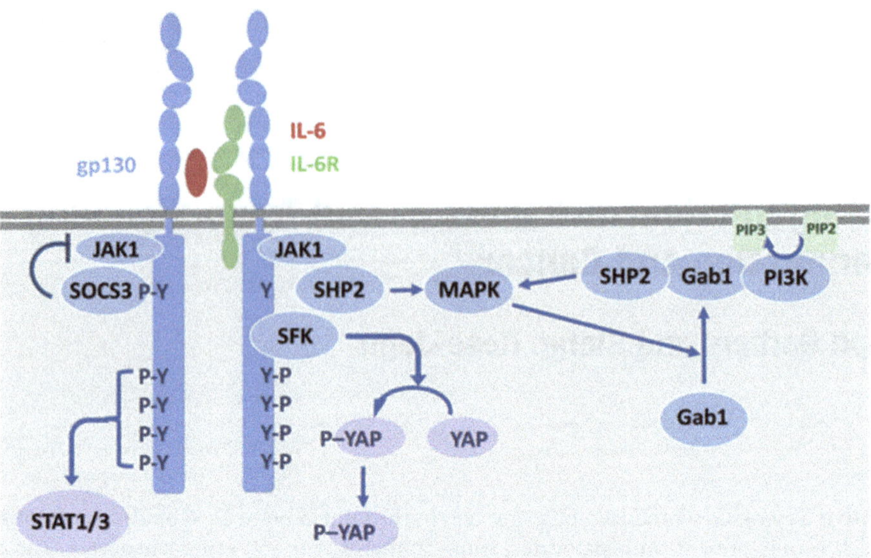

Fig. 1 Signal transduction of gp130. Upon dimerization of gp130, intracellular signaling is initiated by activation of JAK1, which thereupon phosphorylates the five tyrosine residues of the cytoplasmic portion of gp130. The membrane proximal tyrosine is the docking site of the adapter and phosphatase protein SHP2, which stimulates (among others) the MAPK and PI3K pathway. The membrane proximal tyrosine is also targeted by the negative feed-back regulator protein SOCS3, which blocks JAK1 and leads to signal termination. The four membrane distal tyrosine residues are docking sites for STAT1 and STAT3, which are phosphorylated, dimerize and travel to the nucleus to act as transcription factors. Additionally, Src family kinases (SFKs) are activated and phosphorylate YAP, which transfers to the nucleus and associates with transcription factor TEAD

binds to a second receptor subunit, called gp130 [10], which dimerizes and induces intracellular signaling [11] leading to the activation of several signal transduction pathways including the JAK/STAT, MAPK, PI3K and AKT pathways, which occurs via 5 tyrosine residues within its cytoplasmic portion [12]. In addition, the membrane proximal tyrosine is the docking site of SHP2, which is linked to activation of the MAPK and PI3K pathway, and also is essential for binding of the feedback inhibitory protein SOCS3 (Fig. 1).

IL-6 not only acts via the classic signaling pathway mediated by the membrane-bound IL-6R. It has been found that IL-6R-expressing cells can cleave the IL-6R protein, generating a soluble IL-6R (sIL-6R), which is still capable of binding IL-6 [13, 14]. Importantly, the complex of IL-6 and sIL-6R can bind to and dimerize gp130 even on cells which do not express the IL-6R. Such cells even in the presence of IL-6 would not be able to respond to the cytokine since gp130 exhibits no measurable affinity for IL-6. This IL-6 signaling mode has been called IL-6 trans-signaling [15]. Since all cells in the body express gp130 [16], the IL-6

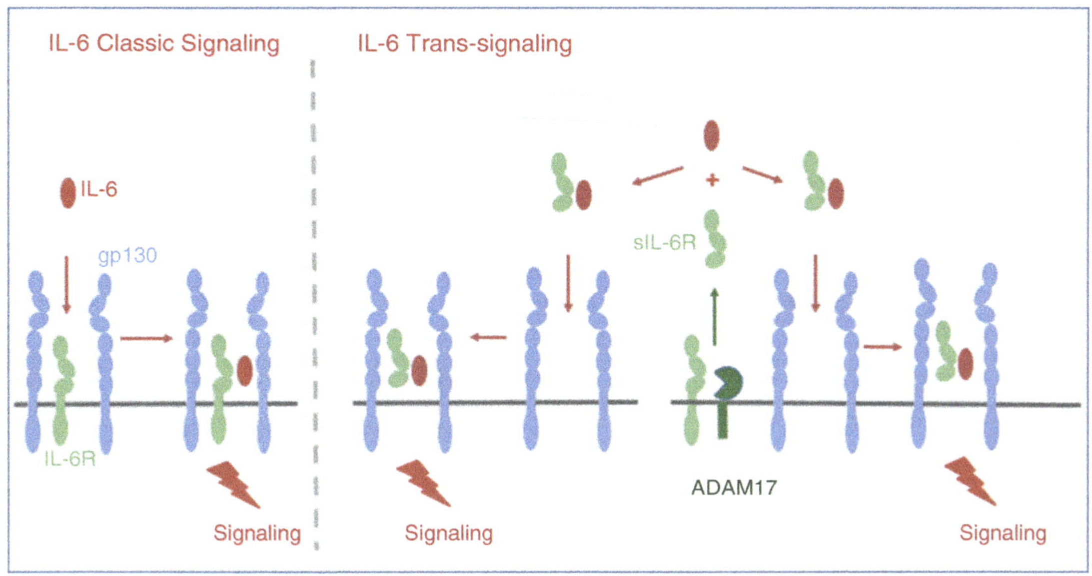

Fig. 2 IL-6 classic- and trans-signaling. In IL-6 classic signaling (left), IL-6 binds to the membrane-bound IL-6R and the complex of IL-6 and IL-6R associates with gp130, which thereupon dimerizes and initiates intracellular signal transduction. In IL-6 trans-signaling, the IL-6R is cleaved by the membrane-bound metalloprotease ADAM17. The resultant soluble IL-6R (sIL-6R) binds IL-6 and the complex of IL-6 and sIL-6R associates with membrane-bound gp130 on the same cell or on a different cell. Binding of IL-6/sIL-6R induces gp130 dimerization and intracellular signal transduction

trans-signaling pathway greatly increases the spectrum of target cells to IL-6 (Fig. 2) [17, 18].

Progress has been made in the past years to understand the complex biology of the cytokine IL-6. This was possible with a couple of molecular tools, which have been generated in our laboratory. In the following we shortly describe their principle, and we will give examples of the application of the described molecular tools in Subheading 2 and 3 in further detail.

We generated a fusion protein of human sIL-6R and human IL-6 in which the two moieties were connected by a linker of 18 flexible amino acids (Fig. 3a) [19]. Since there is no species specificity at the level of gp130 [20], Hyper-IL-6 can be used as a mimic of IL-6 trans-signaling in mouse, rat, human and many other species [21]. The responsiveness of cells to Hyper-IL-6 and IL-6 can be tested side by side to evaluate the requirement of sIL-6R for STAT3 phosphorylation or cellular proliferation. Using Hyper-IL-6 it was shown that embryonic, hematopoietic and neural stem cells, many neural cells and human primary smooth muscle cells depend on IL-6 trans-signaling in their response to IL-6 [22–26]. Moreover, Hyper-IL-6 has been used in vivo to show that IL-6 trans-signaling was needed for liver regeneration [27] and granulocyte generation after exposure to pathogens [28].

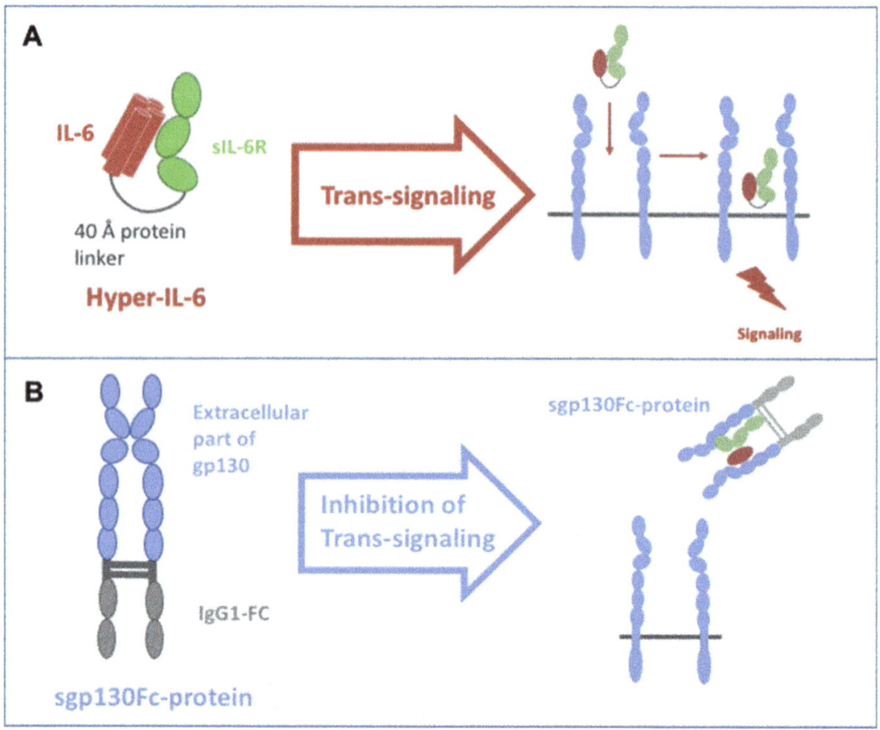

Fig. 3 The molecular tools Hyper-IL-6 and sgp130Fc. (**a**) In Hyper-IL-6, human IL-6 and human sIL-6R are covalently linked by a flexible peptide linker. The Hyper-IL-6 protein can be used in vitro and in vivo to mimic IL-6 trans-signaling. (**b**) The entire extracellular portion of human gp130 is linked to the Fc portion of a human IgG1 antibody. The sgp130Fc protein blocks IL-6 trans-signaling without affecting IL-6 classic signaling

A second protein called sgp130Fc was generated by linking the entire extracellular portion of human gp130 to the Fc portion of human IgG1 (Fig. 3b). The protein bound IL-6 only in the presence of sIL-6R [20]. Consequently, it turned out that sgp130Fc was a specific inhibitor of IL-6 trans-signaling. Since IL-6 showed no measurable affinity to sgp130Fc, classic signaling via the membrane-bound IL-6R was not affected by this protein [20]. Importantly, using the sgp130Fc protein, together with the generation of transgenic mice which express sgp130Fc from a liver promoter, in a myriad of mouse disease models has demonstrated that IL-6 trans-signaling promotes many disease states including inflammatory bowel disease, lupus erythematosus, endotoxemia, pulmonary emphysema, as well as colon and lung cancers (Fig. 4) (Table 1) [5, 20, 29, 34, 36, 39, 48, 49, 52–56].

Recently, we have generated transgenic mice, which express sgp130Fc from the astrocyte specific GFAP promoter. Using these mice, we could demonstrate that most if not all IL-6 signaling in the brain is mediated by IL-6 trans-signaling [45]. Moreover, using these mice, we could show that IL-6 trans-signaling in the brain decreased stress-induced synaptic inhibition/excitation ratio

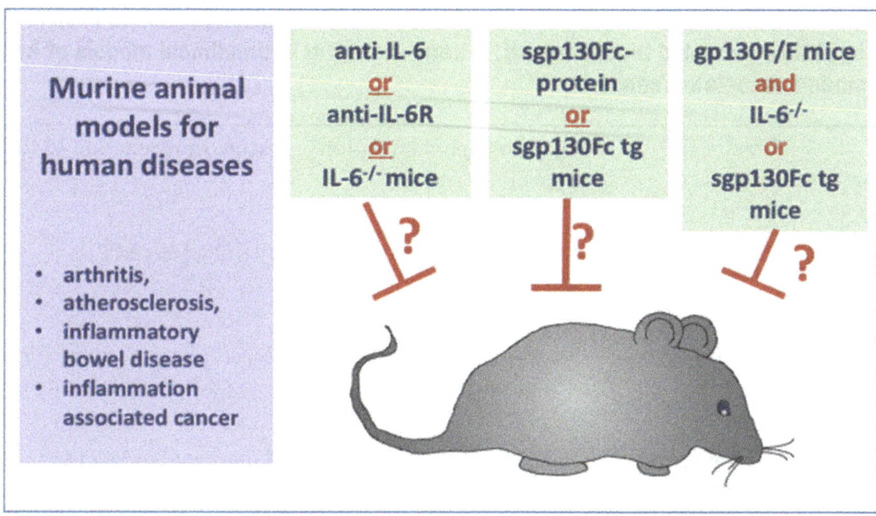

Fig. 4 Evaluation of the role of IL-6 classic- and trans-signaling in vivo. Murine models of human inflammatory diseases are first performed in the presence of IL-6 or IL-6R neutralizing antibodies or in IL-6$^{-/-}$ animals. These experiments show whether a given disease is based on IL-6 activity. In a next set of experiments, the same animal models are performed in the presence of the sgp130Fc protein or in sgp130Fc transgenic mice. These experiments show whether a given disease is dependent on IL-6 trans-signaling. In a final set of experiments, diseases spontaneously occurring in F/F mice are analyzed. F/F mice are crossed to IL-6$^{-/-}$ animals or to sgp130Fc transgenic mice. This set of experiments shows whether the spontaneously occurring diseases are dependent on IL-6 classic- or trans-signaling

[57] and that blockade of central IL-6 trans-signaling affected the sleep architecture [58].

Injection of a cytokine such as IL-6 into a mouse leads to the response of many cell types in various tissues making it impossible to define the specific response of single cells. We have generated at the cDNA level a constitutively active gp130 molecule named L-gp130 by replacing the entire extracellular domain of gp130 with the leucine zipper of the c-fos protein (Fig. 5a) [59]. The resultant cDNA when transfected into IL-6 dependent pre-B-cells led to the proliferation of these cells in the absence of IL-6. Moreover, when transfected into murine embryonic stem cells, these cells highly expressed the Oct4 gene and remained undifferentiated in the absence of LIF [59]. Ectopic expression of the L-gp130 cDNA in bone marrow cells resulted in multiple myeloma development with the characteristics of the human disease including monoclonal gammopathy, bone marrow infiltration with lytic bone lesions and protein deposition in the kidneys [60]. We have recently generated knock-in mice with the L-gp130 cDNA construct in the Rosa26 locus (Fig. 5b). In these mice using appropriate cell-specific cre--transgenic mice, constitutive gp130 activity can be induced in a cell autonomous manner without body-wide cytokine stimulation.

Table 1
Efficacy of sgp130Fc mediated blockade of IL-6 trans-signaling in preclinical models of inflammation and inflammation associated cancer

Intestinal inflammation [29, 30]	Pancreatic cancer [31, 32]	Ovarian hyperstimulation [33]	Acute inflammation [34, 35]
Rheumatoid arthritis [36–38]	Sepsis [4, 5]	Lupus erythematosus [39]	Asthma [40, 41]
Nephrotoxic nephritis [42, 43]	Arterosclerosis [44]	Neuroinflammation and neurodegeneration [45]	Macrophage accumulation in adipose tissue during obesity [3]
Ovarian cancer [5, 46]	Pancreatitis-lung failure [47]	Lung cancer [48]	Lung emphysema [49]
Hepatocellular carcinoma [50]	Colon cancer [6, 51]		

These mice will allow the molecular definition of cellular gp130 responses without the confounding cytokine responses of all other cells responsive to the cytokine.

2 Materials

2.1 Culture of Ba/F3-gp130 and Ba/F3-gp130-IL-6R Cell Lines

1. Cell culture medium: Dulbecco's Modified Eagles Medium (DMEM) supplemented with 10% fetal calf serum (FCS). Ba/F3 cell lines tolerate the addition of 1% penicillin/streptomycin to the medium if this is necessary (termed DMEM +/+) (*see* **Note 1**).
2. Phosphate-buffered saline (PBS, sterile): 137 mM NaCl, 2.7 mM KCl, 1.5 mM KH_2PO_4, 8.1 mM Na_2HPO_4, pH 7.4.
3. 50 ml falcon plastic tubes.
4. 10 ml sterile serological pipets.
5. Sterile petri dishes (90 mm diameter (*see* **Note 2**).
6. Recombinant human IL-6 (*see* **Note 3**).
7. Recombinant human Hyper-IL-6 (*see* **Note 4**).

2.2 Serum Starvation

1. Sterile PBS.
2. Dulbecco's Modified Eagles Medium (DMEM) without any supplements (termed DMEM −/−).
3. Sterile 12-well plates (*see* **Note 5**).

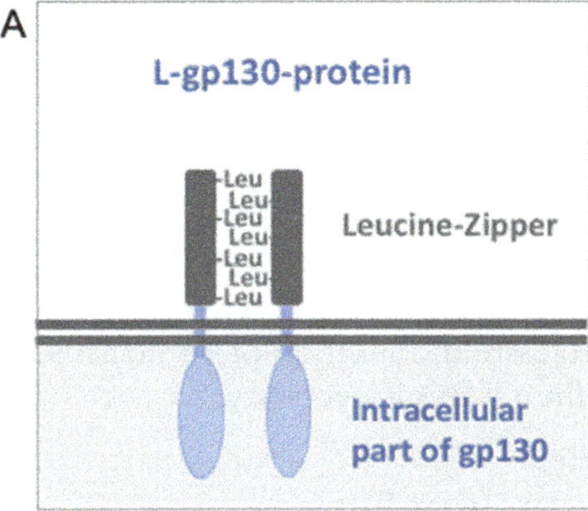

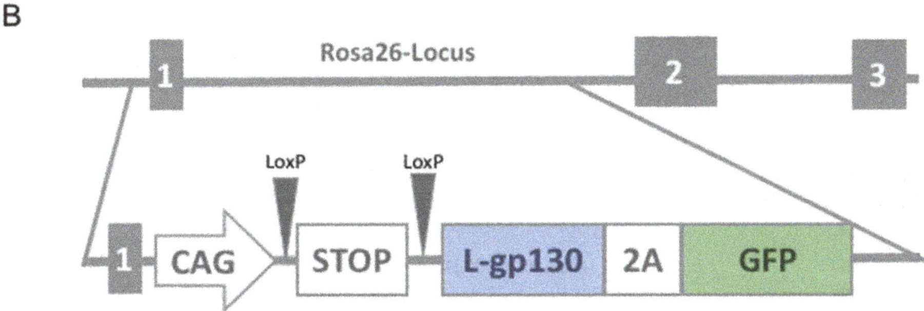

Fig. 5 Constitutively active gp130 and cell-autonomous gp130 stimulation. (**a**) In the L-gp130 protein, the entire extracellular portion of gp130 has been replaced by the leucine zipper of the c-fos protein. Consequently, gp130 is permanently dimerized and activated. (**b**) An L-gp130 coding cDNA has been inserted into the ROSA26 locus of the mouse. Transcription of this locus is blocked by a stop cassette, which can be removed in vivo by crossing the L-gp130 knock-in mice with appropriate cre-transgenic mice. Using these mice, gp130 activity can be induced in a cell autonomous manner in any cell of the mouse to define the cell-specific response to gp130 activation

2.3 Stimulation with IL-6 and Hyper-IL-6

1. Recombinant human IL-6.
2. Recombinant human Hyper-IL-6.
3. Cell lysis buffer: 50 mM Tris–HCl, 150 mM NaCl, 2 mM EDTA, 1 mM NaF, 1 mM Na_3VO_4, 1% Nonidet-P40, 1% Triton-X-100, Complete® protease inhibitor cocktail, pH 7.5 (*see* **Note 6**).

2.4 Measurement of STAT3 Phosphorylation

1. Standard equipment to run an SDS polyacrylamide gel.
2. Standard equipment to transfer the proteins onto a nitrocellulose or polyvinylidene difluoride membrane.
3. Tris-buffered saline (TBS; 10×): 1.5 M NaCl, 0.1 M Tris–HCl, pH 7.4.
4. TBS-T: TBS containing 0.05% Tween-20.
5. Stripping buffer: 62.5 mM Tris–HCl, pH 6.8, 2% SDS, 0.1% β-mercaptoethanol.

6. An antibody directed against phospho-Y705 of STAT3.
7. A pan-STAT3 antibody.

2.5 Measurement of Ba/F3-gp130 (-IL-6R) Cell Viability

1. 96 well-plates (flat bottom).
2. 15 and 50 ml falcon plastic tubes.
3. Cell culture medium: Dulbecco's Modified Eagles Medium (DMEM) supplemented with 10% fetal calf serum (FCS). Ba/F3 cell lines tolerate the addition of 1% penicillin/streptomycin to the medium if this is necessary.
4. Recombinant human IL-6.
5. Recombinant human Hyper-IL-6.
6. CellTiter-Blue® Cell Viability Assay (*see* **Note 7**).

3 Methods

All experiments should be carried out under sterile conditions, e.g., with the help of a laminar flow hood, unless indicated otherwise.

3.1 Permanent Culture of Ba/F3-gp130 and Ba/F3-gp130-IL-6R Cell Lines

1. Grow Ba/F3-gp130 and Ba/F3-gp130-IL-6R cells in 10 ml DMEM +/+ cell culture medium in a standard petri dish.
2. Both cell lines need permanent stimulation by a cytokine and would undergo apoptosis otherwise. Therefore, supplement Ba/F3-gp130 cells with 10 ng/ml Hyper-IL-6 and Ba/F3-gp130-IL-6R cells with 10 ng/ml IL-6 all the time.
3. Ba/F3-gp130 and Ba/F3-gp130-IL-6R cells should be passaged two times a week, e.g., on Mondays and on Thursdays. Here, transfer cells into a 50 ml falcon tube, collect the cells via centrifugation (1300 × *g*, 5 min, room temperature), remove the medium, wash the cells with 10 ml PBS, collect again via centrifugation, and resuspend the cells in 10 ml DMEM +/+. Count the cells and place 250,000 cells in 10 ml DMEM +/+ in a fresh plate. Add the respective cytokines as mentioned above (*see* **Note 8**).

3.2 Serum Starvation and Stimulation with IL-6 or Hyper-IL-6

1. In order to analyze the biological activity of IL-6 and Hyper-IL-6 using the phosphorylation of STAT3 as a readout, Ba/F3-gp130 and Ba/F3-gp130-IL-6R cells are usually serum-starved before applying the cytokines. Therefore, transfer cells into a 50 ml falcon tube, collect the cells via centrifugation (1300 × *g*, 5 min, room temperature), remove the medium and wash the cells with 10 ml PBS. Repeat this washing steps two more times.

2. Count the cells and place 1,000,000 cells in 1 ml DMEM −/− per well into a 12-well plate. Put the plate in an incubator for 90 min (*see* **Note 9**).
3. Stimulate the cells by adding the respective cytokines to the cells. Depending on the experiment, different amounts of the cytokines (usually in the range of 0.1–100 ng/ml) can be used.
4. Put the plate back in the incubator for 15 min (*see* **Note 10**). Afterwards, transfer the cells into 1.5 ml Eppendorf cups and collect the cells via centrifugation (1300 × *g*, 5 min, 4 °C) (*see* **Note 11**).
5. Lyse the pellet in 50 μl cell lysis buffer.

3.3 Measurement of STAT3 Phosphorylation

1. Load an appropriate amount of the protein lysates (e.g., 20 μg total protein) onto a 10% SDS polyacrylamide gel and electrophorese until the dye front arrives at the bottom of the gel. An appropriate protein standard marker should be added to every gel.
2. Transfer the proteins onto a nitrocellulose or polyvinylidene difluoride membrane. Immediately after the transfer, block the membrane with 25 ml of 5% skim milk powder dissolved in TBS-T for at least 60 min at room temperature.
3. Wash the membrane for 10 min with 25 ml TBS-T.
4. Incubate the membrane with the primary antibody, which recognizes the pY705-STAT3 epitope, overnight at 4 °C under constant movement. The antibody should be diluted in 5% BSA dissolved in TBS-T or 5% skim milk powder dissolved in TBS-T depending on the manufacturer's instructions (*see* **Note 12**).
5. Wash the membrane for 3 × 10 min with 25 ml TBS-T.
6. Incubate the membrane for 60 min at room temperature with an appropriate secondary antibody, which should be coupled to a peroxidase or a fluorophore depending on the detection system that is used.
7. Wash the membrane for 3 × 10 min with 25 ml TBS-T and detect the signals afterwards with the system of choice.
8. Having measured phosphorylated STAT3, it is usually beneficial to detect total STAT3 on the same membrane (*see* **Note 13**). In order to do this, the membrane is incubated with 50 ml stripping buffer for 30 min at 65 °C. Afterwards, it is briefly washed in TBS-T, blocked again as described above, and incubated with a pan-STAT3 antibody overnight. Detection of total STAT3 is carried out on the next day as described above.

3.4 Measurement of Ba/F3-gp130 (-IL-6R) Cell Viability

1. Transfer cells into a 50 ml falcon tube, collect the cells via centrifugation (1300 × *g*, 5 min, room temperature), remove the medium and wash the cells with 10 ml PBS.
2. Repeat this washing steps two more times.
3. Count cells and dilute them to a concentration of 62,500 cells per ml in DMEM +/+ medium in a 15 ml falcon tube.
4. Take a 96 well plate and add 80 μl of the cell suspension per well.
5. Add IL-6 and Hyper-IL-6 in different concentrations to the cells (usually in the range of 0.1–100 ng/ml) (*see* **Note 14**).
6. Make sure to include at least one positive and one negative control.
7. Add DMEM +/+ until each well contains 100 μl total volume.
8. Place the 96 well-plate for 48 h into an incubator.
9. Determine cell viability (or proliferation) according to the manufacturer's instruction of the method of choice.

4 Notes

1. In order to minimize the danger of cross-contamination of the different Ba/F3-derived cell lines which are cultured in parallel, it is recommended to use an individual bottle of medium for each cell line.
2. Ba/F3 cells are suspension cells and can in principle be grown in any plastic dish or flask. For the continuous culture of the cells, it is neither necessary nor beneficial to use coated dishes or flasks that are intended for tissue culture and adherent cell lines.
3. IL-6 should be stored at −80 °C for long term storage at concentrations of at least 1 mg/ml for optimal stability. Small aliquots can be stored at 4 °C for 2 weeks without a reduction in biological activity.
4. Hyper-IL-6 should be stored at −80 °C for long term storage at concentrations of at least 1 mg/ml for optimal stability. Small aliquots can be stored at 4 °C for 2 weeks without a reduction in biological activity.
5. For short-time experiments, also coated dishes or flasks that are intended for tissue culture and adherent cell lines can be used.
6. Cell lysis buffer can be stored in small aliquots at −20 °C for longer time periods.
7. Besides the CellTiter-Blue® assay, cell viability and/or cell proliferation can also be determined with any other applicable method or reagent.

8. Ba/F3-gp130 and Ba/F3-gp130-IL-6R start to proliferation cytokine-independent when they grow too dense. Therefore, it is recommended to seed an equal number of cells without cytokine addition in a control plate and to check that these control cells do not proliferate when passaging the cells the next time.
9. Serum-starving of the cells for longer time periods results in increasing number of dying cells, which makes the analysis of intracellular signaling pathways unreliable and should be avoided.
10. STAT3 phosphorylation is rapidly turned on after binding of the cytokines to their receptors, and also rapidly shut down afterwards. At the 15 min time point, STAT3 phosphorylation is easily detectable, whereas it already declines when the cells are collected at later time points.
11. Be sure to carefully collect all cells out of the 12 well plate, which like to adhere to the bottom of the well.
12. Most primary antibodies against pSTAT3 or STAT3 can be used several times, and it works fine to store the diluted antibody at −20 °C until the next use.
13. The detection of total STAT3 on the same membrane can either serve as a loading control, or as a method to get an idea how much of the transcription factor is phosphorylated in response to the cytokine treatment.
14. It is recommended to perform every experiment with three or four biological replicates, which should always be put on the same 96 well plate.

Acknowledgments

This work was supported by the Deutsche Forschungsgemeinschaft (DFG), Bonn, Germany (SFB654, project C5; SFB841, project C1; SFB877, project A1, A10), by the Bundesministerium für Bildung und Forschung www.bmbf.de (grant number InTraSig, project B) and by the German Cluster of Excellence 'Inflammation at Interfaces'.

Competing Interests

S.R.-J. has acted as a consultant and speaker to Chugai, Genentech Roche, AbbVie, Sanofi and Pfizer. He is the inventor of the sgp130Fc protein and he is listed as an inventor on patents owned by CONARIS Research Institute, which develops the sgp130Fc protein (Olamkicept) together with Ferring Pharmaceuticals, and he has stock ownership in CONARIS. C.G. has nothing to disclose.

References

1. Scheller J, Chalaris A, Schmidt-Arras D, Rose-John S (2011) The pro- and anti-inflammatory properties of the cytokine interleukin-6. Biochim Biophys Acta 1813:878–888
2. Harker JA, Lewis GM, Mack L, Zuniga EI (2011) Late interleukin-6 escalates T follicular helper cell responses and controls a chronic viral infection. Science 334:825–829
3. Kraakman MJ, Kammoun HL, Allen TL, Deswaerte V, Henstridge DC, Estevez E et al (2015) Blocking IL-6 trans-signaling prevents high-fat diet-induced adipose tissue macrophage recruitment but does not improve insulin resistance. Cell Metab 21:403–416
4. Barkhausen T, Tschernig T, Rosenstiel P, van Griensven M, Vonberg RP, Dorsch M et al (2011) Selective blockade of interleukin-6 trans-signaling improves survival in a murine polymicrobial sepsis model. Crit Care Med 39:1407–1413
5. Greenhill CJ, Rose-John S, Lissilaa R, Ferlin W, Ernst M, Hertzog PJ et al (2011) IL-6 trans-signaling modulates TLR4-dependent inflammatory responses via STAT3. J Immunol 186:1199–1208
6. Grivennikov S, Karin E, Terzic J, Mucida D, GY Y, Vallabhapurapu S et al (2009) IL-6 and Stat3 are required for survival of intestinal epithelial cells and development of colitis-associated cancer. Cancer Cell 15:103–113
7. Rose-John S, Winthrop KL, Calabrese LH (2017) The role of IL-6 in host defense against infections: immunobiology and clinical implications. Nat Rev Rheumatol 13(7):399–409
8. Bazan JF (1990) Haemopoietic receptors and helical cytokines. Immunol Today 11:350–354
9. Garbers C, Hermanns HM, Schaper F, Muller-Newen G, Grotzinger J, Rose-John S et al (2012) Plasticity and cross-talk of interleukin 6-type cytokines. Cytokine Growth Factor Rev 23:85–97
10. Hibi M, Murakami M, Saito M, Hirano T, Taga T, Kishimoto T (1990) Molecular cloning and expression of an IL-6 signal transducer, gp130. Cell 63:1149–1157
11. Garbers C, Aparicio-Siegmund S, Rose-John S (2015) The IL-6/gp130/STAT3 signaling axis: recent advances towards specific inhibition. Curr Opin Immunol 34:75–82
12. Schaper F, Rose-John S (2015) Interleukin-6: biology, signaling and strategies of blockade. Cytokine Growth Factor Rev 26:475–487
13. Müllberg J, Schooltink H, Stoyan T, Gunther M, Graeve L, Buse G et al (1993) The soluble interleukin-6 receptor is generated by shedding. Eur J Immunol 23:473–480
14. Müllberg J, Schooltink H, Stoyan T, Heinrich PC, Rose-John S (1992) Protein kinase C activity is rate limiting for shedding of the interleukin-6 receptor. Biochem Biophys Res Commun 189:794–800
15. Rose-John S, Heinrich PC (1994) Soluble receptors for cytokines and growth factors: generation and biological function. Biochem J 300(Pt 2):281–290
16. Oberg HH, Wesch D, Grussel S, Rose-John S, Kabelitz D (2006) Differential expression of CD126 and CD130 mediates different STAT-3 phosphorylation in CD4+CD25- and CD25 high regulatory T cells. Int Immunol 18:555–563
17. Jones SA, Scheller J, Rose-John S (2011) Therapeutic strategies for the clinical blockade of IL-6/gp130 signaling. J Clin Invest 121:3375–3383
18. Rose-John S (2012) IL-6 trans-signaling via the soluble IL-6 receptor: importance for the pro-inflammatory activities of IL-6. Int J Biol Sci 8:1237–1247
19. Fischer M, Goldschmitt J, Peschel C, Brakenhoff JP, Kallen KJ, Wollmer A et al (1997) I. A bioactive designer cytokine for human hematopoietic progenitor cell expansion. Nat Biotechnol 15:142–145
20. Jostock T, Müllberg J, Ozbek S, Atreya R, Blinn G, Voltz N et al (2001) Soluble gp130 is the natural inhibitor of soluble interleukin-6 receptor transsignaling responses. Eur J Biochem 268:160–167
21. Appenheimer MM, Girard RA, Chen Q, Wang WC, Bankert KC, Hardison J et al (2007) Conservation of IL-6 trans-signaling mechanisms controlling L-selectin adhesion by fever-range thermal stress. Eur J Immunol 37:2856–2867
22. Humphrey RK, Beattie GM, Lopez AD, Bucay N, King CC, Firpo MT et al (2004) Maintenance of pluripotency in human embryonic stem cells is STAT3 independent. Stem Cells 22:522–530
23. Audet J, Miller CL, Rose-John S, Piret JM, Eaves CJ (2001) Distinct role of gp130 activation in promoting self-renewal divisions by mitogenically stimulated murine hematopoietic stem cells. Proc Natl Acad Sci U S A 98:1757–1762
24. Islam O, Gong X, Rose-John S, Heese K (2009) Interleukin-6 and neural stem cells:

more than gliogenesis. Mol Biol Cell 20:188–199

25. März P, Heese K, Hock C, Golombowski S, Muller-Spahn F, Rose-John S et al (1997) Interleukin-6 (IL-6) and soluble forms of IL-6 receptors are not altered in cerebrospinal fluid of Alzheimer's disease patients. Neurosci Lett 239:29–32
26. Klouche M, Bhakdi S, Hemmes M, Rose-John S (1999) Novel path to activation of vascular smooth muscle cells: up-regulation of gp130 creates an autocrine activation loop by IL-6 and its soluble receptor. J Immunol 163:4583–4589
27. Hecht N, Pappo O, Shouval D, Rose-John S, Galun E, Axelrod JH (2001) Hyper-IL-6 gene therapy reverses fulminant hepatic failure. Mol Ther 3:683–687
28. Walker F, Zhang HH, Matthews V, Weinstock J, Nice EC, Ernst M et al (2008) IL6/sIL6R complex contributes to emergency granulopoietic responses in G-CSF- and GM-CSF-deficient mice. Blood 111:3978–3985
29. Atreya R, Mudter J, Finotto S, Müllberg J, Jostock T, Wirtz S et al (2000) Blockade of interleukin 6 trans signaling suppresses T-cell resistance against apoptosis in chronic intestinal inflammation: evidence in crohn disease and experimental colitis in vivo. Nat Med 6:583–588
30. Mitsuyama K, Matsumoto S, Rose-John S, Suzuki A, Hara T, Tomiyasu N et al (2006) STAT3 activation via interleukin 6 trans-signalling contributes to ileitis in SAMP1/Yit mice. Gut 55:1263–1269
31. Lesina M, Kurkowski MU, Ludes K, Rose-John S, Treiber M, Kloppel G et al (2011) Stat3/Socs3 activation by IL-6 transsignaling promotes progression of pancreatic intraepithelial neoplasia and development of pancreatic cancer. Cancer Cell 19:456–469
32. Goumas FA, Holmer R, Egberts JH, Gontarewicz A, Heneweer C, Geisen U et al (2015) Inhibition of IL-6 signaling significantly reduces primary tumor growth and recurrencies in orthotopic xenograft models of pancreatic cancer. Int J Cancer 137:1035–1046
33. Wei LH, Chou CH, Chen MW, Rose-John S, Kuo ML, Chen SU et al (2013) The role of IL-6 trans-signaling in vascular leakage: implications for ovarian hyperstimulation syndrome in a murine model. J Clin Endocrinol Metab 98:E472–E484
34. Rabe B, Chalaris A, May U, Waetzig GH, Seegert D, Williams AS et al (2008) Transgenic blockade of interleukin 6 transsignaling abrogates inflammation. Blood 111:1021–1028
35. Chalaris A, Rabe B, Paliga K, Lange H, Laskay T, Fielding CA et al (2007) Apoptosis is a natural stimulus of IL6R shedding and contributes to the proinflammatory trans-signaling function of neutrophils. Blood 110:1748–1755
36. Nowell MA, Williams AS, Carty SA, Scheller J, Hayes AJ, Jones GW et al (2009) Therapeutic targeting of IL-6 trans signaling counteracts STAT3 control of experimental inflammatory arthritis. J Immunol 182:613–622
37. Nowell MA, Richards PJ, Horiuchi S, Yamamoto N, Rose-John S, Topley N et al (2003) Soluble IL-6 receptor governs IL-6 activity in experimental arthritis: blockade of arthritis severity by soluble glycoprotein 130. J Immunol 171:3202–3209
38. Richards PJ, Nowell MA, Horiuchi S, McLoughlin RM, Fielding CA, Grau S et al (2006) Functional characterization of a soluble gp130 isoform and its therapeutic capacity in an experimental model of inflammatory arthritis. Arthritis Rheum 54:1662–1672
39. Tsantikos E, Maxwell MJ, Putoczki T, Ernst M, Rose-John S, Tarlinton DM et al (2013) Interleukin-6 trans-signaling exacerbates inflammation and renal pathology in lupus-prone mice. Arthritis Rheum 65:2691–2702
40. Doganci A, Eigenbrod T, Krug N, De Sanctis GT, Hausding M, Erpenbeck VJ et al (2005) The IL-6R alpha chain controls lung CD4+CD25+ treg development and function during allergic airway inflammation in vivo. J Clin Invest 115:313–325
41. Ullah MA, Revez JA, Loh Z, Simpson J, Zhang V, Bain L et al (2015) Allergen-induced IL-6 trans-signaling activates gammadelta T cells to promote type 2 and type 17 airway inflammation. J Allergy Clin Immunol 136:1065–1073
42. Luig M, Kluger MA, Goerke B, Meyer M, Nosko A, Yan I et al (2015) Inflammation-Induced IL-6 functions as a natural brake on macrophages and limits GN. J Am Soc Nephrol 26:1597–1607
43. Braun GS, Nagayama Y, Maruta Y, Heymann F, van Roeyen CR, Klinkhammer BM et al (2016) IL-6 trans-signaling drives murine crescentic GN. J Am Soc Nephrol 27:132–142
44. Schuett H, Oestreich R, Waetzig GH, Annema W, Luchtefeld M, Hillmer A et al (2012) Transsignaling of interleukin-6 crucially contributes to atherosclerosis in mice. Arterioscler Thromb Vasc Biol 32:281–290

45. Campbell IL, Erta M, Lim SL, Frausto R, May U, Rose-John S et al (2014) Trans-signaling is a dominant mechanism for the pathogenic actions of interleukin-6 in the brain. J Neurosci 34:2503–2513
46. Lo CW, Chen MW, Hsiao M, Wang S, Chen CA, Hsiao SM et al (2011) IL-6 trans-signaling in formation and progression of malignant ascites in ovarian cancer. Cancer Res 71:424–434
47. Zhang H, Neuhofer P, Song L, Rabe B, Lesina M, Kurkowski MU et al (2013) IL-6 trans-signaling promotes pancreatitis-associated lung injury and lethality. J Clin Invest 123:1019–1031
48. Brooks GD, McLeod L, Alhayyani S, Miller A, Russell PA, Ferlin W et al (2016) IL6 trans-signaling promotes KRAS-driven lung carcinogenesis. Cancer Res 76:866–876
49. Ruwanpura SM, McLeod L, Dousha LF, Seow HJ, Alhayyani S, Tate MD et al (2016) Therapeutic targeting of the IL-6 trans-signalling/mTORC1 axis in pulmonary emphysema. Am J Respir Crit Care Med 194:1494–1505
50. Bergmann J, Muller M, Baumann N, Reichert M, Heneweer C, Bolik J et al (2017) IL-6 trans-signaling is essential for the development of hepatocellular carcinoma in mice. Hepatology 65:89–103
51. Matsumoto S, Hara T, Mitsuyama K, Yamamoto M, Tsuruta O, Sata M et al (2010) Essential roles of IL-6 trans-signaling in colonic epithelial cells, induced by the IL-6/soluble-IL-6 receptor derived from lamina propria macrophages, on the development of colitis-associated premalignant cancer in a murine model. J Immunol 184:1543–1551
52. Becker C, Fantini MC, Schramm C, Lehr HA, Wirtz S, Nikolaev A et al (2004) TGF-beta suppresses tumor progression in colon cancer by inhibition of IL-6 trans-signaling. Immunity 21:491–501
53. Sodenkamp J, Waetzig GH, Scheller J, Seegert D, Grötzinger J, Rose-John S et al (2012) Therapeutic targeting of interleukin-6 trans-signaling does not affect the outcome of experimental tuberculosis. Immunobiology 217:996–1004
54. Hoge J, Yan I, Jänner N, Schumacher V, Chalaris A, Steinmetz OM et al (2013) IL-6 controls the innate immune response against Listeria monocytogenes via classical IL-6 signaling. J Immunol 190:703–711
55. Jenkins BJ, Grail D, Nheu T, Najdovska M, Wang B, Waring P et al (2005) Hyperactivation of Stat3 in gp130 mutant mice promotes gastric hyperproliferation and desensitizes TGF-beta signaling. Nat Med 11:845–852
56. Judd LM, Alderman BM, Howlett M, Shulkes A, Dow C, Moverley J et al (2004) Gastric cancer development in mice lacking the SHP2 binding site on the IL-6 family co-receptor gp130. Gastroenterology 126:196–207
57. Garcia-Oscos F, Pena D, Housini M, Cheng D, Lopez D, Borland MS et al (2015) Vagal nerve stimulation blocks interleukin 6-dependent synaptic hyperexcitability induced by lipopolysaccharide-induced acute stress in the rodent prefrontal cortex. Brain Behav Immun 43:149–158
58. Oyanedel CN, Kelemen E, Scheller J, Born J, Rose-John S (2015) Peripheral and central blockade of interleukin-6 trans-signaling differentially affects sleep architecture. Brain Behav Immun 50:178–185
59. Stuhlmann-Laeisz C, Lang S, Chalaris A, Krzysztof P, Enge S, Eichler J et al (2006) Forced dimerization of gp130 leads to constitutive STAT3 activation, cytokine-independent growth, and blockade of differentiation of embryonic stem cells. Mol Biol Cell 17:2986–2995
60. Dechow T, Steidle S, Gotze KS, Rudelius M, Behnke K, Pechloff K et al (2014) GP130 activation induces myeloma and collaborates with MYC. J Clin Invest 124:5263–5274

Part II

Experimental Techniques

Chapter 12

Laser Microdissection of Cellular Compartments for Expression Analyses in Cancer Models

Tae-Su Han and Masanobu Oshima

Abstract

Cancer tissues are composed of various cell types including cancer cells, cancer-associated fibroblasts (CAFs), tumor-associated macrophages (TAMs) and endothelial cells. These surrounding stromal cells form the tumor microenvironment, partly through the inflammatory response, which plays an important role in the development and malignant progression of cancer. It is therefore important to examine the expression profiles and protein modifications of each cellular component independently to decipher the interaction between the tumor cells and the microenvironment. We herein describe a protocol for laser microdissection, which allows for the individual cellular compartments to be collected separately. This will allow us to perform real-time RT-PCRs and microarray analyses of specific cell types in tumor tissues.

Key words Laser microdissection, Cancer model, Frozen section, Paraffin-embedded section, RNA extraction, DNA extraction

1 Introduction

It has been established that the tumor microenvironment, which consists of bone marrow-derived inflammatory cells and activated residential cells, supports cancer development [1]. CAFs and TAMs are major components of the tumor microenvironment, and play important roles, not only in the early stage of tumorigenesis, but also in the process of malignant progression, including metastasis and relapse [2, 3]. Recent studies have also indicated that innate immune responses through Toll-like receptors (TLRs) are activated both in the immune cells and in cancer cells, and that TLR signaling in both types of cells is essential for tumorigenesis through the activation of independent pathways [4, 5]. Moreover, there is heterogeneity within the same tumor tissue; for example, EMT cells or cancer stem cells may be present at the invasion front [6, 7]. Accordingly, it is important to examine the expression in different cellular compartments within tumor tissues by sampling

Brendan J. Jenkins (ed.), *Inflammation and Cancer: Methods and Protocols*, Methods in Molecular Biology, vol. 1725, https://doi.org/10.1007/978-1-4939-7568-6_12, © Springer Science+Business Media, LLC 2018

the respective cell types separately, without contamination of other types of cells.

Previously, in situ hybridization (ISH) of specific mRNA was the standard method for determining the types of cells expressing specific genes. However, it was difficult to estimate the expression levels by ISH. In contrast, the collection of specific cells under a microscope by laser microdissection (LMD) allows us to prepare samples for both a real-time RT-PCR and a transcriptome analysis of mRNA and microRNA (miRNA), or next generation DNA sequencing. Recent studies that have applied the LMD technique have revealed useful information about the heterogeneity of tumor tissues [8, 9]. In our laboratory, we have examined the tumor cell-specific expression of inflammation-related genes and miRNAs in gastric tumors [10] and the induction of tumor suppressor-related genes in the invasion front of intestinal tumors using LMD (unpublished). We herein describe the method that is routinely used in our laboratory to collect specific cellular compartments of tumor tissues from mouse gastric and intestinal tumors by LMD for use in real-time RT-PCRs, and miRNA microarray and genomic DNA analyses.

2 Materials

For the preparation of all solutions, use ultrapure water (prepared by purifying deionized water). Store all reagents at room temperature unless indicated otherwise. Diligently follow all waste disposal regulations when disposing of waste materials. It is recommended that commercial extraction kits be used for the extraction of RNA, miRNA, or DNA from small amounts of microdissected tissue.

2.1 Frozen Sections and Staining

1. Phosphate buffered saline (PBS) pH 7.4: Dilute 10× PBS Buffer with ultrapure water.
2. Aluminum foil cups for embedding tissues (Fig. 1) (*see* **Note 1**).
3. O.C.T. compound for embedding tissues.
4. LMD membrane slides covered with PEN-membrane 2.0 μm (Leica), pretreated for RNase free before use (*see* **Note 2**).
5. Fixation solution, 19:1 mixture of ethanol:acetic acid (*see* **Note 3**).
6. 0.05% Toluidine blue solution, pH 7.0, for staining frozen sections.

2.2 Paraffin-Embedded Sections and Staining

1. 4% paraformaldehyde in 0.1 M phosphate-buffer (pH 7.4) (*see* **Note 4**).
2. Paraffin-embedded tissue blocks with fixed tissues.
3. LMD membrane slides covered with PEN-membrane (2.0 μm; Leica), coated with poly-L-lysine (*see* **Note 5**).

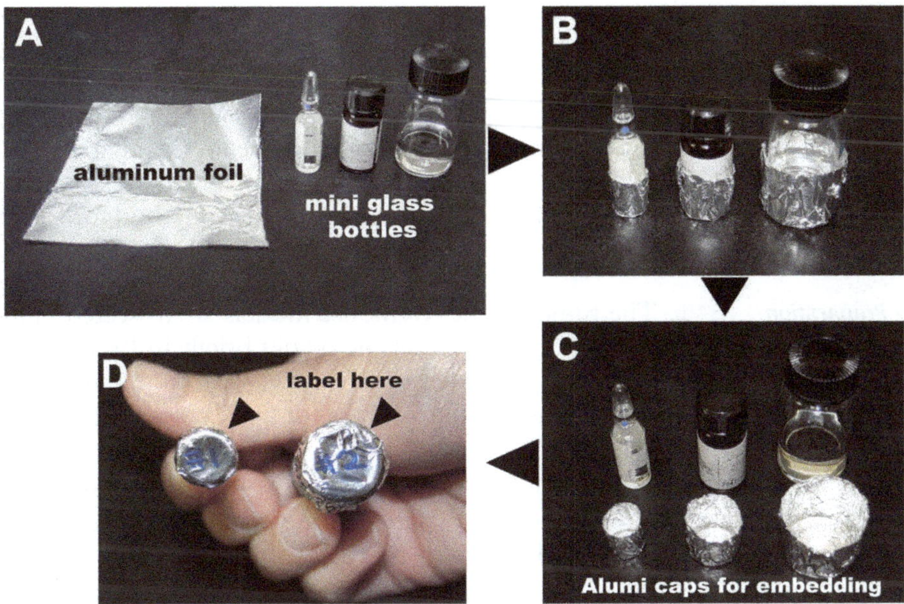

Fig. 1 The preparation of aluminum foil cups for embedding frozen tissue in O.C.T. compound. (**a**) Prepare square-cut aluminum foil and various sizes of mini glass bottles. (**b**, **c**) Make aluminum foil cups using the bottom of the glass bottles, as indicated. (**d**) Label the bottom of the aluminum cups to identify the tissues

4. Xylene deparaffinization solution and rehydration solutions (100% ethanol, 95% ethanol, 70% ethanol, and ultrapure water) (*see* **Note 6**).
5. Mayer's hematoxylin solution for staining paraffin-embedded sections.

2.3 Laser Microdissection

1. Laser microdissection microscope system with UV-laser.
2. Collection tubes: autoclaved 0.2 mL PCR tubes with a flat cap (*see* **Note 7**).

2.4 RNA/DNA Extraction Kits

1. RNeasy Plus Micro Kit (Qiagen) for total RNA extraction.
2. miRNeasy Micro kit (Qiagen) for miRNA extraction.
3. High Pure PCR Template Preparation Kit (Roche) for genomic DNA extraction.
4. Qubit RNA HS Assay Kit (Invitrogen) for the measurement of RNA.

3 Methods

To achieve better results in the expression analysis using LMD samples, frozen sections of fresh tissues should be used (rather than formalin-fixed paraffin-embedded sections). This will preserve the nucleic acids from degradation. We use flash-frozen tissues to extract RNA and miRNA from LMD samples. For genomic DNA analyses (cell-type specific genotyping), formalin-fixed paraffin-embedded sections are routinely used. The microdissection methods differ according to the microscope system that is used. Please follow the manual provided by the manufacturer for the precise microdissection method. We describe the method for LMD for the Leica LMD 7000.

3.1 The Preparation of Frozen Sections for RNA or miRNA Extraction

1. The tumor tissues of mouse models are dissected immediately after euthanasia. Wash the tissues briefly in PBS in a petri dish, immerse the tissue specimen in O.C.T. compound, and place it into an aluminum foil cup with O.C.T. compound (Fig. 2) (*see* **Note 8**).
2. Freeze the O.C.T. compound-embedded tissues in liquid nitrogen (LN_2) and store the sections in a deep freezer at −80 °C (Fig. 2) (*see* **Note 9**).
3. Adjust the temperature of the O.C.T. compound-embedded tissue block to −20 °C. Cut the frozen block into 10 μm-thick

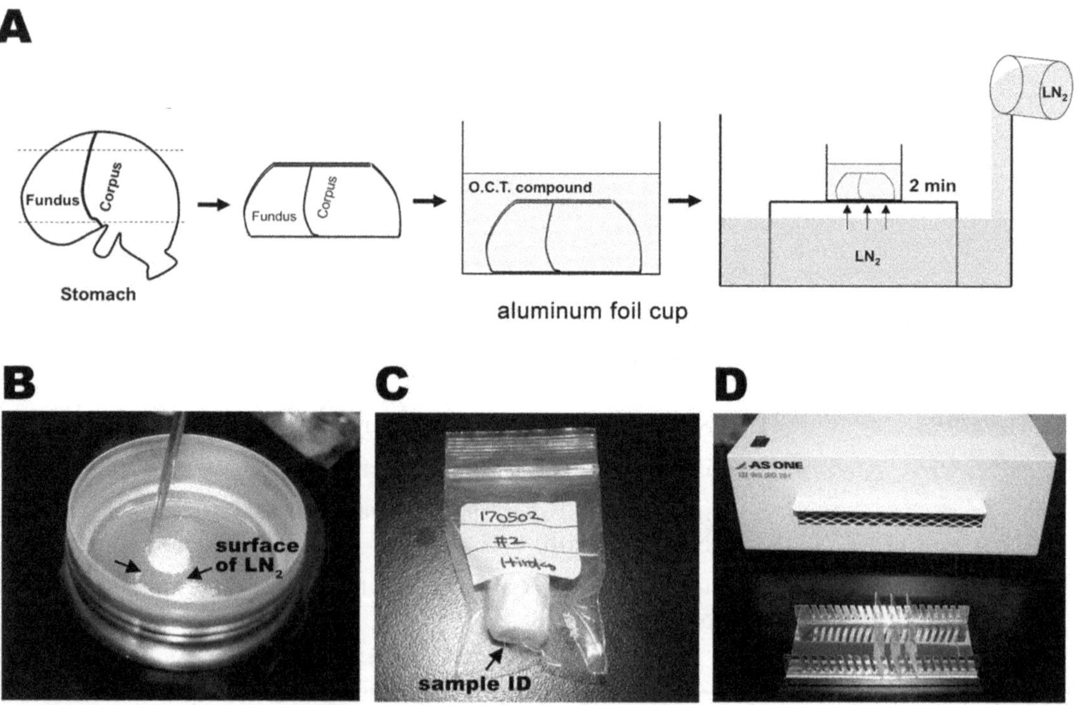

Fig. 2 The preparation of O.C.T. compound-embedded frozen sections. After cutting and wash with PBS, the tissue is placed in O.C.T. compound in an aluminum foil cup and then gradually frozen in LN_2, as described in the Methods (**a**), without directly touching the LN_2 or (**b**) by soaking initially only the bottom of the aluminum cup. (**c**) O.C.T. compound-embedded tissues should be stored in plastic bags at −80 °C. (**d**) Dry the frozen sections using slide glass dryer

slices using a cryostat, and immediately place each section on the RNase-free membrane of an LMD membrane slide (*see* **Note 10**). Let the frozen sections thaw to adhere to the membrane. If the cut sections are not used immediately, they can be stored at −80 °C.

3.2 The Fixation and Staining of Frozen Sections

1. Fix the frozen sections on the membrane slides in an ice-cold 19:1 solution of ethanol:acetic acid for 3 min on ice by soaking in a 50 mL tube. Then, wash the sections in ultrapure water for 1 min on ice.
2. Proceed to stain the fixed sections in 0.05% Toluidine blue (pH 7.0) (*see* **Note 11**), and wash twice in ultrapure water for 1 min on ice.
3. Dry the fixed and stained sections using a slide glass dryer or hair dryer until the tissues are completely dried (Fig. 2). It usually takes less than 5 min. If the dried sections are not used immediately, they can be stored at −80 °C.

3.3 Microdissection from Frozen Sections

We herein describe the method for LMD using a Leica LMD 7000.

1. Add 20 μL of lysis buffer from an RNeasy Micro Kit or miRNeasy Micro Kit mixed with 1% volume of β-mercaptoethanol (β-ME) (mix 10 μL of β-ME in 1 mL of extraction buffer) inside the caps of autoclaved PCR tubes, and place them in an appropriate location for LMD (Fig. 3). The buffer is selected according to the purpose of the experiment.
2. Determine all of the cell compartments of interest, i.e., stromal cells, cancer cells, or adjacent normal cells. Draw a line around

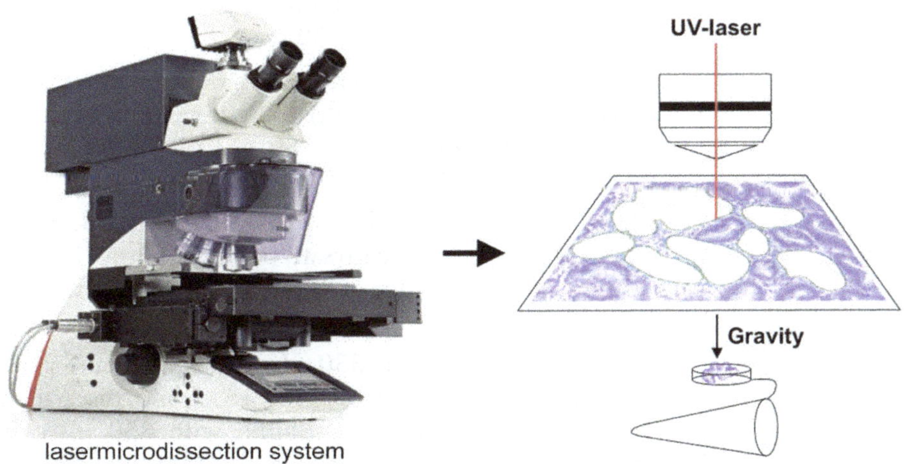

Fig. 3 An image of LMD sample preparation. When the Leica LMD 7000 is used, dissected tissue samples are collected inside the cap of a 0.2 mL PCR tube by gravity. Thus, lysis buffer or extraction buffer should be added to the inside of the cap before LMD

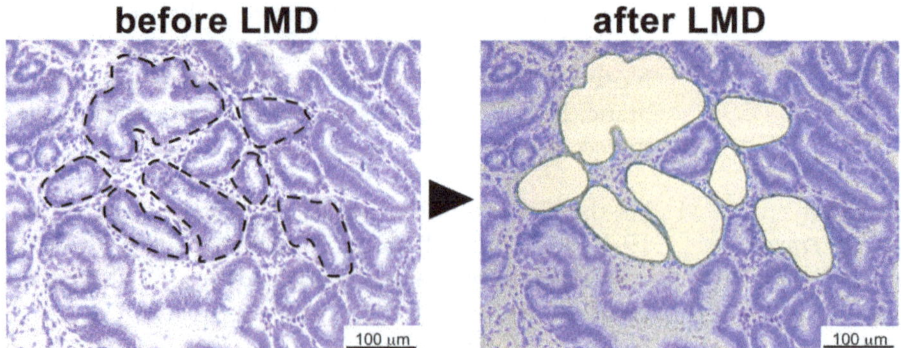

Fig. 4 Photographs of frozen sections before LMD (left) and after LMD (right). These photographs are particularly important to confirm and record the cellular compartments by LMD

the cell clusters of interest on the monitor screen, and cut the cell cluster out using a UV-laser. The dissected cells are then collected by gravity in the extraction buffer in the PCR tube cap (Fig. 3) (*see* **Note 12**). Take photographs of the tissue sections before and after microdissection to confirm the cell-types that were collected (Fig. 4). If a fluorescent LMD system is used, then LMD should be performed after fluorescence immunohistochemistry, which allows for the collection of more specific cell-types, including (but not limited to) Ki-67-positive proliferating cells, and F4/80-expressing TAMs.

3.4 The Extraction of mRNA from Frozen LMD Samples

The extraction of mRNA is performed using an RNeasy Plus Micro Kit. All steps are performed at room temperature. The indicated buffers and columns are included in the kit.

1. Transfer solution including dissected cells from the PCR tube cap to a 1.5 mL tube containing 75 μl of lysis buffer (RLT), and mix well using a vortex for 30 s.
2. Transfer the lysate to a genomic DNA eliminator spin column (gDNA Eliminator column) to remove genomic DNA, and centrifuge at 8000 × *g* for 30 s. Collect the flow-through containing total RNA.
3. Add 75 μL of 70% ethanol to RNA solution, mix well by pipetting. Apply the cell lysate to the column (MinElute spin column), and centrifuge at 8000 × *g* for 15 s. Discard the flow-through.
4. Wash the column with 350 μL of washing buffer (RW1) by centrifugation at 8000 × *g* for 15 s, and discard the flow-through. Then, wash the column with 350 μL of washing buffer (RPE) by centrifugation at 8000 × *g* for 15 s, and discard the flow-through.
5. Wash the column with 500 μL of 80% ethanol by centrifugation at 8000 × *g* for 15 s, and discard the flow-through. After that,

Table 1
The size of frozen section that are required for each of the experiments

Area (μm^2)	Concentration (ng/μL)	RNA amount (ng)	Purpose
200,000	0.05–0.2	0.5–2	miRNA qPCR
1,000,000	1–3	10–30	mRNAs qPCR
40,000,000	40–60	400–600	Microarray and RNA sequencing
70,000,000	180–210	1800–2100	

centrifuge again at 12,000 × *g* for 2 min, and discard the flow-through.

6. Add 10 μL of autoclaved ultrapure water and elute total RNA by centrifugation at 12,000 × *g* for 1 min.
7. Measure the RNA concentration using Qubit RNA HS Assay Kits and a Qubit 3.0 Fluorometer. The amount of RNA that can be expected to be extracted from LMD sections is indicated in Table 1.

3.5 The Extraction of miRNA from Frozen LMD Samples

The purification of miRNA is performed using a miRNeasy Micro Kit. Perform all steps at room temperature. The indicated buffers and columns are included in the kit.

1. Add 200 μL of QIAzol Lysis Reagent in a 0.2 mL PCR tube containing dissected cells and mix well using vortex for 30 s.
2. Transfer the homogenized cell solution in the 1.5 mL tube and add 500 μL of QIAzol Lysis Reagent and mix well by vortexing for 30 s.
3. Add 140 μL chloroform to the tube and shake the tube vigorously for 15 s and centrifuge at 12,000 × *g* for 15 min at 4 °C.
4. Transfer the upper aqueous phase to a new 1.5 mL tube and add 525 μL (1.5 volume) of 100% ethanol and mix vigorously for 15 s.
5. Apply the sample to a column (RNeasy MinElute spin column) in a 2 mL tube and centrifuge at 8000 × *g* for 15 s at room temperature.
6. Add 700 μL of Buffer RWT to the column and centrifuge at 8000 × *g* for 15 s at room temperature.
7. Add 500 μL of Buffer RPE to the column and centrifuge at 8000 × *g* for 15 s at room temperature.
8. Wash the column with 500 μL of 80% ethanol by centrifuge for 2 min at 8000 × *g* and discard the flow-through and centrifuge at 12,000 × *g* for 5 min.

9. Add 10 μL of RNase-free water and elute the total RNA including the miRNA by centrifugation at 12,000 × *g* for 2 min and measure the RNA concentration. The amount of RNA that can be expected to be extracted from LMD sections is indicated in Table 1.

3.6 Paraffin-Embedded Sections for Genomic DNA Extraction

1. Using 4% paraformaldehyde-fixed paraffin-embedded blocks, cut paraffin into 4 μm thick sections using a microtome, and put the section on the poly-L-lysin-coated LMD membrane slide.
2. Dry the sections overnight on a hotplate set to 37 °C.
3. Deparaffinize the paraffin sections by soaking in xylene (5 min × 3 times), and then rehydrate the sections by soaking in 100% ethanol (5 min), 95% ethanol (5 min), 70% ethanol (5 min), and water (5 min).
4. Stain the sections with Mayer's hematoxylin solution for 5 min and wash the sections with water.
5. Dry the stained sections overnight on a hotplate set to 37 °C (*see* **Note 12**).

3.7 Microdissection and Extraction of Genomic DNA

This is a protocol for the isolation of genomic DNA from paraffin-embedded sections for genotyping by a PCR.

1. Add 20 μL of DNA extraction buffer from a High Pure PCR template purification kit to the cap of an autoclaved PCR tube, and place the tube in an appropriate location for laser microdissection (Fig. 3).
2. Determine the cell compartments of interest in the stained section, and draw lines around the cell clusters on the monitor screen, then cut the cell clusters out using a UV-laser. The dissected cells are then collected by gravity in extraction buffer in a PCR tube cap. Take photographs of the tissue sections before and after microdissection to confirm the cell-types that were collected.
3. Incubate the sections overnight with proteinkinase K at 5 mg/mL at 55 °C to remove of proteins, including nuclease contamination; then inactivate proteinase K by incubation at 99 °C for 10 min.
4. Add RNase at 1% vol and incubate at 37 °C for 10 min to remove RNA, and then inactivate RNase by incubation at 70 °C for 5 min.
5. Extract DNA according to the protocol provided by manufacturer. Usually, LMD samples from 3 to 5 sections are sufficient for the extraction of genomic DNA for genomic PCR by amplification of 200–300 bases.

4 Notes

1. O.C.T. compound embedding cups can be made from aluminum foil using various small bottles as templates (Fig. 1). After making the O.C.T. compound embedding cups, label the sample on the bottom of the aluminum cup for the purpose of identification. Without labeling, it is difficult to identify the tissues that are embedded inside the compound.
2. It is recommended that the LMD membrane slide be wiped with an RNase-removing solution to protect the frozen sections from RNase. RNase-free LMD membrane slides are also commercially available.
3. The fixation solution is made by adding 38 mL of ethanol and 2 ml of acetic acid to a 50 mL conical plastic tube and mixing well. Two slide glasses (back-to-back) can be directly placed in this tube for fixation.
4. To make 0.1 M sodium phosphate buffer (pH 7.4), add 3.1 g of $NaH_2PO_4{\cdot}H_2O$ and 10.9 g of Na_2HPO_4 to 1 L of distilled water. The pH should be adjusted to 7.4. Pour 100 mL of 0.1 M sodium phosphate buffer into a flask containing 4 g of paraformaldehayde. Cover with parafilm and put the flask in a 70 °C water bath and mix until completely dissolved. This fixation solution should be freshly made.
5. Place a drop of Poly-L-lysin on the membrane of the LMD membrane slide and coat the surface with Kim wipes.
6. Pour xylene, 100% ethanol, 95% ethanol, 70% ethanol and ultrapure water into independent staining glass jars with lids. Prepare three sets of xylene.
7. These PCR tubes are required for the collection of microdissected tissues when using a Leica LMD 7000 (Fig. 3). Please follow the manual provided by the manufacturer for other LMD systems.
8. When you plan to make frozen tissue sections of stomach and intestine, the inside of the tissues should be washed with PBS using a 10 mL syringe with a needle, and then filled with O.C.T. compound using a 10 mL syringe without a needle. This process is particularly important for tissues from the gastrointestinal tract, as it avoids the development of bubbles in the embedded frozen blocks, which is a common issue in sectioning.
9. O.C.T. compound can be cracked by liquid nitrogen if the O.C.T. compound-containing aluminum foil cup is rapidly frozen in LN_2. To avoid cracking, prevent direct contact between the liquid nitrogen and the O.C.T. compound, O.C. T compound should be gradually frozen from outside for the

first 2 min; then, the whole cup should be placed in LN_2 to ensure that it freezes completely (Fig. 2a). Alternatively, it is acceptable to only soak the bottom of the aluminum cup in LN_2 for the first 30 s, and then freeze the whole cup (Fig. 2b). Store the embedded frozen blocks at −80 °C after labeling the bottom of the aluminum cups with indelible marker pen.

10. It is recommended that normal slide glass be used (not LMD membrane slide) for the first section to check the tissue morphology and to confirm that the required cellular compartments are contained within the section by Toluidine blue staining. After confirmation, cut the section, place it on a slide, and thaw it to adhere. We usually place three to five serial frozen sections on the same LMD membrane slide, depending on the sample size. In the case of a real-time RT-PCR, two slides (namely, up to 6–10 sections) are sufficient to analyze the expression levels of several independent genes. In contrast, more than five slides are required to extract a sufficient amount of RNA for a microarray.
11. It is crucial to check the Toluidine blue staining time because it can be difficult to observe the cell morphology in weakly or strongly stained sections. In the case of mouse stomach specimens, the slide should be loaded in Toluidine blue for 10 min to distinguish normal epithelial cells, tumor epithelial cells and stromal cells.
12. Paraffin sections should be dried completely before LMD because contamination with residual water will affect the amount of recoverable DNA.

References

1. Shalapour S, Karin M (2015) Immunity, inflammation, and cancer: an eternal fight between good and evil. J Clin Invest 125:3347–3355
2. Orimo A, Weinberg RA (2006) Stromal fibroblasts in cancer: a novel tumor-promoting cell type. Cell Cycle 5:1597–1601
3. Lewis CE, Harney AS, Pollard JW (2016) The multifaced role of perivascular macrophages in tumors. Cancer Cell 30:18–25
4. Tye H, Kennedy CL, Najdovska M, McLeod L, McCormack W, Hughes N, Dev A, Sievert W, Ooi CH, Ishikawa TO, Oshima H, Bhathai PS, Parker AE, Oshima M, Tan P, Jenkins BJ (2012) STAT3-driven upregulation of TLR2 promotes gastric tumorigenesis independent of tumor inflammation. Cancer Cell 22:466–478
5. Maeda Y, Echizen K, Oshima H, Yu L, Sakulsak N, Hirose O, Yamada Y, Taniguchi T, Jenkins BJ, Saya H, Oshima M (2016) Myeloid differentiation factor 88 signaling in bone marrow-derived cells promotes gastric tumorigenesis by generation of inflammatory microenvironment. Cancer Prev Res 9:253–263
6. Shibue T, Weinberg RA (2017) EMT, CSC, and drug resistance: the mechanistic link and clinical implications. Nat Rev Clin Oncol 14 (10):611–629. https://doi.org/10.1038/nrclinonc.2017.44. (published online)
7. De Sousa e Melo F, Kurtova AV, Harnoss JM, Kljavin N, Hoeck JD, Hung J, Anderson JE, Storm EE, Modrusan Z, Koeppen H, Dijkgraaf GJP, Piskol R, de Sauvage FJ (2017) A distinct role for Lgr5+ stem cells in primary and metastatic colon cancer. Nature 543:676–680
8. Refinetti P, Arstad C, Thilly WG, Morgenthaler S, Ekstrom PO (2017) Mapping mitochondrial heteroplasmy in a Leydig tumor

by laser capture microdissection and cycling temperature capillary electrophoresis. BMC Clin Pathol 17:6

9. Großerueschkamp F, Bracht T, Diehl HC, Kuepper C, Ahrens M, Kallenbac-Thieltges A, Mosig A, Eisenacher M, Marcus K, Behrens T, Brüning T, Theegarten D, Sitek B, Gerwert K (2017) Spatial and molecular resolution of diffuse malignant mesothelioma heterogeneity by integrating label-free FTIR imaging, laser capture microdissection and proteomics. Sci Rep 7:44829

10. Oshima H, Ishikawa T, Yoshida GJ, Naoi K, Maeda Y, Naka K, Ju X, Yamada Y, Minamoto T, Mukaida N, Saya H, Oshima M (2014) TNF-α/TNFR1 signaling promotes gastric tumorigenesis through induction of Noxo1 and Gna14 in tumor cells. Oncogene 33:3820–3829

Chapter 13

Tissue Processing for Stereological Analyses of Lung Structure in Chronic Obstructive Pulmonary Disease

Mohamed Saad and Saleela M. Ruwanpura

Abstract

Quantitative data on lung structure, such as volume, surface area and length, are used for assessment of the functional performance of the lung during normal development and inflammatory-related diseases such as chronic obstructive pulmonary disorder (COPD), and carcinogenesis, in animal models. Stereology is considered as the gold standard to obtain quantitative data on lung structure, with a key advantage being to quantify irregular three-dimensional structures on the basis of measurement made on two-dimensional sections. Therefore, preservation of original tissue dimensions without shrinkage is vital for stereology.

Three steps, fixation, sampling and embedding, are essential requirements to minimise tissue shrinkage to obtain theoretically unbiased estimates of stereological parameters of lung structures. Perfusion fixation by intratracheal instillation with 1.5% glutaraldehyde/1.5% formaldehyde at a pressure of 25 cm fluid column is considered as one of the best methods. A systematic uniform random sampling scheme is then applied to the fixed lung to ensure each and every part of the lung is analysed, irrespective of homogeneity or heterogeneity of the structural distribution. The sampled tissue sections are then embedded in glycol methacrylate to minimise further tissue shrinkage. Here we describe the accurate fixation, sampling and embedding for stereological methods to quantify lung structures in mice.

Key words Fixation, Intratracheal instillation, Glutaraldehyde, Sampling, Glycol methacrylate, Tissue shrinkage

1 Introduction

The quantitative lung structural data attempt to understand the important structural designs in the lung such as volume of airspaces, surface of parenchyma, which determine the physiological function of the lung. The quantitative structural changes in the lung are highly applied for phenotypic characterization in animal models of lung inflammatory-related diseases and carcinogenesis, as the analyses of systemic gene and/or protein expression levels are not sufficient to characterize the pathology and disturbances of functional performance [1, 2]. For example, structural changes such as increase volume of airspaces and loss of parenchymal surface tissues result in airspace enlargement, leading to poor gas exchange

Brendan J. Jenkins (ed.), *Inflammation and Cancer: Methods and Protocols*, Methods in Molecular Biology, vol. 1725, https://doi.org/10.1007/978-1-4939-7568-6_13, © Springer Science+Business Media, LLC 2018

during breathing which is a hallmark of emphysema, the major debilitating component of COPD [3]. State-of-the-art stereology is a well-established method for obtaining quantitative data on lung structure, which provides unbiased mathematical estimates of lung parameters based on two-dimensional lung sections extracted from three-dimensional lung [4]. In that regard, the whole lung should be adequately inflated, sampled to represent every part of the lung and processed correctly to avoid any shrinkage that may alter structural dimensions and thus interpretation of lung pathophysiology.

The first step of tissue processing for lung stereology is the fixation of lung with sufficient degree of inflation. A fixed lung at a well-defined state of inflation prevents contraction of the lung during the sectioning that may have effects on analyses of the volume of air space and surface area of parenchyma [4, 5]. Perfusion fixation by intratracheal instillation of fixative at a constant pressure of 20–25 cm fluid column results in quick and uniform preservation of lung and is considered to be the best method of fixation [6]. The choice of fixative should be able to well-stabilize lung tissues to prevent lung from collapsing during the processing. Since popular fixatives such as formaldehyde alone is inadequate, glutaraldehyde-based fixative is used [7–9].

The fixed lung is then sampled to obtain representative sections of the whole organ. This step is important in many disease models, especially in emphysema where characteristic lesions are heterogeneously distributed [10]. A systematic, uniform random sampling (SURS) scheme is applied to the fixed lung to ensure that each and every part of the lung is sufficiently analysed. The final step prior to stereological assessment is embedding and this should be well controlled, standardised and monitored for shrinkage affects. Routinely used embedding reagent paraffin usually leads to considerable shrinkage of about 40% of lung [7], therefore other embedding reagents such as glycol methacrylate or epoxy resins are used for tissue processing stereology to avoid catastrophic shrinkage. Here, we provide detailed instructions for fixation with glutaraldehyde-based fixative via instillation, SURS scheme and embedding in glycol methacrylate of mouse lung for stereological assessments which can be employed in inflammatory-related and carcinogenic disease states of the lung.

2 Materials

Personal protection wear (lab coats), laboratory safety gloves, eye protection wear and laboratory masks should be worn during the preparation of all the materials and procedures. Prepare and store all reagents at room temperature in a fume hood (unless indicated otherwise). Diligently follow all waste disposal regulations when disposing waste materials.

2.1 Fixation

1. Euthanasia: Pentobarbital sodium anaesthetic at a dose of 100 mg per kilogram of mouse weight (*see* **Note 1**).
2. 22 gauge cannula.
3. Surgical sutures.
4. Fixative: 1.5% glutaraldehyde/1.5% paraformaldehyde mixture in 0.04 M phosphate buffer solution (PBS) [9]. First prepare 0.04 M PBS by adding 400 mL of 0.1 M of stock PBS to 600 mL ultrapure water (prepared by purifying deionized water, to attain a sensitivity of 18 MΩ-cm at 25 °C) (*see* **Note 2**). Then weigh 15 g of paraformaldehyde into a conical flask or a beaker, add 0.04 M PBS to a volume of 1 L and seal with parafilm. On a heated stirrer, mix until the milky solution turns colourless. Allow to cool before handling and store at 4 °C for long term usage. As the final step of the fixative preparation (prepare fresh prior to use), add 30 mL of glutaraldehyde in 50% solution to a beaker or a glass bottle and then make up volume to 1 L with 1.5% paraformaldehyde mixture in 0.04 M PBS.
5. A fixative reservoir with a starting fixative level about 25 cm above the table (*see* **Note 3**).

2.2 Sampling

1. Sharp tissue cutting knives.
2. 4% agar: Add 4 g of agar into 100 mL of deionized water in a beaker and boil in a microwave until it dissolves.

2.3 Embedding

1. 70, 90 and 100% acetone: dilute acetone in deionized water.
2. Technovit® Glycol Methacrylate (GMA) embedding kits (7100 or 8100) developed by Kulzer in Germany. These kits consist of glycol methacrylate monomer, hardener I and hardener II (*see* **Note 4**).
3. Plastic embedding moulds to hold 1 mL of solution.
4. Technovit® 3040 is a two-component resin based on methyl methacrylate which is used for making backing blocks for glycol methacrylate embedded tissues blocks.

3 Methods

Carry out all procedures at room temperature unless otherwise specified.

3.1 Perfusion Fixation with Glutaraldehyde-based Fixative via Instillation

1. Euthanize the mouse by intraperitoneal injection of pentobarbital sodium anaesthetic and place the mouse on a sloped platform.

2. Shave the ventral part of the neck area (also disinfect the neck area with 70% alcohol), make a small surgical incision in the neck and with forceps gently pull the skin and muscles in the neck until exposure of the trachea.
3. Make an incision in the trachea proximal to the larynx, and then insert the 22 gauge cannula via the incision (about 5 mm). Loosely tie up the trachea around the cannula using sutures (or use an artery clip) to prevent movement of the cannula during the fixation procedure.
4. Carefully open the thorax and peritoneal cavity with a midline incision and induce a bilateral pneumothorax by carefully making insertions on both side of the diaphragm. Remove the diaphragm and lateral chest plate carefully to expose the lung (*see* **Note 5**).
5. Connect the cannula to the three way stop cock tap of the fixative reservoir containing 1.5% glutaraldehyde/1.5% paraformaldehyde mixture in 0.04 M PBS. Set the top surface of fixative 25 cm above the level of the mouse (make sure no air bubbles in the fixation tubing by running fixative).
6. Open the stopcock to inflate the lungs with 1.5% glutaraldehyde/1.5% paraformaldehyde mixture in 0.04 M PBS. Leave the lungs under pressure until the flow has finished (*see* **Note 6**).
7. Tie off the trachea while removing cannula simultaneously. Then dissect out the intact lungs, heart and thymus, by gently tugging on the trachea while cutting away connective tissue (Fig. 1).

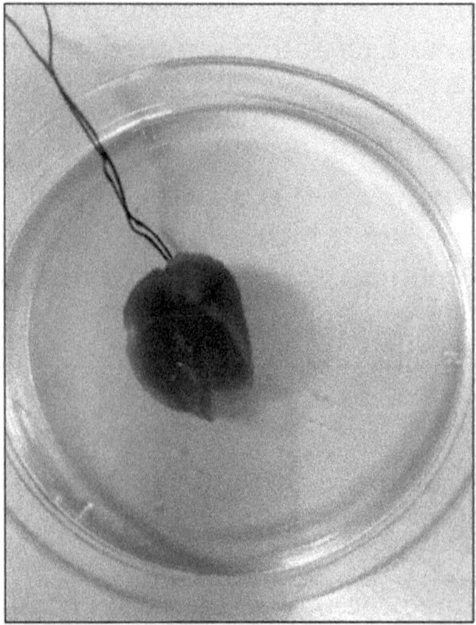
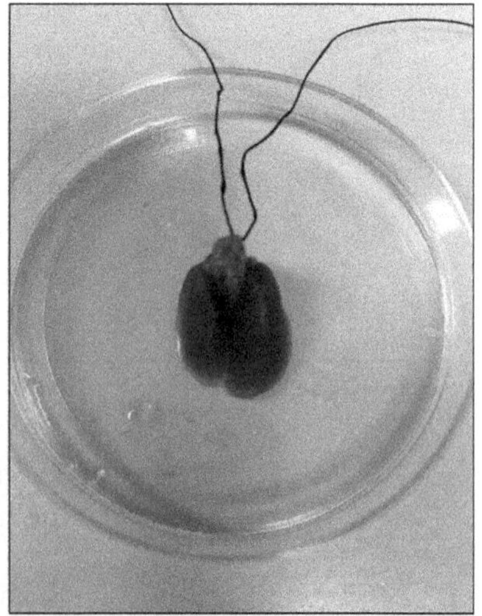

Fig. 1 The dissected lung after perfusion fixation via tracheal instillation. Trachea is tied off with sutures to prevent escape of any fixative. Heart, thymus and trachea are intact with lungs

8. Place the intact lungs in a container filled with the fixative 1.5% glutaraldehyde/1.5% paraformaldehyde mixture in 0.04 M PBS for least 16 h (or overnight) at 4 °C. Measure the fixed lung volume (using water displacement method) before further histological processing (not described in this chapter).

3.2 Sampling of the Fixed Lung Using SURS

1. Remove as much non lung tissue as possible from the fixed lung (trachea, heart, thymus, connective tissues).
2. Embed the lung in 4% agar, ensuring that the tissue is completely immersed in agar. When the agar has hardened, measure the length of the lung and cut the lung into slabs of roughly the same thickness (the average thickness is the lung length divided by the number of slabs) (Fig. 2) (*see* **Note 7**).
3. Separate and arrange the agar slabs between right and left lung always facing the same cut face pointing upwards. Remove the

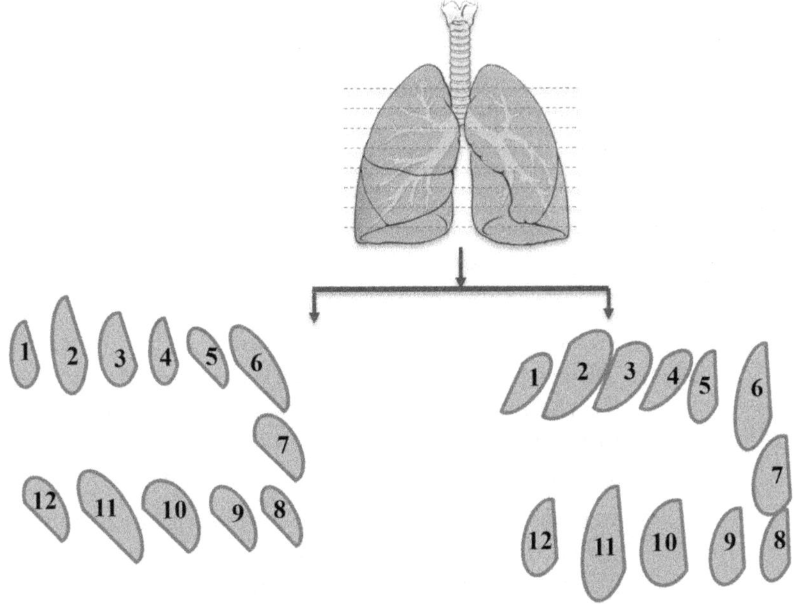

Arrange slabs first sectioned to last sectioned

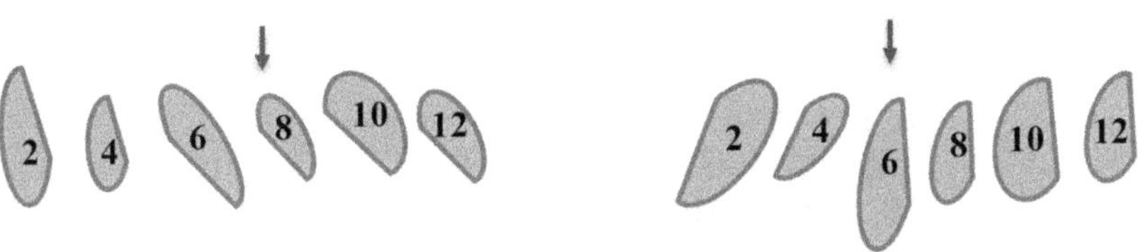

Every second piece of slab from a random start is assigned for embedding

Fig. 2 The agar-embedded lung is cut into slabs roughly the same thickness. The agar slabs are separated and arranged between right and left lung facing same cut face pointing upwards. Every second slab from a random starting position is assigned for glycol methacrylate embedding

surrounding agar and enumerate all slabs from the first to last one sectioned. Assign every X^{th} slab for embedding with a random start in the interval from 1-X (Fig. 2) (*see* **Note 8**).

3.3 Dehydration of the Sampled Fixed Lung Slabs

The sampled fixed lung slabs to be embedded are placed into 5 mL plastic containers with screw cap lids and placed on a roller to gently agitate tissue during the processing.

1. Place fixed lung slabs in 70% acetone, followed by 90% acetone for 1 h each.
2. Place fixed lungs slabs in 100% acetone for three times for 1 h each, followed by one time for 3 h.
3. After the final dehydration step, remove acetone and follow the embedding (*see* **Note 9**).

3.4 Embedding of the Sampled Fixed Lung Slabs in Glycol Methacrylate

1. Prepare infiltration solution from the Technovit® 7100 GMA kit by dissolving 1 g of Hardener I in 100 mL of Glycol Methacrylate monomer. This solution is agitated by hand until the hardener is dissolved.
2. Incubate the dehydrated sampled lung slabs in a 1 mL of infiltration solution on the roller for at least 48 h (*see* **Note 10**).
3. Place the sampled lung slabs into moulds for embedding. The lung slabs are oriented so that the largest area faces towards the bottom of the mould, hence forming the cutting face.
4. Prepare embedding solution by adding 1 mL of Hardener II to 15 mL of the infiltration solution.
5. Working quickly, fill the moulds with embedding solution using a pipette. It is necessary to watch the lung tissue blocks for the next 15–20 min and ensure that the lung slabs remain properly positioned, as often they float to the top. The blocks are left to polymerise at least overnight.
6. In order to allow proper placement of blocks in the microtome for sectioning, backing blocks are adhered to the GMA blocks prior to their removal from the moulds.
7. Prepare backing blocks separately in the same moulds as are used for GMA blocks. Using Technovit® 3040 at a ratio of 2:1 powder to liquid, quickly prepare the mixture and pour into the moulds. While the blocks are setting, use a stick to scrape away excess resin from around each block, otherwise it will be difficult to remove when fully set. Let the moulds stand for 10 min and then pop out the blocks (*see* **Note 11**).
8. Weigh out 5 g of powder and add to 2.5 mL of liquid (Technovit® 3040, at a time), pour this mixture over the back of all the set lung blocks, and then put on the backing block. Allow to harden for about 10 min before removing the whole block. Store blocks at room temperature in a container containing silica gel desiccant beads (Fig. 3).

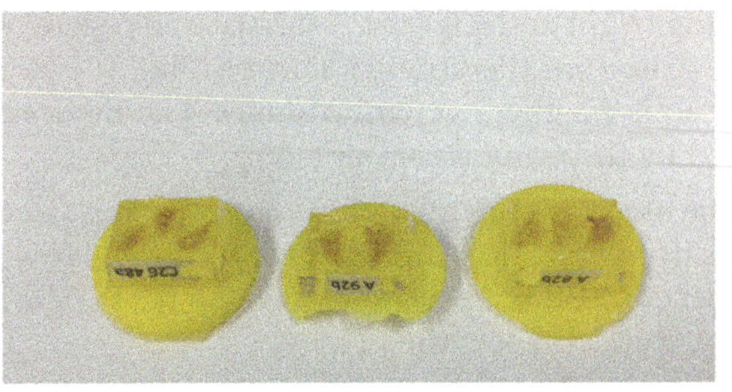

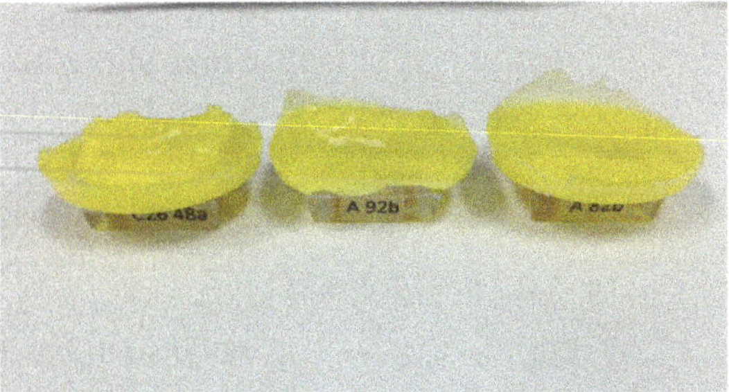

Fig. 3 The illustrations of glycol methacrylate embedded sampled fixed lung tissues with back blocks

4 Notes

1. Use 27 gauge on 1 mL syringes on pharmaceutical grade Pentobarbital sodium anaesthetic.
2. There are many different ways to prepare 0.1 M stock PBS with or without potassium. One of the most common preparations is addition of 80 g NaCl, 2 g KCl, 14.2 g disodium phosphate and 2.4 g monopotassium phosphate to 1 L of ultrapure water. However when diluted to 0.04 M PBS, mix well and adjust pH to 7.4.
3. To build a fixative reservoir, attached a funnel to the free end of a 25 cm tubing with a three way stop cock tap. Then use a stand to keep the tubing above the table.
4. Technovit® 7100 GMA is less sensitive to oxygen during polymerization, thus no sealing of the molds is required.
5. It is important not to accidently hit the lungs while making an insertion to the diaphragm or removal of chest plate. Use saline (or 0.9% NaCl solution) to flush the pleural cavity to eliminate and prevent any pleural adhesion.
6. To keep the lungs under 25 cm pressure during the fixation, top up the fixative reservoir to 25 cm continuously, until the flow has finished. It will take about 30 s to 1 min for flow to finish. From our experience delays can lead to sticking of the fixed lungs to surrounding tissues due to glutaraldehyde, therefore removing the lung immediately after the fixation is critical.
7. Use a millimetre ruler or a tissue slicer for cutting as those enable homogenous and smooth slabs of agar embedded lung. Each slab is then used for the estimation of the total lung volume based on the Cavalieri method (not discussed in this chapter).
8. To determine *X*, divide the number of slabs by the desired amount of samples. We usually randomly select about 4–6

slabs from each lung (right and left) and 8–12 slabs all together from whole lung (based on the arrangement on Fig. 2, every second piece of slab is assigned for embedding). The random start is determined by throwing a coin or a dice.

9. Ethanol can also be used as the dehydration solvent, as it is safer than acetone (less flammable, less injurious to the user). However, ethanol appears to cause tissue shrinkage of up to 10%, while such has not seen with acetone [11].
10. Some protocols suggest overnight incubation of dehydrated fixed tissues with a mixture of infiltration and acetone in equal amounts, followed by 48 h of incubation with just the infiltration solution [7]. However, we do 8 h of dehydration through a series of acetone, therefore fixed lung tissues are immediately transferred to the infiltration solution following the final dehydration step.
11. Backing blocks must be made before embedding, usually the day before during the dehydration procedure. Weigh 10 g of powder and add 5 mL of liquid from Technovit® 3040 kit at once for preparation of backing blocks. This resin sets to stiff consistency in about 1 min, therefore the procedure must be very rapid.

References

1. Weibel ER, Hsia CC, Ochs M (2007) How much is there really? Why stereology is essential in lung morphometry. J Appl Physiol 102:459–467
2. Muhlfeld C, Hegermann J, Wrede C, Ochs M (2015) A review of recent developments and applications of morphometry/stereology in lung research. Am J Physiol Lung Cell Mol Physiol 309:L526–L536
3. Ochs M (2014) Estimating structural alterations in animal models of lung emphysema. Is there a gold standard? Ann Anat 196:26–33
4. Ochs M (2016) A brief update on lung stereology. J Microsc 222:188–200
5. Soutiere SE, Mitzner W (2004) On defining total lung capacity in the mouse. J Appl Physiol 96:1658–1664
6. Bur S, Bachofen H, Gehr P, Weibel ER (1985) Lung fixation by airway instillation: effects on capillary hematocrit. Exp Lung Res 9:57–66
7. Schneider JP, Ochs M (2014) Alterations of mouse lung tissue dimensions during processing for morphometry: a comparison of methods. Am J Physiol Lung Cell Mol Physiol 306:L341–L350
8. Ruwanpura SM, McLeod L, Dousha LF, Seow HJ, Alhayyani S, Tate MD, Deswaerte V, Brooks GD, Bozinovski S, MacDonald M, Garbers C, King PT, Bardin PG, Vlahos R, Rose-John S, Anderson GP, Jenkins BJ (2016) Therapeutic targeting of the IL-6 trans-signaling/mechanistic target of rapamycin complex 1 axis in pulmonary emphysema. Am J Respir Crit Care Med 194:1494–1505
9. Ruwanpura SM, McLeod L, Miller A, Jones J, Bozinovski S, Vlahos R, Ernst M, Armes J, Bardin PG, Anderson GP, Jenkins BJ (2011) Interleukin-6 promotes pulmonary emphysema associated with apoptosis in mice. Am J Respir Cell Mol Biol 45:720–730
10. Ito S, Ingenito EP, Arold SP, Parameswaran H, Tgavalekos NT, Lutchen KR, Suki B (2004) Tissue heterogeneity in the mouse lung: effects of elastase treatment. J Appl Physiol 97:204–212
11. Page SG, Huxley HE (1963) Filament lengths in striated muscle. J Cell Biol 19:369–390

Chapter 14

Quantifying Caspase-1 Activity in Murine Macrophages

Dave Boucher, Amy Chan, Connie Ross, and Kate Schroder

Abstract

The caspase-1 protease is a core component of multiprotein inflammasome complexes, which play a critical role in regulating the secretion of mature, bioactive pro-inflammatory cytokines interleukin (IL)-1β and IL-18. The activity of caspase-1 is often measured indirectly, by monitoring cleavage of cellular caspase-1 substrates, processing of caspase-1 itself, or by quantifying cell death. Here we describe methods for eliciting caspase-1 activity in murine macrophages, via activation of the NLRP3, NAIP/NLRC4 or AIM2 inflammasomes. We then describe a simple fluorogenic assay for directly quantifying cellular caspase-1 activity.

Key words Inflammasome, Inflammatory caspases, Biochemistry, Protease

1 Introduction

Inflammasomes are key regulators of innate immune system function [1]. Inflammasomes are large signalling platforms that assemble upon recognition of various stress or danger-associated signals by inflammasome sensor proteins [e.g., Nod-like receptors (NLRs), absent in melanoma-2 (AIM2) or pyrin] [2, 3]. Canonical inflammasomes enable the activation of the zymogen protease, caspase-1, by facilitating caspase-1 clustering and proximity-induced autoactivation upon the signalling complex. In turn, caspase-1 cleaves gasdermin D, which elicits a form of rapid osmotic cell lysis, termed pyroptosis [4–6]. Caspase-1 also activates interleukin (IL)-1β and IL-18, which are then secreted to regulate inflammatory responses. Caspase-1 also cleaves other substrates [7] but the molecular and cellular function that are modulated by such cleavage events are poorly characterised.

Several canonical inflammasomes have been characterised. The NLRP3 inflammasome [8] assembles in response to cell stress signals (e.g., potassium efflux, reactive oxygen species), which can also be induced by pathogen-derived proteins (e.g., bacterial toxins such as nigericin). Experimentally, NLRP3 function can be blocked

Brendan J. Jenkins (ed.), *Inflammation and Cancer: Methods and Protocols*, Methods in Molecular Biology, vol. 1725, https://doi.org/10.1007/978-1-4939-7568-6_14, © Springer Science+Business Media, LLC 2018

by culturing cells in potassium-rich media, or by treating cells with the NLRP3-specific inhibitor, MCC950 [9]. The NAIP/NLRC4 inflammasome is triggered by cytosolic bacterial components, such as flagellin from *Salmonella* [10, 11]. Flagellin is directly recognized by the NLR protein NAIP, which recruits NLRC4 to assemble the NAIP/NLRC4 inflammasome [12, 13]. The NLRP1 inflammasome is activated by *Bacillus anthraxis* lethal toxin and by *Taxoplasma gondii* [14, 15]. The AIM2 inflammasome assembles upon AIM2 sensing of cytosolic double-stranded DNA [16–18]. The pyrin inflammasome is activated upon bacterial modifications of host RhoA GTPase [3]. Inflammasome formation requires a priming signal (signal 1) to upregulate components of the inflammasome pathway and to induce the expression of pro-interleukin (IL)-1β [19, 20]. The priming signal can derive from Toll-like receptor (TLR) ligation, e.g., TLR4 binding to bacterial lipopolysaccharide (LPS) [21]. Following priming, a triggering stimulus (signal 2) is required for inflammasome formation.

The activation of inflammatory caspases is generally assessed indirectly by monitoring cellular outcomes of their activity. These indicators include caspase self-cleavage, cell death, and pro-inflammatory cytokine release. Techniques for quantifying such outcomes are described by others [22, 23]. Here, we discuss a protocol for direct monitoring of caspase-1 activity in murine primary macrophages. This method involves a direct fluorogenic assay for substrate cleavage, and takes advantage of the well characterised, preferred cleavage sequence of caspase-1 [24].

2 Materials

2.1 Generation of Murine Bone Marrow-Derived Macrophages (BMDM)

1. Mice (*see* **Note 1**).
2. Ice.
3. Sterile complete macrophage media (CMM), warmed to 37 °C: RPMI-1640 supplemented with 1% Glutamax, 10% Fetal Calf Serum (FCS) (*see* **Note 2**).
4. 150 ng/mL final concentration of recombinant colony stimulating factor-1 (CSF-1) (*see* **Note 3**).
5. Surgical scissors and forceps (sterilized in 70% ethanol).
6. 70% ethanol solution.
7. Sterile 50 mL Falcon tubes.
8. Sterile 100 μm cell strainers.
9. Sterile 10 mL syringe bodies.
10. Sterile 18, 21 and 27 gauge needles.
11. Sterile 10 cm square bacteriological dish (e.g., Sterillin, i.e., not tissue culture coated plastic).

12. Sterile 6-well plate/cell culture dish (tissue culture grade).
13. Low-lint tissue (Kimwipes™).
14. Sterile red blood cell ACK lysis buffer: 150 mM NH_4Cl, 1 mM $KHCO_3$, 50 μM EDTA, in sterile distilled water, filter-sterilized.
15. Sterile Dulbecco's Phosphate-Buffered Saline (DPBS).
16. Trypan blue solution.
17. Hemocytometer.
18. Sterile 1.5 mL Eppendorf tubes.
19. Tissue culture-grade dimethyl sulfoxide (DMSO).
20. Cell freezing media (90% FCS, 10% DMSO).

2.2 Inflammasome Priming and Triggering

1. Sterile 96-well plate, black (fluorescence grade).
2. Eppendorf tubes.
3. Sterile distilled water.
4. 1 mg/mL stock solution of Ultrapure LPS from K12 *E. coli*, prepared in sterile distilled water.
5. 5 mM stock solution (in ethanol) of Nigericin sodium salt.
6. 1 mg/mL stock solution of DNA from Calf Thymus (CT DNA) in sterile distilled water).
7. 100 μg/mL stock solution of recombinant flagellin, ultrapure grade in sterile distilled water.
8. Lipofectamine 2000.
9. Lipofectamine LTX.
10. Opti-MEM media.
11. 10 mM stock solution (in water) of MCC950 (*see* **Note 4**).
12. 50 mM stock solution (in DMSO) of VX-765 (*see* **Note 4**).

2.3 Cellular Caspase Activity Assay

1. Sterile 96-well plate, black (fluorescence grade).
2. Fluorescence plate reader (*see* **Note 5**).
3. 1 M solution Dithiothreitol (DTT) in ultrapure water, filter sterilized.
4. 100 mM stock solution (in DMSO) of acYVAD-afc (*see* **Note 6**).
5. 2× Caspase activity buffer: 100 mM HEPES pH 8.0, 400 mM NaCl, 100 mM KCl) (*see* **Note 7**).
6. Digitonin.

3 Methods

3.1 Generation of BMDM

1. Euthanize a mouse using a CO_2 euthanasia chamber or by cervical dislocation (*see* **Note 8**). Check that the blink reflex is absent by touching the eyes to confirm euthanasia.
2. Place the mouse on its back on a polystyrene foam board, and immobilize the extended limbs by pinning with 21 gauge needles.
3. Spray the abdomen with 70% ethanol. Make a small incision on the abdominal skin with scissors. From this incision, cut the skin towards the knee and ankle of each leg to expose the muscle surrounding the tibia and femur. Cut each leg at the hip joint and at the ankle. Remove the intact tibiae and the femurs and soak them in 2 mL of 70% ethanol for 15–30 seconds (s). Immediately proceed to the next step to avoid prolonged incubation of bones in ethanol.

   All the following steps should be performed in a biohazard tissue culture hood.

4. For each mouse to be sacrificed, add 3 mL of 70% ethanol to one well and 3 mL CMM to the adjacent well of a 6-well plate.
5. Remove the remaining muscle from the bones by rubbing the muscle away with a low-lint tissue. When each bone is cleaned, dip the bone in the well containing 70% ethanol for 5 s and then place in the well containing CMM.
6. Cut each bone proximal to each joint with sterilized scissors.
7. With a 10 mL syringe containing CMM attached to a 27 gauge needle, flush the bone marrow cavity from each end into a 50 mL falcon tube via a cell strainer to prevent bone fragments from collecting in the tube. Continue flushing the bone marrow until the cavity appears white.
8. Rinse the cell strainer with 5 mL of CMM to maximise cell recovery.
9. Centrifuge the cells at 500 × g for 5 min.
10. Aspirate the media, and gently resuspend the cell pellet in ACK buffer (2 mL per mouse) to lyse red blood cells. Incubate the cells for 5 min at room temperature. Quench with 10 mL of CMM.
11. Centrifuge at 500 × g for 5 min (*see* **Note 9**).
12. Aspirate the media, and resuspend the cell pellet in CMM. Distribute the cells in 10 cm square plastic plates in a final volume of 12 mL of CMM per plate (6–8 dishes per mouse). Supplement media with 150 ng/mL CSF-1.

13. Place cells in a 37 °C incubator venting 5% CO_2 to allow the cells to differentiate over 5 days.
14. On day 5, add 5 mL of fresh CMM supplemented with 150 ng/mL CSF-1 to each plate.
15. On day 6, aspirate the media and add 10 mL of cold DPBS to each plate. Incubate the cells for 5 min at room temperature.
16. Using an 18 gauge needle and a 10 mL syringe, harvest the cells by gently spraying attached cells with cold DBPS. Transfer cells to 50 mL Falcon tube. Rinse the plates with DPBS and transfer the remaining cells to the 50 mL Falcon tube.
17. Centrifuge the cells at 500 × *g* for 5 min.
18. Remove the supernatant and resuspend the cell pellet in warm CMM.
19. Take a small sample of the cells and stain with 0.2% (final concentration) trypan blue. Count live (trypan blue-excluded) cells using a hemocytometer.
20. Adjust the volume of the cell stock with warm CMM (supplemented with 150 ng/mL CSF-1) to yield a 1 × 10^6 cells/mL cell suspension (*see* **Note 10**).

3.2 Activation of the NLRP3 Inflammasome

1. Add 1 × 10^6 cells/mL of differentiated BMDM (day 6) to a black 96-well plate (100 μL/well). Include triplicate wells for each of the following samples:

   Unprimed control.

   LPS only (primed control).

   Nigericin only (unprimed control).

   LPS + nigericin (priming + treatment).

   LPS + VX-765 + nigericin (Caspase inhibitor negative control).

   LPS + MCC950 + nigericin (NLRP3 inhibitor negative control).

   See Fig. 1 for a schematic of how cells can be plated.
2. Place the cells in a 37 °C incubator venting 5% CO_2 overnight.
3. On the following morning, add 100 ng/mL of ultrapure K12 LPS (from 100 μg/mL working stock; *see* **Note 11**), to all samples to receive LPS (not unprimed controls). Return the cells to the 37 °C cell incubator for 3 h.
4. Add 5 μL of 500 μM VX-765 (prepared in CMM from a 50 mM stock solution) or 5 μL of 200 μM MCC950 (prepared in CMM) to the negative control inhibitor samples. Return the cells to the 37 °C cell incubator for an additional 1 h.
5. Prepare a fresh 50 μM nigericin working solution by diluting 1 μL of the 5 mM stock solution in 99 μL of CMM.

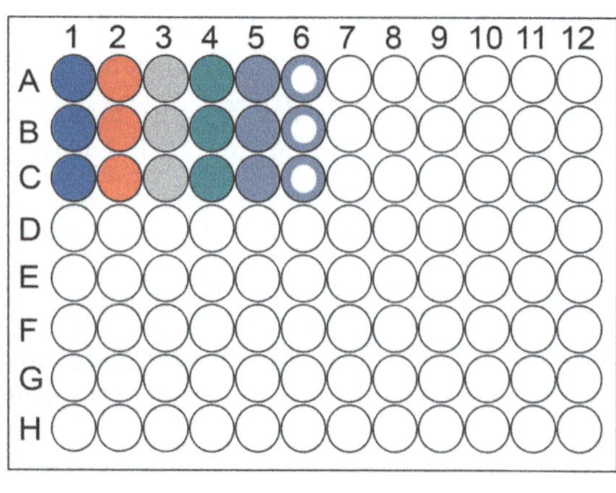

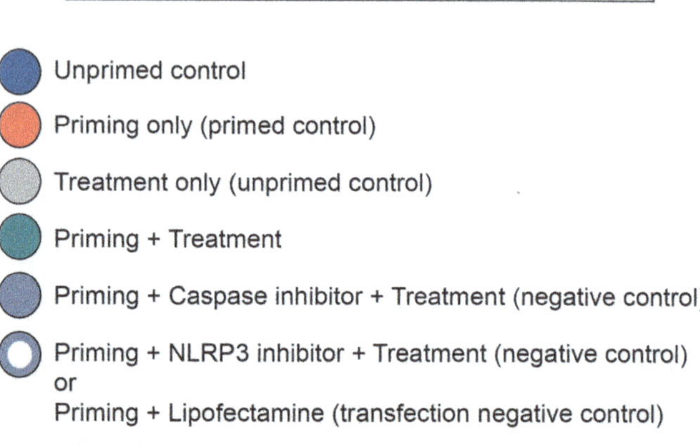

Fig. 1 Sample plating guide for inflammasome activation in triplicate wells of a 96-well plate. For activation of the NLRP3 inflammasome (Subheading 3.2): treatment = nigericin, negative controls = Caspase inhibitor VX-765 and NLRP3 inhibitor MC9950. For activation of the AIM2 inflammasome (Subheading 3.3): treatment = DNA transfection, negative controls = VX-765 Caspase inhibitor and Lipofectamine 2000 transfection control. For activation of the NAIP/NLRC4 inflammasome (Subheading 3.4): treatment = Flagellin transfection, negative controls = VX-765 Caspase inhibitor and Lipofectamine LTX transfection control

6. Retrieve the cells from the incubator 4 h after LPS priming commenced. Remove 10 μL of media from the samples to receive nigericin treatment, and replace it with 10 μL of the 50 μM nigericin working solution. Swirl the plate gently to mix.
7. Return the cells to the 37 °C cell incubator for 30 min.
8. The cells are ready for the caspase activity assay (Subheading 3.5).

3.3 Activation of the AIM2 Inflammasome

1. Add 1×10^6 cells/mL of differentiated BMDM (day 6) to a black 96-well plate (100 μL/well). Include triplicate wells for each of the following samples:

Unprimed control.

LPS only (primed control).

DNA transfection (unprimed control).

LPS + DNA transfection (priming + treatment).

LPS + VX-765 + DNA Transfection (Caspase inhibitor negative control).

LPS + Lipofectamine 2000 (transfection negative control).

See Fig. 1 for a schematic of how cells can be plated.

2. Place cells in a 37 °C incubator venting 5% CO_2 overnight.
3. The following morning, add 100 ng/mL of ultrapure K12 LPS (from 100 μg/mL working stock; *see* **Note 1**), to all samples to receive LPS (not unprimed controls). Return the cells to the 37 °C cell incubator for 3 h.
4. Add 5 μL of 500 μM VX-765 (prepared in CMM from a 50 mM stock solution) to the negative control samples to receive VX-765 inhibitor. Return the cells to the 37 °C cell incubator for an additional 1 h.
5. Prepare the DNA transfection mix in one Eppendorf tube by adding 250 μL of tepid Opti-MEM and 2.5 μL of 0.25% (final concentration) Lipofectamine 2000. Incubate at room temperature for 5 min. Add 1 μg of CT DNA to the tube.
6. Prepare the control transfection mix in another Eppendorf tube by adding 125 μL of tepid Opti-MEM and 1.25 μL of Lipofectamine 2000.
7. Incubate both transfection mixes for 20 min at room temperature.
8. Add Opti-MEM to a final volume of 1 mL for the DNA transfection tube, and to a final volume of 500 μL for the control transfection tube (lipofectamine only). Add 150 ng/mL (final concentration) of CSF-1 to both samples.
9. Remove 350 μL of the DNA transfection mix and place into a new tube. Add 0.18 μL of 50 mM (stock-solution) VX-765. This reaction mix will be used for the VX-765 inhibited negative control column.
10. Retrieve the cells from the incubator 4 h after LPS priming commenced. Aspirate media from the cells to be transfected (all treatment samples and transfection negative control, columns 3–6, Fig. 1), and replace the media with 100 μL of the appropriate transfection mix prepared above. For the remaining control samples that are not to be transfected (columns 1–2, Fig. 1), aspirate the media and replace it with 100 μL Opti-MEM (supplemented with 150 ng/mL CSF-1).
11. Centrifuge the plate at 500 × *g* for 5 min at room temperature.

12. Return the cells to the 37 °C cell incubator for 30 min.
13. The cells are ready for the caspase activity assay (Subheading 3.5).

3.4 Activation of the NAIP/NLRC4 Inflammasome

1. Add 1×10^6 cells/mL of differentiated BMDM (day 6) to a black 96-well plate (100 μL/well). Include triplicate wells for each of the following samples:

   Unprimed control.

   LPS only (primed control).

   Flagellin transfection (unprimed control).

   LPS + flagellin transfection (priming + treatment).

   LPS + VX-765 + flagellin transfection (Caspase inhibitor negative control).

   LPS + Lipofectamine LTX (transfection negative control).

   See Fig. 1 for a schematic of how cells can be plated.
2. Place cells in a 37 °C incubator venting 5% CO_2 overnight.
3. On the following morning, add 100 ng/mL of ultrapure K12 LPS (from 100 μg/mL working stock; *see* **Note 11**), to all samples to receive LPS (not unprimed controls). Return the cells to the 37 °C cell incubator for 3 h.
4. Add 5 μL of 500 μM VX-765 (prepared in CMM from a 50 mM stock solution) to the negative control samples to receive VX-765 inhibitor. Return the cells to the cell incubator for an additional 1 h at 37 °C.
5. Prepare the flagellin transfection mix in 1 Eppendorf tube by adding 250 μL of tepid Opti-MEM and 4 μL of Lipofectamine LTX (final concentration of 0.40%). Incubate at room temperature for 5 min. Add 1.5 μL of 100 μg/mL recombinant flagellin to the tube.
6. Prepare the control transfection mix in another Eppendorf tube by adding 125 μL of tepid Opti-MEM and 2 μL of Lipofectamine LTX.
7. Incubate both transfection mixes for 20 min at room temperature.
8. Add Opti-MEM to a final volume of 1 mL for the flagellin transfection tube, and to a final volume of 500 μL for the control transfection tube (lipofectamine only). Add 150 ng/mL CSF-1 (final concentration) to both samples.
9. Remove 350 μL of the flagellin transfection mix and place into a new tube. Add 0.18 μL of 50 mM stock-solution of VX-765. This reaction mix will be used for the VX-765 inhibited negative control column.

10. Retrieve the cells from the incubator 4 h after LPS priming commenced. Aspirate media from the cells to be transfected (all treatment samples and transfection negative control, columns 3–6, Fig. 1), and replace the media with 100 μL of the appropriate transfection mix prepared above. For the remaining control samples that are not to be transfected (columns 1–2, Fig. 1), aspirate the media and replace it with 100 μL OptiMem (supplemented with 150 ng/mL CSF-1).
11. Centrifuge the plate at 500 × *g* for 5 min at room temperature.
12. Return the cells to the 37 °C cell incubator for 30 min.
13. The cells are ready for the caspase activity assay (Subheading 3.5).

3.5 Cellular Caspase Activity Assay

1. During cell stimulation, prepare the 1× caspase activity buffer. Prepare 100 μL/well of buffer for the different treatment conditions. Freshly supplement the buffer with 100 μg/mL digitonin, 10 mM DTT and 100 μM YVAD-afc. For example, for a 2 mL working stock, add 1 mL of 2× caspase activity buffer, 978 μL of sterile distilled water, 200 μg of digitonin, 20 μL of 1 M DTT, and 2 μL of 100 mM YVAD-afc. Warm the buffer to 37 °C and pre-heat the fluorescence plate reader to 37 °C.
2. 30 min after the inflammasome agonist was added to cells, remove the cells from the incubator.
3. Using a multichannel pipette, transfer the cell culture media from the black 96-well plate to a new 96-well plate. Retain the media on ice for future use (*see* **Note 12**). Add 100 μL of 1× caspase activity buffer to each well of the black plate containing cells, to lyse the cells.
4. Quickly transfer the plate to the fluorescence plate reader. Read the fluorescence at excitation $\lambda = 405$ nm and emission $\lambda = 510$ nm for 30 min in kinetics mode, taking readings every 15 s.
5. Save the resulting data as a Microsoft Excel file.

3.6 Analysis of Caspase Activity

1. Open the Microsoft Excel file. For each well, subtract the first kinetic reading from every other reading for this well (i.e., perform background subtraction for each well, setting the initial fluorescence reading to 0). This will facilitate comparison between different samples.
2. Using data analysis software (e.g., GraphPad Prism), plot the corrected fluorescence value (obtained in Subheading 3.6, **step 1**) as a function of time. An example of the generated graphical output is shown in Fig. 2.
3. Identify a section on the curve where the slope is linear (*see* **Note 13**). Calculate the slope to determine the reaction speed

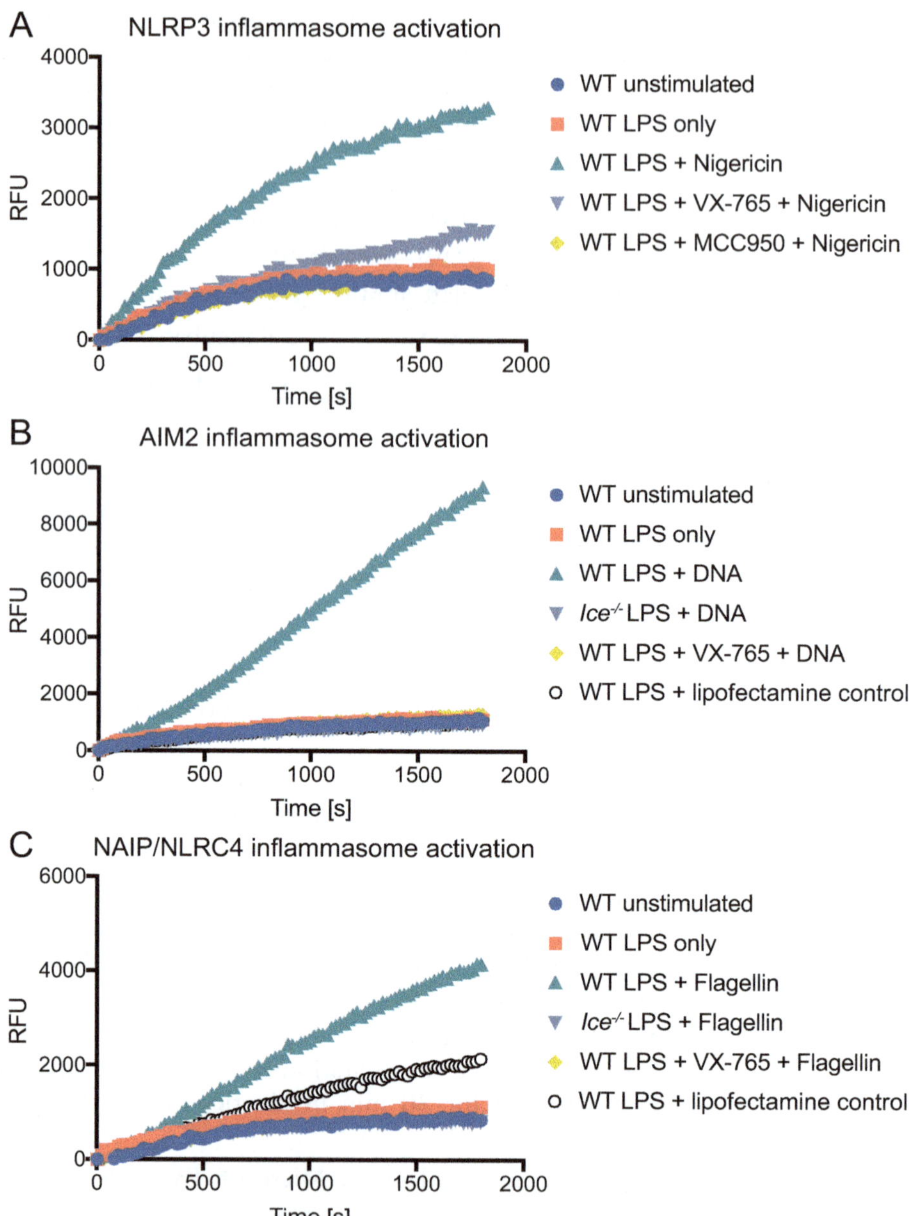

Fig. 2 Representative data obtained with the cellular caspase activity assay following inflammasome activation. (**a**) Activation of the NLRP3 inflammasome with nigericin (Subheading 3.2). (**b**) Activation of the AIM2 inflammasome upon DNA transfection (Subheading 3.3). (**c**) Activation of the NAIP/NLRC4 inflammasome upon flagellin transfection (Subheading 3.4)

using the formula: speed = $(y_2-y_1)/(x_2/x_1)$ as measured in mRFU/s (*see* **Note 14**). In this equation, y_2 and y_1 are fluorescence (mRFU) value of the curve generated in Subheading 3.6, **step 2** where the curve is linear and x_1 and x_2 are the time (in seconds) corresponding to the fluorescence values selected (y_2 and y_1). *See* Fig. 3 for an example.

1. Trace the graph using normalised data

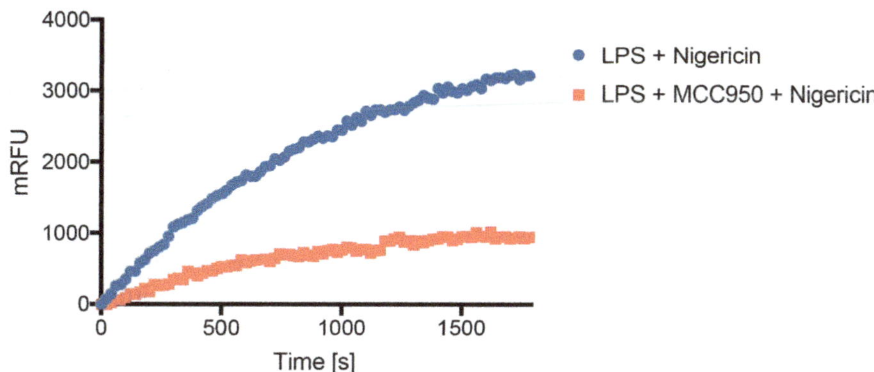

2. Define an area where the curve is linear
Identify the coordinate at the extremity of the linear region

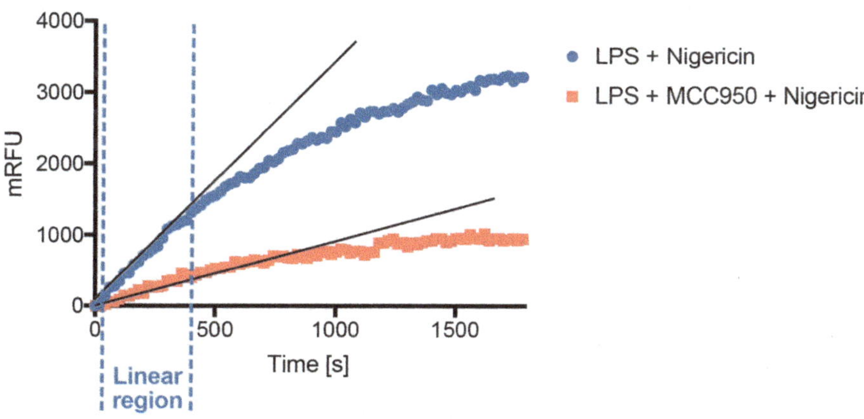

3. Calculate the slope to determine caspase activity

X1 = 0
X2 = 480

Nigericin: Y1 = 0 ; Y2 = 1532
Nigericin + MCC950: Y1 = 0; Y2 = 505

Formula: speed = (Y2-Y1) / (X2-X-1)

Nigericin: speed = (1532-0) / (480-0) = 3.2 mRFU/sec
Nigericin + MCC950: speed = (505-0) / (480-0) = 1.1 mRFU/sec

Fig. 3 Example of the calculations required to determine caspase-1 activity (Subheading 3.6)

4 Notes

1. Various knockout mice are available for studying inflammasome signalling pathways. Mice deficient in caspase-1/11 (*Ice* [25]) and other signalling components (e.g., *Nlrp3, Nlrc4, Aim2, Asc*) are available, and cells derived from these mice are valuable as assay controls.
2. FCS should be carefully selected when culturing BMDM. Serum lots should be screened for the presence of endotoxin and other microbial components that can affect BMDM differentiation and behaviour.
3. We use recombinant human CSF-1 (endotoxin-free) produced in-house in insect cells. CSF-1 is also commercially available. We recommend titrating CSF-1 for optimal BMDM yield and differentiation state (assessed by screening for presence of the F4/80 surface marker), as different sources of CSF-1 can exhibit variable potency.
4. Caspase-1 inhibitors, like zVAD-fmk and VX-765 [26], are commonly used as negative controls. MCC950 can also be used to inhibit NLRP3-dependent caspase-1 activation [9].
5. We recommend using a heat-controlled plate reader that will accommodate time-point measurements, as caspase activity assays involve kinetic measurement at 37 °C. We routinely use a TECAN M1000 Pro to perform these assays.
6. Substrates should be carefully selected when monitoring the activity of specific caspases. For example, caspase-1 efficiently cleaves acYVAD-afc. Fluorophores other than afc (e.g., amc; 7-Amino-4-Methylcoumarin), or chromophores (e.g., pNA; p-nitroaniline) can also be used. As DMSO can affect caspase activity, we recommend preparing concentrated substrate stock solutions (100 mM in DMSO), so that DMSO is diluted during caspase assays.
7. Other caspase activity buffers can be used to monitor caspase activity (e.g., activity assays with recombinant enzyme) and have been described elsewhere [27]. However, for cell-based assays, we recommend the buffer described in this protocol.
8. We routinely use 6–10 week old mice. Mouse age and sex can affect BMDM yield and inflammasome responses. We recommend keeping mouse age and sex consistent throughout a study.
9. It is possible to freeze excess of BMDM progenitor at this stage using freezing media. We routinely freeze half the bone marrow of a mouse in 1 mL of freezing media.

10. This procedure yields 60–150 × 10^6 BMDM per mouse, depending on mouse age and sex. On day 6 of their differentiation, excess macrophages can be preserved and frozen in freezing media for future experiments.
11. LPS tends to aggregate, and requires vigorous vortexing before use.
12. The cell culture media can be used at this step to evaluate the extent of cell death (e.g., by measuring the release of lactate dehydrogenase) and/or cytokine secretion [22].
13. The selection of a linear slope is important to obtain an accurate comparison between samples. Substrate depletion can lead to decreased apparent caspase activity over time.
14. The speed can also be determined in nM/s of substrate degraded instead of mRFU/s. To do so, the substrate and the spectrophotometer need to be calibrated. Such calibration is not described in this chapter but the detailed procedure can be found elsewhere [27].

Acknowledgments

This work was supported by a Project Grant (DP160102702) from the Australian Research Council to KS. DB was supported by Postdoctoral Fellowships from the Fonds de Recherche du Québec en Santé and the University of Queensland. AC was supported by an Australian Postgraduate Award. KS was supported by an Australian Research Council Future Fellowship (FT130100361).

References

1. Schroder K, Tschopp J (2010) The inflammasomes. Cell 140:821–832
2. Xiao TS (2015) The nucleic acid-sensing inflammasomes. Immunol Rev 265:103–111
3. Xu H, Yang J, Gao W, Li L, Li P, Zhang L, Gong YN, Peng X, Xi JJ, Chen S, Wang F, Shao F (2014) Innate immune sensing of bacterial modifications of Rho GTPases by the Pyrin inflammasome. Nature 513:237–241
4. Man SM, Karki R, Kanneganti TD (2017) Molecular mechanisms and functions of pyroptosis, inflammatory caspases and inflammasomes in infectious diseases. Immunol Rev 277:61–75
5. Shi J, Zhao Y, Wang K, Shi X, Wang Y, Huang H, Zhuang Y, Cai T, Wang F, Shao F (2015) Cleavage of GSDMD by inflammatory caspases determines pyroptotic cell death. Nature 526:660–665
6. Kayagaki N, Stowe IB, Lee BL, O'Rourke K, Anderson K, Warming S, Cuellar T, Haley B, Roose-Girma M, Phung QT, Liu PS, Lill JR, Li H, Wu J, Kummerfeld S, Zhang J, Lee WP, Snipas SJ, Salvesen GS, Morris LX, Fitzgerald L, Zhang Y, Bertram EM, Goodnow CC, Dixit VM (2015) Caspase-11 cleaves gasdermin D for non-canonical inflammasome signalling. Nature 526:666–671
7. Agard NJ, Maltby D, Wells JA (2010) Inflammatory stimuli regulate caspase substrate profiles. Mol Cell Proteomics 9:880–93
8. He Y, Hara H, Nunez G (2016) Mechanism and regulation of NLRP3 inflammasome activation. Trends Biochem Sci 41:1012–1021
9. Coll RC, Robertson AA, Chae JJ, Higgins SC, Munoz-Planillo R, Inserra MC, Vetter I, Dungan LS, Monks BG, Stutz A, Croker DE, Butler MS, Haneklaus M, Sutton CE, Nunez G, Latz E, Kastner DL, Mills KH, Masters SL,

Schroder K, Cooper MA, O'Neill LA (2015) A small-molecule inhibitor of the NLRP3 inflammasome for the treatment of inflammatory diseases. Nat Med 21:248–255

10. Miao EA, Alpuche-Aranda CM, Dors M, Clark AE, Bader MW, Miller SI, Aderem A (2006) Cytoplasmic flagellin activates caspase-1 and secretion of interleukin 1beta via Ipaf. Nat Immunol 7:569–575

11. Franchi L, Amer A, Body-Malapel M, Kanneganti TD, Ozoren N, Jagirdar R, Inohara N, Vandenabeele P, Bertin J, Coyle A, Grant EP, Nunez G (2006) Cytosolic flagellin requires Ipaf for activation of caspase-1 and interleukin 1beta in salmonella-infected macrophages. Nat Immunol 7:576–582

12. Zhao Y, Yang J, Shi J, Gong YN, Lu Q, Xu H, Liu L, Shao F (2011) The NLRC4 inflammasome receptors for bacterial flagellin and type III secretion apparatus. Nature 477:596–600

13. Kofoed EM, Vance RE (2011) Innate immune recognition of bacterial ligands by NAIPs determines inflammasome specificity. Nature 477:592–595

14. Levinsohn JL, Newman ZL, Hellmich KA, Fattah R, Getz MA, Liu S, Sastalla I, Leppla SH, Moayeri M (2012) Anthrax lethal factor cleavage of Nlrp1 is required for activation of the inflammasome. PLoS Pathog 8:e1002638

15. Witola WH, Mui E, Hargrave A, Liu S, Hypolite M, Montpetit A, Cavailles P, Bisanz C, Cesbron-Delauw MF, Fournie GJ, McLeod R (2011) NALP1 influences susceptibility to human congenital toxoplasmosis, proinflammatory cytokine response, and fate of Toxoplasma gondii-infected monocytic cells. Infect Immun 79:756–766

16. Roberts TL, Idris A, Dunn JA, Kelly GM, Burnton CM, Hodgson S, Hardy LL, Garceau V, Sweet MJ, Ross IL, Hume DA, Stacey KJ (2009) HIN-200 proteins regulate caspase activation in response to foreign cytoplasmic DNA. Science 323:1057–1060

17. Fernandes-Alnemri T, Yu JW, Datta P, Wu J, Alnemri ES (2009) AIM2 activates the inflammasome and cell death in response to cytoplasmic DNA. Nature 458:509–513

18. Hornung V, Ablasser A, Charrel-Dennis M, Bauernfeind F, Horvath G, Caffrey DR, Latz E, Fitzgerald KA (2009) AIM2 recognizes cytosolic dsDNA and forms a caspase-1-activating inflammasome with ASC. Nature 458:514–518

19. Zhu Q, Kanneganti TD (2017) Cutting edge: distinct regulatory mechanisms control proinflammatory cytokines IL-18 and IL-1beta. J Immunol 198:4210–4215

20. Bauernfeind FG, Horvath G, Stutz A, Alnemri ES, MacDonald K, Speert D, Fernandes-Alnemri T, Wu J, Monks BG, Fitzgerald KA, Hornung V, Latz E (2009) Cutting edge: NF-kappaB activating pattern recognition and cytokine receptors license NLRP3 inflammasome activation by regulating NLRP3 expression. J Immunol 183:787–791

21. Poltorak A, He X, Smirnova I, Liu MY, Van Huffel C, Du X, Birdwell D, Alejos E, Silva M, Galanos C, Freudenberg M, Ricciardi-Castagnoli P, Layton B, Beutler B (1998) Defective LPS signaling in C3H/HeJ and C57BL/10ScCr mice: mutations in Tlr4 gene. Science 282:2085–2088

22. Gross O (2012) Measuring the inflammasome. Methods Mol Biol 844:199–222

23. Broz P, Monack DM (2013) Measuring inflammasome activation in response to bacterial infection. Methods Mol Biol 1040:65–84

24. Thornberry NA, Rano TA, Peterson EP, Rasper DM, Timkey T, Garcia-Calvo M, Houtzager VM, Nordstrom PA, Roy S, Vaillancourt JP, Chapman KT, Nicholson DW (1997) A combinatorial approach defines specificities of members of the caspase family and granzyme B. Functional relationships established for key mediators of apoptosis. J Biol Chem 272:17907–17911

25. Kuida K, Lippke JA, Ku G, Harding MW, Livingston DJ, Su MS, Flavell RA (1995) Altered cytokine export and apoptosis in mice deficient in interleukin-1 beta converting enzyme. Science 267:2000–2003

26. Linton SD (2005) Caspase inhibitors: a pharmaceutical industry perspective. Curr Top Med Chem 5:1697–1717

27. Boucher D, Duclos C, Denault JB (2014) General in vitro caspase assay procedures. Methods Mol Biol 1133:3–39

Chapter 15

Analysis of Histone Modifications in Acute Myeloid Leukaemia Using Chromatin Immunoprecipitation

Benjamin J. Shields, Andrew Keniry, Marnie E. Blewitt, and Matthew P. McCormack

Abstract

Chromatin Immunoprecipitation (ChIP) using antibodies specific for histone modifications is a powerful technique for assessing the epigenetic states of cell populations by either quantitative PCR (ChIP-PCR) or next generation sequencing analysis (ChIP-Seq). Here we describe the procedure for ChIP of histone marks in myeloid leukaemia cell lines and the subsequent purification of genomic DNA associated with repressive and activating histone modifications for further analysis. This procedure can be widely applied to a variety of histone marks to assess both activating and repressive modifications in the context of myeloid leukaemia.

Key words Epigenetics, Immunoprecipitation, Chromatin, Histone modifications, Acute myeloid leukaemia

1 Introduction

Recent advances in decoding the layer of gene regulation written by epigenetic modifying enzymes have been made possible by Chromatin Immunoprecipitation (ChIP) techniques that facilitate the isolation of genomic DNA associated with antibodies which detect specific histone amino acid modifications [1]. These modifications include methylation, ubiquitination and acetylation and are recognized by epigenetic readers as being marks of activated or repressed chromatin [2–4].

In this chapter, we describe a methodology for stable cross-linking of protein-DNA interactions and the purification of nuclei and subsequent shearing of genomic DNA for ChIP of histone modifications in myeloid leukaemia cell lines. We have successfully applied this technique to assess marks catalyzed by the epigenetic writers PRC2 (H3K27Me3) and MLL (H3K4Me3) in mouse myeloid leukaemia cell lines [5] by both ChIP-Seq and ChIP-PCR, as well as in wild-type myeloid progenitors by ChIP-PCR

Brendan J. Jenkins (ed.), *Inflammation and Cancer: Methods and Protocols*, Methods in Molecular Biology, vol. 1725, https://doi.org/10.1007/978-1-4939-7568-6_15,

(Lin$^-$Sca1$^+$Kit$^+$ cells expanded in vitro for 5 days [6] (*see* **Note 1**)). However, by empirical testing of different antibodies in the immunoprecipitation, this technique can potentially be applied to assess any histone modification. Moreover, with modifications in fixation and sonication, the technique can potentially be applied to any cell type.

2 Materials

2.1 Formaldehyde Fixation of Cultured Cells

1. Up to 1×10^7 MLL-ENL Acute Myeloid Leukaemia (AML) or hematopoietic progenitor cells (*see* **Note 1**) in a final volume of 1 mL Iscove's Modified Dulbecco's Medium (IMDM) without added serum.
2. 37% Formaldehyde (*see* **Note 2**).
3. 1 M Glycine stock solution: Weigh 7.5 g Glycine and add 100 mL water.
4. Phosphate-buffered saline (pH 7.4, Mg^{2+}, Ca^{2+} free).

2.2 Chromatin Immunoprecipitation (ChIP)

1. Immunoprecipitation (IP) Buffer: 50 mM Tris–HCl (pH 7.5), 150 mM NaCl, 5 mM EDTA, 0.5% (v/v) NP40, 1% (v/v) TritonX-100 (*see* **Note 3**), 1× Roche Complete Protease Inhibitor Cocktail (*see* **Note 4**).
2. Rabbit anti-sera for immunoprecipitations: antibodies against histones, such as 2 μg/mL final concentration rabbit-raised anti-histone H3K27Me3 and H3K4Me3. For control antibodies, use 2 μg/mL final concentration isotype-matched Normal Rabbit IgG (*see* **Note 5**).
3. 50% slurry of protein-A-sepharose beads (*see* **Note 6**).
4. 2 μg/mL RNAse A.
5. 20 μg/μL proteinase K.
6. Elution Buffer: 1% (w/v) Sodium Dodecyl Sulfate (SDS; w/v), 0.1 M $NaHCO_3$ (*see* **Note 7**).
7. Qiagen Qiaquick PCR Purification kit (*see* **Note 8**).

3 Methods

3.1 Formaldehyde Fixation of Cultured Cells

1. Aliquot 1×10^7 cultured cells (*see* **Note 9**) in 1 mL IMDM into a 10 mL tube. Add 40 μL of 37% Formaldehyde solution to the side of the tube then mix through immediately by vortexing (final concentration 1.4%). Incubate at room temperature for 10 min on a rolling platform to facilitate efficient mixing of the sample.

2. Add 141 μL 1 M Glycine to fixed cells (final concentration 125 mM) to quench any unreacted Formaldehyde. Incubate at room temperature for 5 min on a rolling platform to facilitate efficient mixing of the sample.
3. To remove traces of Formaldehyde, wash cells twice with PBS. Pellet fixed cells by centrifugation in a benchtop swing out bucket centrifuge at 2000 × *g* for 5 min.
4. Remove supernatant using a p1000 pipette and disrupt the cell pellet by gently flicking the tube.
5. Using a 10 mL pipette add 10 mL PBS to tube and mix by inversion.
6. Pellet fixed cells by centrifugation in a benchtop swing out bucket centrifuge (2000 × *g* for 5 min) and pour off supernatant.
7. Repeat **steps 6** and 7 to complete second wash, then re-suspend cell pellet in residual PBS and transfer to 1.5 mL Eppendorf tube.
8. Pellet cells in a benchtop swing out bucket centrifuge (2000 × *g* for 5 min) and remove final traces of PBS from cell pellet using a p200 pipette (*see* **Note 10**).
9. At this point in the procedure the fixed cell pellet can be snap frozen in liquid nitrogen and stored at −80 °C for short periods (up to 1 week), or processed immediately for ChIP (Subheading 3.2). Note that chromatin yields are best from freshly fixed cell pellets.

3.2 ChIP Assay

DAY 1.

1. If using frozen fixed cell pellets, allow samples to thaw on ice.
2. Lyse the cells with 1 mL of chilled IP buffer by pipetting up and down ten times then incubate the sample on ice for 10 min.
3. Pellet cell nuclei by centrifugation at 12,000 × *g* for 1 min at 4 °C in a benchtop fixed angle centrifuge.
4. Remove supernatant and being careful not to disturb the pellet, wash nuclei with 1 mL IP buffer by pipetting up and down ten times.
5. Pellet cell nuclei (12,000 × *g* for 1 min at 4 °C) and re-suspend in 130 μL of IP buffer and transfer the entire sample to a CoVaris Microtube (*see* **Note 11**).
6. Sonicate the sample using the following settings on the CoVaris S220 system (*see* **Note 12**):
   (a) Duty cycle = 10%.
   (b) Peak power = 125.
   (c) Burst/cycles = 200.
   (d) Time = 30 min.

7. Carefully remove the lysate from the CoVaris Microtube using a p200 pipette and transfer to a pre-chilled Eppendorf tube (*see* **Notes 13** and **14**).
8. Clear the sample of any particulate matter by centrifuging at 12,000 × *g* for 10 min at 4 °C and transfer the supernatant to a pre-chilled Eppendorf tube.
9. Transfer 10 μL of the sample (Whole Cell Extract (WCE)) to a new Eppendorf tube, snap freeze in liquid nitrogen and store at −20 °C (*see* **Note 15**).
10. Dilute the remaining sample with IP buffer so that each immunoprecipitation is performed with 100 μL of cleared chromatin. For example, if 4 immunoprecipitations are to be performed then dilute the sample to 400 mL.
11. Transfer 100 μL of the diluted chromatin to a new pre-chilled Eppendorf tube and add 900 μL of IP buffer.
12. Add 2 μg of either IgG (control) or H3K27Me3 and H3K4Me3 antibodies to each sample and incubate on a rolling platform in a cold room overnight.

DAY 2.

13. Clear the sample of any particulate matter by centrifuging at 12,000 × *g* for 10 min at 4 °C.
14. Equilibrate the requisite amount of protein-A-sepharose beads for 20 μL for each IP by washing the beads three times in 1 mL cold IP buffer (*see* **Note 16**).
15. Re-suspend the beads in the amount of IP buffer equal to the original volume (to make a 50% slurry) and aliquot 20 μL into pre-chilled Eppendorf tubes (*see* **Note 17**).
16. Add the top 900 μL of cleared chromatin to the pre-washed beads and incubate on a rolling platform in a cold room for 1 h. Beads require six washes with 1 mL IP buffer to remove contaminating proteins.
17. Centrifuge the sample at 300 × *g* for 2 min at 4 °C and remove supernatant (*see* **Note 18**).
18. Wash the beads by gently re-suspending them in 1 mL IP buffer then centrifuge the sample at 300 × *g* for 2 min at 4 °C and remove supernatant (*see* **Note 18**).
19. Repeat this step five times.
20. To elute the DNA, after the final wash step re-suspend the beads in 250 μL freshly prepared Elution Buffer and place Eppendorf tubes on a rotating wheel at room temperature for 15 min.
21. Centrifuge the sample at 300 × *g* for 2 min at 4 °C and remove the supernatant to a fresh Eppendorf Tube (*see* **Note 19**).

22. Add a second volume (250 μL) freshly prepared Elution Buffer and place Eppendorf tubes on a rotating wheel at room temperature for 15 min.
23. Centrifuge the sample at 300 × *g* for 2 min at 4 °C and add the supernatant to the first volume (total 500 μL; *see* **Note 19**).
24. Remove WCE sample from −20°C storage (from **step 9**) and make up to 500 μL with Elution buffer.
25. From this point in the ChIP procedure treat all samples in the same manner. To reverse DNA-protein crosslinks add 20 μL of 5 M NaCl to each sample.
26. To degrade contaminating RNA, add 2 μL of RNAse A to each sample.
27. Incubate samples on a heat block at 65 °C for 4 h.
28. To degrade proteins, add 1 μL of proteinase K and incubate on a heat block at 65 °C for 1 h.
29. Extract the DNA using the Qiaquick PCR Purification kit (*see* **Note 20**). The purified DNA is now able to be used in DNA sequencing (ChIP-Seq) or quantitative PCR (ChIP-PCR).

3.3 Quantitative PCR (ChIP-PCR) and DNA Sequencing (ChIP-Seq)

1. Quantitative qPCR reactions are performed using Promega GoTaq qPCR mix and run on a LightCycler 480 Real-Time PCR System to determine the percentage of input chromatin that is precipitated in each sample [5].
2. ChIP-Seq DNA libraries can be constructed using Illumina TruSeq Nano DNA sample preparation according to the manufacturer's instructions and sequenced on an Illumina NextSeq 500. For chromatin wide differential analysis of chromatin marks, at least 20 million 150 bp single-end reads should ideally be obtained for bioinformatic analysis as described [5].

4 Notes

1. For fetal liver derived HSPC ChIP-seq experiments, as few as 250,000 cells have been used [7, 8]. For in vitro cultured myeloid progenitors [6], to obtain sufficient cells for ChIP, flow cytometry sorted and purified LSKs were expanded in IMDM +10% FCS in the presence of IL-3 (10 ng/mL) and SCF (25 ng/mL) for 5 days prior to analysis. LSK: L = Lineage negative (bone marrow depleted for mature blood cells using antisera specific for CD4, CD8, B220, CD19, Gr1, Mac1 and Ter119 markers), S = Sca1 positive, K = Kit positive.
2. Formaldehyde is a possible carcinogen and should be used in a fume hood to avoid inhalation of vapors.

3. Allow at least 2 h when making up stock solutions of NP40 and TritonX-100 in 50 mL tubes. To avoid generating bubbles, place mixtures on rolling platform and allow mixing to occur slowly.
4. Protease inhibitors are purchased as tablets from Roche and inhibit a broad range of serine, cysteine, and metalloproteases, as well as calpains. Protease inhibitors should be added to freshly prepared IP buffer.
5. The IgG control is useful in ChIP-qPCR as a negative control.
6. Protein-A-Sepharose beads should be equilibrated in the desired buffer prior to use. Follow the manufacturer's instructions to reconstitute the beads and wash the beads in 1 mL IP buffer at least three times prior to use. Alternatively, Protein A/G conjugated-magnetic beads (e.g., ChIP-Grade Protein G Magnetic Beads) can be used in place of Sepharose beads.
7. SDS is an irritant by inhalation. To avoid breathing dust, SDS should be weighed out in a fume cupboard and a respirator should be worn. Elution Buffer should be made up freshly from stock solutions before use.
8. Alternatively, the Zymo ChIP DNA Clean and Concentrator kit can be used for DNA purification and removal of SDS and 0.1 M $NaHCO_3$.
9. The viability of the AML cells should be tested prior to proceeding with the ChIP protocol. Best results are expected when viability of cells is 80% or greater. It is recommended that cell lines be passaged 1 or 2 days prior to the day of the experiment so that cell density is optimal for viability (i.e., $2–3 \times 10^6$ cells per 10 mL culture).
10. For efficient cell lysis all traces of PBS should be removed from the pellet. Care should be taken at this point to avoid aspirating cells in the last few microliters of PBS.
11. The Covaris Microtube is available with re-sealable pre-cut septa lids to make loading and removal of the small sample volume easier and to minimize sample loss. To add the sample to the tube, load a p200 pipette tip with 130 μL sample using a p200 pipette and push the tip through the pre-cut septa lid. Push the tip to the bottom of the tube, then as the sample is dispensed, slowly withdraw the tip from the tube. This will minimize the incorporation of trapped air in the tube which reduces the amount of sample that can be loaded and alters the efficacy of sonication.
12. This protocol has been optimized for DNA fragmentation of mouse Bone-Marrow derived MLL-ENL AML cell lines and LSK cultures using the Covaris S220 system. The optimal technical parameters for DNA fragmentation of cell lines

from other sources and/or with alternative sonicators will need to be determined by the user. The Covaris S220 system was utilized for sample preparation because it prevents sample overheating and facilitates shearing of genomic DNA into approximately nucleosome sized fragments (~150–300 bp), which provides the highest resolution possible for histone ChIP.

13. To remove the sample from the Covaris Microtube, use a p200 pipette. Push the tip through the pre-cut septa lid and aspirate the sample whilst pushing the tip into the tube.
14. The sample can be analysed on a 1% agarose (w/v) gel or Tapestation device (Agilent technologies) or similar Bioanalyser, to determine the size range of sheared chromatin. To do this, treat the sample as described for the WCE. If using a different cell type, determine the minimum sonication time that will facilitate shearing of the genomic DNA to approximately nucleosome sized fragments (~150–300 bp on average).
15. The Whole Cell Extract (WCE) chromatin sample is the pre-IP material. When processed as described in **steps 25–29**, it is used as baseline control in qPCR analysis to calculate the relative amount of signal for a given amplicon pre- and post-IP (i.e., % enrichment post IP) and used to make a library of the total input genomic DNA for next generation sequencing analysis.
16. Wash steps are performed using IP buffer without added protease inhibitors.
17. To enable accurate aliquoting of small volumes of Protein-A-Sepharose beads, we recommend that the end 2 mm of the p200 tip be removed with a clean pair of scissors.
18. When aspirating the wash fractions, it is recommended that a suction device with a long Pasteur pipette with a p200 tip attached be used to avoid inadvertently disturbing the beads.
19. Take care when removing the supernatant not to disturb the pelleted Protein-A-Sepharose beads.
20. A large volume of Binding Buffer (PB) is required. The Qiaquick PCR Purification kit protocol stipulates that 5 volumes of PB buffer are required to add to the sample to be purified, which in this case is 200 μL (5 × 200 μL = 1 mL). The loading capacity of the purification columns used in the kit is ~800 μL, so 750 μL of each sample is loaded, centrifuged at 17,900 × *g* for 1 min and the supernatant discarded and this procedure repeated again until the entire sample is run through.

References

1. Nelson JD, Denisenko O, Sova P, Bomsztyk K (2006) Fast chromatin immunoprecipitation assay. Nucleic Acids Res 34:e2
2. Dawson MA, Kouzarides T (2012) Cancer epigenetics: from mechanism to therapy. Cell 150:12–27
3. Kouzarides T (2007) Chromatin modifications and their function. Cell 128:693–705
4. Tan M, Luo H, Lee S, Jin F, Yang JS, Montellier E, Buchou T, Cheng Z, Rousseaux S, Rajagopal N, Lu Z, Ye Z, Zhu Q, Wysocka J, Ye Y, Khochbin S, Ren B, Zhao Y (2011) Identification of 67 histone marks and histone lysine crotonylation as a new type of histone modification. Cell 146:1016–1028
5. Shields BJ, Jackson JT, Metcalf D, Shi W, Huang Q, Garnham AL, Glaser SP, Beck D, Pimanda JE, Bogue CW, Smyth GK, Alexander WS, McCormack MP (2016) Acute myeloid leukemia requires Hhex to enable PRC2-mediated epigenetic repression of Cdkn2a. Genes Dev 30:78–91
6. Jackson JT, Shields BJ, Shi W, Di Rago L, Metcalf D, Nicola NA, McCormack MP (2017) Hhex regulates hematopoietic stem cell self-renewal and stress hematopoiesis via repression of Cdkn2a. Stem Cells 35(8):1948–1957
7. Kinkel SA, Galeev R, Flensburg C, Keniry A, Breslin K, Gilan O, Lee S, Liu J, Chen K, Gearing LJ, Moore DL, Alexander WS, Dawson M, Majewski IJ, Oshlack A, Larsson J, Blewitt ME (2015) Jarid2 regulates hematopoietic stem cell function by acting with polycomb repressive complex 2. Blood 125:1890–1900
8. Flensburg C, Kinkel SA, Keniry A, Blewitt ME, Oshlack A (2014) A comparison of control samples for ChIP-seq of histone modifications. Front Genet 5:329

Chapter 16

Analysis of DNA Methylation in Tissues Exposed to Inflammation

Naoko Hattori and Toshikazu Ushijima

Abstract

Induction of aberrant DNA methylation is one of the most important mechanisms mediating the effect of inflammation on cancer development. Aberrant methylation of promoter CpG islands of tumor suppressor genes can silence their downstream genes, and that in cancer tissues is associated with prognosis or therapeutic effects. In addition, aberrant methylation can occur in tissues exposed to specific types of inflammation, producing a so-called "epigenetic field for cancerization," and its accumulation is correlated with cancer risk. Thus, aberrant methylation at specific loci is an important biomarker and mediator of the carcinogenic effect of inflammation. DNA methylation at specific genomic regions can be analyzed by various methods based upon bisulfite-mediated DNA conversion, which specifically converts unmethylated cytosines into uracils under appropriate conditions. Methylation-specific PCR (MSP), quantitative MSP, and bisulfite sequencing are widely used, and this chapter provides protocols for bisulfite-mediated conversion, quantitative MSP, and bisulfite sequencing.

Key words DNA methylation, Bisulfite-mediated conversion, Methylation-specific PCR (MSP), Bisulfite sequencing

1 Introduction

Aberrant DNA methylation is involved in cancer development and progression because DNA methylation patterns are inherited with high fidelity in somatic cells and DNA methylation of promoter CpG islands can silence its downstream genes [1, 2]. In cancer, methylation silencing of tumor suppressor genes is one of the major mechanisms of their inactivation, along with mutations and chromosomal losses (Fig. 1). Aberrant methylation at a specific locus is associated with patient prognosis and therapeutic effects in specific types of cancers [3]. In addition, aberrant methylation occurs in non-cancerous tissues, particularly inflammation-associated cancers, and produces a so-called "epigenetic field for cancerization" [4]. The epigenetic field for cancerization is characterized by accumulation of aberrant methylation of various genes in a tissue

Brendan J. Jenkins (ed.), *Inflammation and Cancer: Methods and Protocols*, Methods in Molecular Biology, vol. 1725, https://doi.org/10.1007/978-1-4939-7568-6_16, © Springer Science+Business Media, LLC 2018

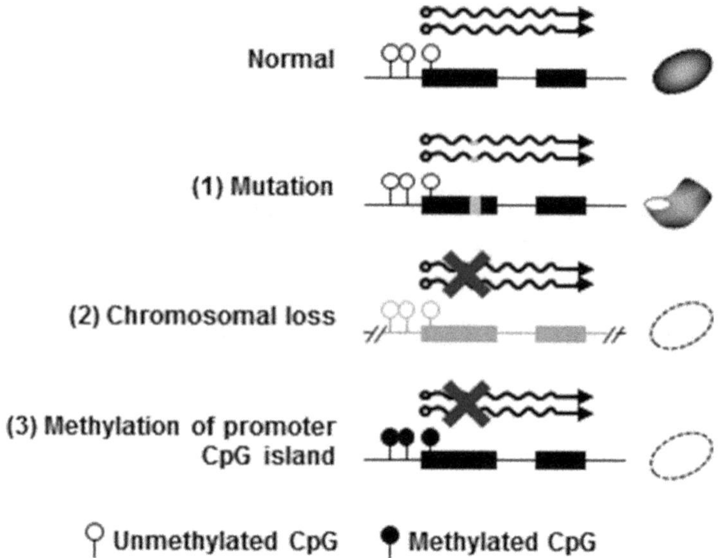

Fig. 1 Mechanisms for inactivation of a tumor suppressor gene. There are three major mechanisms for inactivating a tumor suppressor gene: mutation, chromosomal loss, and aberrant DNA methylation of its promoter CpG island

without clonal lesions and its severity is correlated with cancer risk [5, 6]. These lines of evidence demonstrate the importance of analyzing aberrant methylation at specific regions.

For region-specific methylation analysis, a variety of methods are available. Most widely used methods depend on bisulfite-mediated conversion, which converts unmethylated cytosine (C) into uracil (U) rapidly but methylated C extremely slowly [7] (Fig. 2). Therefore, differences in methylation status can be interpreted as differences in DNA sequence by bisulfite-mediated conversion. Differences in DNA sequences can be readily detected by various methods, such as sequencing (bisulfite sequencing), PCR [methylation-specific PCR (MSP) and quantitative MSP], restriction enzyme digestion (combined bisulfite restriction analysis), and other single nucleotide difference-detection methods (pyrosequencing and MassARRAY® analysis).

Among these methods, conventional and quantitative MSP and bisulfite sequencing are widely used because of their flexibility for selecting a genomic region to analyze and their technical simplicity. Conventional and quantitative MSP detect the methylation statuses of multiple CpG sites at PCR primer sites by using primers specific to methylated or unmethylated sequences [8] (Fig. 3a). The amounts of PCR products indicate methylated and unmethylated DNA. Bisulfite sequencing can analyze individual CpG sites between PCR primers by sequencing a PCR product amplified using bisulfite-converted DNA and PCR primers common to methylated and unmethylated sequences (Fig. 4) [9]. A combination of bisulfite sequencing and

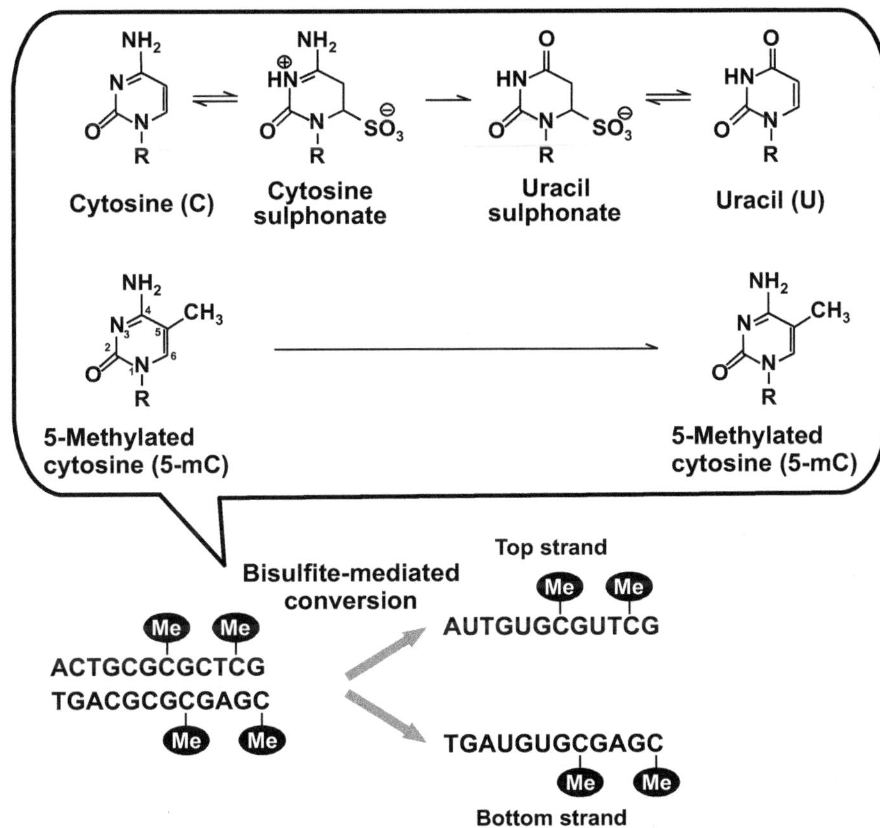

Fig. 2 Principles of DNA methylation detection by bisulfite-mediated conversion. Unmethylated cytosines are converted rapidly into uracil by deamination, whereas methylated cytosines are converted extremely slowly. The difference in methylation status of a CpG site can be converted into a difference of sequence, UpG or CpG. After bisulfite-mediated conversion, the upper and lower strands are no longer complementary

next-generation sequencing (AmpliconBS) enables analysis of a large number of molecules, and accurately detects methylation levels [10, 11] (Fig. 4c). The number of sequence reads with cytosine and thymine at a CpG site indicates the numbers of methylated and unmethylated C, respectively, in the original DNA.

In this chapter, we provide protocols and tips necessary to perform bisulfite-mediated conversion, quantitative MSP, and bisulfite sequencing, which are the most popular methods for evaluating gene-specific DNA methylation.

2 Materials

2.1 Bisulfite-Mediated Conversion

Bisulfite-mediated conversion involves DNA denaturation, bisulfite conversion, DNA purification, and desulfonation. The reagents for all steps can be prepared in the laboratory, but multiple companies provide kits for all of the steps.

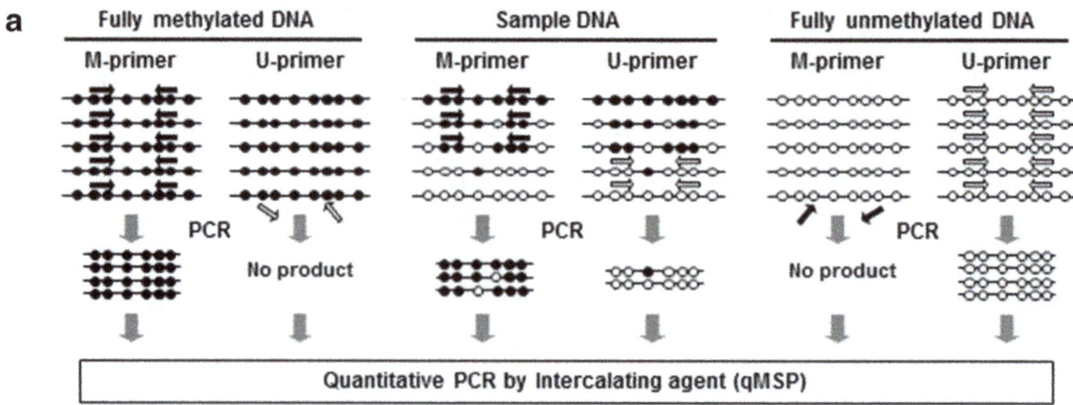

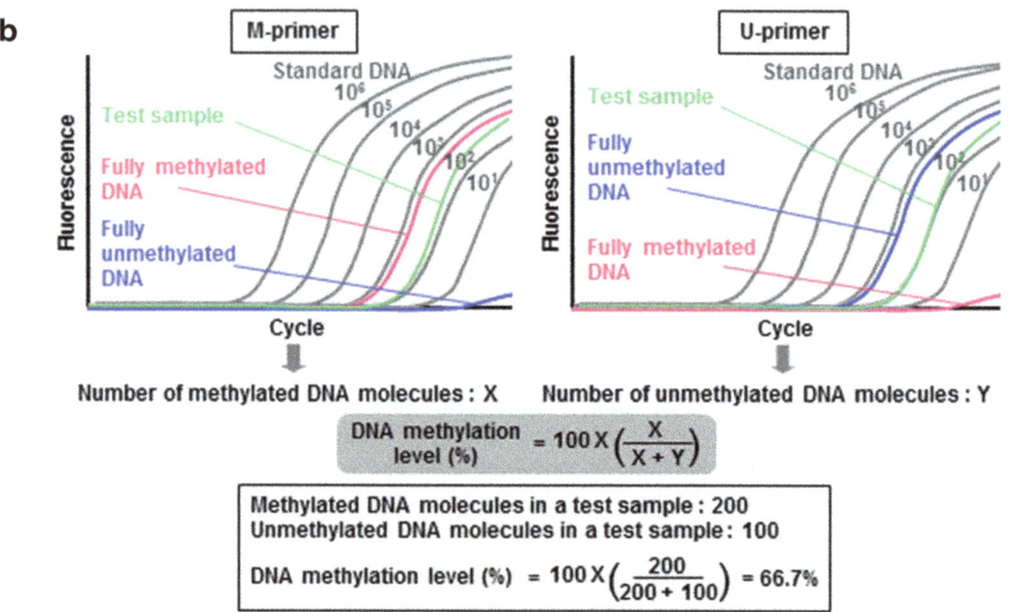

Fig. 3 Principle of MSP and strategies for quantifying methylation levels. (**a**) Principles of quantitative MSP. Methylation statuses at several CpG sites within primer sequences are evaluated by performing PCR with primers specific to methylated or unmethylated sequence (M-primer and U-primer). Methylated and unmethylated CpG sites are shown with *closed* and *open circles*, respectively. (**b**) Quantification of methylated and unmethylated DNA molecules using standard DNA samples. A test sample, control DNA samples (fully methylated DNA and fully unmethylated DNA), and standard DNA samples are amplified with M-primer or U-primer. Numbers of methylated or unmethylated DNA molecules can be quantified by comparing the amplification curve of the test sample with those of standard DNA samples containing known numbers of DNA molecules. Methylation level is calculated using the following formula; methylation level (%) $= 100 \times$ (number of methylated DNA molecules)/(number of methylated DNA molecules + number of unmethylated DNA molecules)

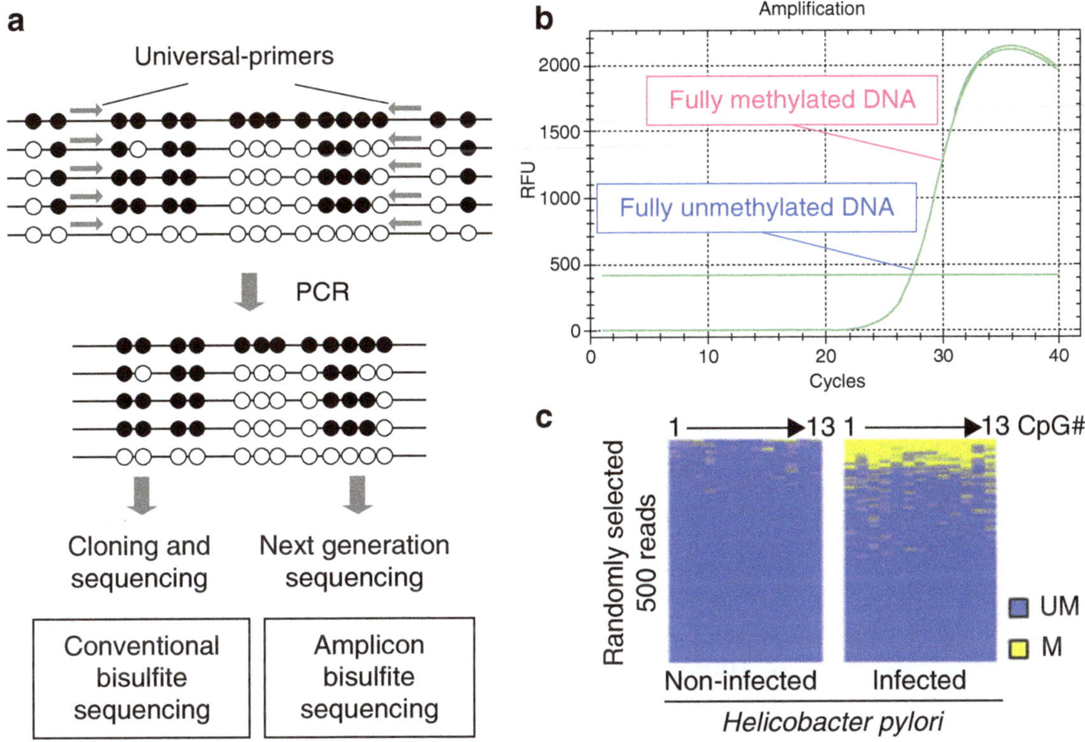

Fig. 4 Bisulfite sequencing. (**a**) Principle of bisulfite sequencing. Bisulfite-converted DNA is amplified by PCR with primers covering no CpG sites (universal-primers). For conventional bisulfite sequencing, the PCR product is cloned and then individual clones are sequenced. Combining this method with next-generation sequencing is known as amplicon bisulfite sequencing, which leads to more accurate assessment of methylation levels. (**b**) Optimization of bisulfite sequencing. The influence of primers on PCR efficiency was examined by amplifying fully methylated DNA and fully unmethylated DNA by real-time PCR. (**c**) Representative data of amplicon bisulfite sequencing. Amplicon bisulfite sequencing can evaluate DNA methylation level of numerous DNA clones. Aberrant methylation of a CpG island was induced by *Helicobacter pylori* infection in gastric mucosae of Mongolian gerbil. The data was adopted from our previous report [11]

2.1.1 Conventional Protocol for Bisulfite-Mediated Conversion

1. 6 M NaOH: Prepare fresh. Dissolve 3 g of NaOH (pellet) in 12.1 mL of distilled water. This will make 15 mL of 6 M NaOH.
2. Sodium metabisulfite ($Na_2S_2O_5$).
3. 4.04 M sodium bisulfate ($NaHSO_3$): Prepare fresh. Dissolve 1.92 g of sodium metabisulfite in 4.4 mL of distilled water. This will make 5 mL of 4.04 M $NaHSO_3$.
4. 10 mM hydroquinone (HQ): Prepare fresh. Dissolve 11 mg of hydroquinone in 10 mL of distilled water. This will make 10 mL of 10 mM HQ.
5. 1 μg of genomic DNA (*see* **Note 1**).
6. Thermal cycler.
7. DNA Purification kit, and 80% ethanol.

8. 1× Tris-EDTA (TE) buffer (pH 8.0): 10 mM Tris–HCl (pH 8.0) and 1 mM EDTA (pH 8.0).

2.1.2 Bisulfite-Mediated Conversion Using a Kit

1. EZ DNA Methylation™ Kit (*see* **Note 2**).
2. 1 μg of genomic DNA (*see* **Note 1**).
3. Thermal cycler.

2.2 Preparation of Control DNA

PCR conditions, including optimal primers and the optimal annealing temperature, should be determined using fully methylated and fully unmethylated DNA controls [12].

2.2.1 Preparation of Fully Unmethylated DNA

1. Genomic DNA from normal cells, such as blood DNA, from a healthy individual.
2. Illustra GenomiPhi HY Kit.
3. Sample Buffer and Reaction Buffer: Supplied with GenomiPhi HY Kit.
4. Phenol, saturated with TE buffer (pH 7.9).
5. Chloroform.
6. 100%/70% ethanol.
7. 1× Tris–EDTA (TE) buffer (pH 8.0): 10 mM Tris–HCl (pH 8.0) and 1 mM EDTA (pH 8.0).
8. 3 M sodium acetate, pH 5.2.

2.2.2 Preparation of Fully Methylated DNA

1. CpG methyltransferase (M. *Sss*I).
2. 200× *S*-Adenosylmethionine [SAM] (*see* **Note 3**). Supplied with *Sss*I methylase.
3. 10× *Sss*I buffer (*see* **Note 4**): 500 mM NaCl, 100 mM Tris–HCl (pH 7.9), and 100 mM EDTA.

2.3 Preparation of Standard DNA for Quantitative MSP

To estimate the degree of DNA degradation during bisulfite conversion and to quantify DNA methylation levels by quantitative MSP, standard DNA with known numbers of DNA molecules is necessary (Fig. 3b). This sample can be prepared in two ways. First, the PCR product can be conveniently purified with a gel-filtration column to remove unreacted nucleotides and primers. Second, the PCR product is cloned into a plasmid, and the plasmid is linearized by a restriction enzyme to produce accurate amounts of standard DNA. Because the protocol for standard DNA is not specific for quantitative MSP but is widely used for real-time PCR, we do not provide the detailed protocol.

2.4 Quantitative MSP

1. AmpliTaq Gold (*see* **Note 5**).
2. 10× PCR and dNTPs: Supplied with AmpliTaq Gold.
3. SYBR Green I: Prepare by dissolving 10,000× concentrate SYBR® Green I in DMSO. Dispense into small aliquots in light-shielding tubes, and store at −20 °C.
4. Real-time PCR machine.

2.5 Bisulfite Sequencing

Bisulfite-converted DNA is amplified by PCR using primers located in genomic regions lacking CpG sites. In conventional bisulfite sequencing, the PCR product is sequenced after cloning. In amplicon bisulfite sequencing, the PCR product is used to prepare a library for next-generation sequencing.

2.5.1 Conventional Bisulfite Sequencing

1. AmpliTaq Gold (*see* **Note 5**).
2. 10× PCR and dNTPs: Supplied with AmpliTaq Gold.
3. PCR cloning kit: e.g., pGEM®-T Easy Vector Systems.
4. Competent *Escherichia coli*: e.g., XL1-blue.
5. Agar medium for transformation containing IPTG, X-gal, and appropriate antibiotics.
6. Reagents and equipment for Sanger sequencing.
7. Web tool for analysis of methylation data: e.g., QUMA (http://quma.cdb.riken.jp/top/index.html); BiQ Analyzer (http://biq-analyzer.bioinf.mpi-inf.mpg.de).

2.5.2 Amplicon Bisulfite Sequencing Using a Next-Generation Sequencer

1. AmpliTaq Gold: (*see* **Note 5**).
2. 10× PCR and dNTPs: Supplied with AmpliTaq Gold.
3. Purification kit of PCR product.
4. Reagents for a DNA library preparation: Depends on the next-generation sequencer platform being used.
5. Tool to map bisulfite-converted sequence reads and determine cytosine methylation status: e.g., Bismark (Babraham Bioinformatics) (https://www.bioinformatics.babraham.ac.uk/projects/bismark/).

3 Methods

3.1 Bisulfite-Mediated Conversion

During bisulfite-mediated conversion, DNA degradation is induced and the number of DNA molecules that can serve as a PCR template decreases to 5–10% of the original DNA [13]. Therefore, two important issues in bisulfite-mediated conversion are (1) avoiding DNA degradation as much as possible and (2) achieving complete conversion of unmethylated cytosine to uracil.

3.1.1 Conventional Protocol for Bisulfite-Mediated DNA Conversion

1. Prepare the following reaction mixture. This will make 120 μL of solution (3.6 M sodium bisulfite and 0.6 mM HQ, pH 5.0).

4.04 M sodium bisulfite	107 μL
10 mM HQ	7 μL
6 M NaOH	6 μL

2. Add 1 μL of 6 M NaOH to 19 μL of a DNA solution containing 1 μg of DNA.
3. To denature DNA, incubate at 37 °C for 15 min.
4. Add the reaction mixture prepared in **step 1** to the denatured DNA solution.
5. Incubate the sample under condition of 15 cycles of 30 s at 95 °C and 15 min at 50 °C.
6. To purify the converted DNA using a Zymo-spin column, transfer the DNA solution to a new tube.
7. Add 600 μL of M-Binding Buffer and then mix.
8. Load the sample into a Zymo-spin column and centrifuge at full speed for 1 min. Discard the flow-through. Repeat this step to centrifuge the remaining sample.
9. Add 200 μL of 80% ethanol and centrifuge at full speed for 1 min. Discard the flow-through.
10. For desulfonation, prepare the following mixture of NaOH and ethanol.

Distilled water	10 μL
100% ethanol	100 μL
6 M NaOH	1.7 μL

11. Add 100 μL of the mixture of NaOH and ethanol and let the mixture stand at room temperature for 15 min.
12. After incubation, centrifuge at full speed for 1 min.
13. Add 200 μL of 80% ethanol and centrifuge at full speed for 1 min. Discard the flow-through.
14. Add another 200 μL of 80% ethanol and centrifuge for an additional 3 min. Remove the 80% ethanol completely.
15. Place the column into a 1.5 mL tube. Add 22 μL of TE Buffer directly to the column and let the tube stand at room temperature for 1 min.
16. To elute the DNA, centrifuge at full speed for 1 min.
17. Repeat **steps 15** and **16**.
18. The DNA can be stored at −20 °C (*see* **Note 6**).

3.1.2 Bisulfite-Mediated Conversion Using a Kit

Bisulfite-mediated conversion and DNA purification should be conducted according to the manufacture's protocol. The storage condition of the converted DNA is important (*see* **Note 6**).

3.2 Preparation of Control DNA (Fully Unmethylated and Fully Methylated DNA)

Fully unmethylated DNA is prepared by amplifying normal cell DNA, such as blood DNA from a healthy individual, 1000 times twice with the GenomiPhi DNA amplification system. Because DNA methylation is not introduced during in vitro amplification, amplification by 10^6 times eliminates virtually all DNA methylation in the original DNA from normal cells.

Fully methylated DNA should be prepared from the fully unmethylated DNA using *Sss*I methylase. This will eliminate the concern that fully unmethylated and methylated DNA are present in different copy numbers at individual genomic loci.

3.2.1 Preparation of Fully Unmethylated DNA

1. Prepare the DNA solution by adding of 10 ng of genomic DNA in 2.5–22.5 μL of Sample Buffer.
2. Incubate at 95 °C for 3 min to denature the DNA and then place the sample on ice immediately.
3. Prepare the following enzyme mixture.

Reaction buffer	22.5 μL
Enzyme mix	2.5 μL

4. Mix the DNA solution (**step 1**) and enzyme mixture.
5. Incubate the mixture at 30 °C for 4 h.
6. Place the mixture at 65 °C for 10 min to inactivate the enzyme.
7. Perform phenol extraction twice and chloroform extraction twice and then precipitate the DNA by ethanol precipitation.
8. Dissolve the pellet in 100 μL of TE.
9. Quantify the DNA concentration.
10. Repeat **steps 1–7**. Prepare multiple tubes for reaction.
11. Dissolve the pellet in 30 μL of TE.
12. Quantify the DNA concentration (*see* **Note 7**).

3.2.2 Preparation of Fully Methylated DNA

1. Prepare the following reaction mixture.

GenomiPhi-amplified DNA	20 μg
32 mM SAM (thaw fresh)	1.5 μL
*Sss*I methylase (4 U/μL)	15 μL

Nuclease-free water to a final volume of 300 μL

2. Incubate at 37 °C for 15 min.

3. Add 1.5 μL of 32 mM SAM and 15 μL of *Sss*I methylase.
4. Incubate at 37 °C for 1 h.
5. Extract DNA with phenol twice, chloroform twice, and ethanol precipitation.
6. After ethanol precipitation, dissolve the DNA pellet in 50 μL of TE.
7. Repeat **steps 1–5**.
8. Dissolve the DNA pellet in 50 μL of TE.
9. Quantify the solution.

3.3 Primer Design for MSP

Primers (M-primer to amplify methylated DNA and U-primer to amplify unmethylated DNA) can be designed using software [e.g., Methyl Primer Express® (Applied Biosystems) (www.appliedbiosystems.jp/website/methylprimerexpress.html), BiSearch (http://bisearch.enzim.hu), MethPrimer (http://www.urogene.org/cgi-bin/methprimer)].

The following issues should be noted for the design of primers with high specificity using a top strand. If designing good primers using the top strand is difficult, the bottom strand can be used. However, note that C (or T) recognized by a specific primer will shift from C to G at a CpG site.

- Length of PCR product: 85–150 bp.
- 3′ terminal of upper primer: C at a CpG site.
- 3′ terminal of lower primer: G at a CpG site.
- G + C content before bisulfite conversion: 50%.
- Number of CpG sites: 2–5 sites per primer.
- M- and U-primers are ideally located at the same positions, but may be shifted to share some positions.

3.4 Optimization of Real-Time MSP

Quantitative MSP enables accurate, sensitive, and quantitative assessment of DNA methylation levels. Under appropriate conditions, DNA methylation levels obtained by quantitative MSP show $\leq$20% variation in the methylation level. The specificity of M-primers and U-primers is the most important issue. The annealing temperature and magnesium ion concentration should be optimized using fully methylated and fully unmethylated DNA controls (Fig. 3b).

1. Prepare the reaction mixture. Fully methylated and fully unmethylated DNA samples are used as template DNA.

10× PCR buffer (15 mM $MgCl_2$)	5 μL
2 mM dNTPs	5 μL (final conc. 0.2 mM)
10 μM Forward primer	1 μL (final conc. 0.2 μM)
10 μM Reverse primer	1 μL (final conc. 0.2 μM)
AmpliTaq Gold (5 U/μL)	0.2 μL
Bisulfite-converted DNA	1 μL
SYBR Green I	0.1 μL

Nuclease-free water to a final volume of 50 μL

2. Perform the PCR under the following condition (*see* **Note 8**).

Stage	Step	Temperature	Time
Holding	Initial denaturation	95 °C	10 min
Cycling (×40)	Denaturation	95 °C	30 s
	Annealing	53–60 °C	30 s
	Extension	72 °C	30 s
Cycling	Dissociation	50 → 95 °C	

3. Determine an optimal condition based on the amplification curve (Fig. 3b) and melting curve. The amplification curve under appropriate conditions shows a steep increase during an early PCR cycle, and a flat plateau for target methylated (or unmethylated) DNA. The derivative of the melting curve of the target DNA should show a single sharp peak. Non-target DNA should not be amplified in early cycles, and the derivative of PCR products produced in late cycles, if any, should not overlap with that of the target DNA.
4. The PCR product showing good amplification can be used as the template for standard DNA.

3.5 Quantitative MSP Using Test Samples

DNA methylation level of test samples can be estimated by real-time MSP using standard DNAs, test samples, control DNA samples (fully methylated DNA and fully unmethylated DNA), and a negative control (nuclease-free water).

1. Prepare the reaction mixture. PCR should be performed separately using M-primer or U-primer, which may require different conditions.

10× PCR buffer (15 mM $MgCl_2$)	5 μL
2 mM dNTPs	5 μL (final conc. 0.2 mM)
10 μM Forward primer	1 μL (final conc. 0.2 μM)
10 μM Reverse primer	1 μL (final conc. 0.2 μM)
AmpliTaq Gold (5 U/μL)	0.2 μL
Bisulfite-converted DNA	1 μL
SYBR Green I	0.1 μL

Nuclease-free water to a final volume of 50 μL

2. Perform the PCR under the following condition.

Stage	Step	Temperature	Time
Holding	Initial denaturation	95 °C	10 min
Cycling (×40)	Denaturation	95 °C	30 s
	Annealing	x °C[a]	30 s
	Extension	72 °C	30 s
Cycling	Dissociation	50 → 95 °C	

[a]The annealing temperature is determined in Subheading 3.4.

3. Make a calibration curve using standard DNA samples.
4. Calculate the absolute copy number of test samples by comparing the amplification curve of the test samples with those of standard DNA samples. Methylation level is calculated using the following formula;

$$\text{Methylation level } (\%) = 100 \times (\text{number of methylated DNA molecules}) / (\text{number of methylated DNA molecules} + \text{number of unmethylated DNA molecules}).$$

3.6 Primer Design for Bisulfite Sequencing

The primers for bisulfite sequencing can be designed using software [e.g., Methyl Primer Express®, BiSearch (http://bisearch.enzim.hu), MethPrimer (http://www.urogene.org/cgi-bin/methprimer)].

The following issues should be noted for designing primers with high specificity:

- No CpG sites in the primer sequence.
- Inclusion of C of the original DNA in the primer sequence.
- The length of primer: 25–40 mer.
- G + C contents before bisulfite conversion: ~40%.
- Length of the PCR product: 100–300 bp.

3.7 Optimization of PCR for Bisulfite Sequencing

For bisulfite sequencing, depending on the PCR conditions, PCR bias may lead to preferential amplification of either unmethylated or methylated DNA [14]. To avoid PCR bias, a PCR condition that amplifies fully methylated and fully unmethylated DNA controls equally should be established by selecting optimal primers and an optimal annealing temperature (Fig. 3b). Additionally, PCR cycles should be minimized if a sufficient amount of PCR product for cloning is obtained. Excessive PCR cycles cause denaturation of the PCR product in the absence of Taq polymerase activity and produce an amplification of chimeric products not present in the template DNA. Excessive PCR cycles also exaggerate the differences in PCR efficiency between methylated and unmethylated DNA.

To optimize PCR condition and cycles, real-time PCR is preferable using fully methylated and fully unmethylated DNA as template DNA.

1. Prepare the following reaction mixture.

10× PCR buffer (15 mM $MgCl_2$)	5 μL
2 mM dNTPs	5 μL (final conc. 0.2 mM)
10 μM Forward primer	1 μL (final conc. 0.2 μM)
10 μM Reverse primer	1 μL (final conc. 0.2 μM)
AmpliTaq Gold (5 U/μL)	0.2 μL
Bisulfite-converted DNA	1 μL
SYBR Green I	0.1 μL

Nuclease-free water to a final volume of 50 μL

2. Perform the PCR under the following conditions (*see* **Note 8**).

Stage	Step	Temperature	Time
Holding	Initial denaturation	95 °C	10 min
Cycling (×40)	Denaturation	95 °C	30 s
	Annealing	53–60 °C	30 s
	Extension	72 °C	30 s
Cycling	Dissociation	50 → 95 °C	

3.8 Bisulfite Sequencing and Data Analysis

3.8.1 Conventional Protocol for Bisulfite Sequencing

1. After determining the best PCR conditions, perform PCR using the sample.
2. For cloning, mix the reactions by pipetting.

2× Rapid Ligation Buffer, T4 DNA Ligase	5 μL
50 ng pGEM®-T East Vector	0.2 μL
PCR product	3.8 μL
T4 DNA Ligase	1.0 μL

Nuclease-free water to a final volume of 10 μL

3. Incubate the reactions for 1 h at room temperature.
4. Transform high-efficiency competent cells (e.g., XL1-blue).
5. After overnight incubation, pick at least 24 white colonies.
6. Isolate the plasmid DNA and sequence the DNA with a Sanger sequencer.
7. Analyze DNA methylation status by comparing the sequencing data with the sequence before bisulfite conversion. This comparison can be automatically conducted using web tools.

3.8.2 Protocol for Amplicon Bisulfite Sequencing Using a Next-Generation Sequencer

1. Perform PCR using a sample and stop the PCR before the amplification reaches a plateau.
2. Purify the PCR products following the manufacturer's protocol.
3. Prepare a DNA library using the reagents for a next-generation sequencer.
4. Perform sequencing with a next-generation sequencer.
5. Convert the sequences obtained to CpG methylation statuses using a tool such as Bismark.
6. Calculate the fraction of methylated molecules in the total number of DNA molecules (methylated molecules plus unmethylated molecules).

4 Notes

1. Quantify after restriction digestion (avoid a site that affects PCR using your primers) and removal of RNA by RNase A treatment. Fragmented or low-grade DNA does not require digestion by a restriction enzyme.
2. Among commercially available kits, we found this kit to be most suitable by assessing both the maintenance of DNA integrity (number of DNA molecules remaining as a PCR template) and conversion efficiency (rate of conversion of unmethylated cytosines to uracils).
3. Dispense into 5 μL of aliquot after the first melting of a purchased solution and store at −80 °C because SAM is very unstable. Do not use again after melting the aliquot.
4. This buffer is more effective than the buffer provided by the manufacture.
5. The most suitable polymerase may differ depending on the G + C content and length of the regions analyzed, and several enzymes should be tested.
6. Bisulfite-converted DNA should be stored at −20 °C. To avoid repeated freeze-thaw cycles, DNA should be aliquoted.

7. Because the DNA amplified using this kit does not contain methylated cytosine, it can be used as fully unmethylated DNA. This kit amplifies approximately 5 ng DNA into approximately 5 μg DNA. We typically perform the amplification step twice to dilute methylated DNA in the original DNA sufficiently and to obtain a large amount of DNA. If the amount of DNA after amplification is less than expected, amplification can be performed using another 5 ng DNA.
8. The annealing temperature can be estimated based on the Tm of each primer set. However, we recommend performing gradient PCR using a 2 °C difference to determine the optimal annealing temperature.

References

1. Ushijima T (2005) Detection and interpretation of altered methylation patterns in cancer cells. Nat Rev Cancer 5:223–231
2. Feinberg AP, Koldobskiy MA, Gondor A (2016) Epigenetic modulators, modifiers and mediators in cancer aetiology and progression. Nat Rev Genet 17:284–299
3. Hattori N, Ushijima T (2016) Epigenetic impact of infection on carcinogenesis: mechanisms and applications. Genome Med 8:10
4. Ushijima T (2007) Epigenetic field for cancerization. J Biochem Mol Biol 40:142–150
5. Asada K, Nakajima T, Shimazu T et al (2015) Demonstration of the usefulness of epigenetic cancer risk prediction by a multicentre prospective cohort study. Gut 64:388–396
6. Maeda M, Nakajima T, Oda I et al (2017) High impact of methylation accumulation on metachronous gastric cancer: 5-year follow-up of a multicentre prospective cohort study. Gut 66 (9):1721–1723
7. Hayatsu H, Wataya Y, Kazushige K (1970) The addition of sodium bisulfite to uracil and to cytosine. J Am Chem Soc 92:724–726
8. Herman JG, Graff JR, Myohanen S et al (1996) Methylation-specific PCR: a novel PCR assay for methylation status of CpG islands. Proc Natl Acad Sci U S A 93:9821–9826
9. Clark SJ, Harrison J, Paul CL et al (1994) High sensitivity mapping of methylated cytosines. Nucleic Acids Res 22:2990–2997
10. Bock C, Halbritter F, Carmona FJ et al (2016) Quantitative comparison of DNA methylation assays for biomarker development and clinical applications. Nat Biotechnol 34:726–737
11. Takeshima H, Niwa T, Toyoda T et al (2017) Degree of methylation burden is determined by the exposure period to carcinogenic factors. Cancer Sci 108:316–321
12. Warnecke PM, Stirzaker C, Song J, Grunau C, Melki JR, Clark SJ (2002) Identification and resolution of artifacts in bisulfite sequencing. Methods 27:101–107
13. Munson K, Clark J, Lamparska-Kupsik K et al (2007) Recovery of bisulfite-converted genomic sequences in the methylation-sensitive QPCR. Nucleic Acids Res 35:2893–2903
14. Shen L, Guo Y, Chen X, Ahmed S, Issa JJ (2007) Optimizing annealing temperature overcomes bias in bisulfite PCR methylation analysis. BioTechniques 42:48–58

Chapter 17

A Comprehensive Protocol Resource for Performing Pooled shRNA and CRISPR Screens

Leonie A. Cluse, Iva Nikolic, Deborah Knight, Piyush B. Madhamshettiwar, Jennii Luu, Karla J. Cowley, Timothy Semple, Gisela Mir Arnau, Jake Shortt, Ricky W. Johnstone, and Kaylene J. Simpson

Abstract

This chapter details a compendium of protocols that collectively enable the reader to perform a pooled shRNA and/or CRISPR screen—with methods to identify and validate positive controls and subsequent hits; establish a viral titer in the cell line of choice; create and screen libraries, sequence strategies, and bioinformatics resources to analyze outcomes. Collectively, this provides an overarching resource from the start to finish of a screening project, making this technology possible in all laboratories.

Key words Pooled shRNA, Pooled CRISPR, Lentivirus, Drop out screen

1 Introduction

This collection of protocols is designed to provide the reader with sufficient resources to be able to perform a pooled short hairpin RNA (shRNA) or CRISPR screen, to identify hits from these screens through bioinformatics strategies and to validate the targets identified from the screen in a high throughput manner. There are many published screens available, but the fine detail is often lost in a mainstream publication where the biological consequences of depletion or deletion of the target genes is more important. Screens such as these are quite complex to perform, particularly on a large scale but represent the direction many laboratories are taking to discover new targets for the biological process under investigation. The protocols presented here were derived whilst performing a comparative shRNA versus CRISPR screen study to identify genes regulating cell viability in OPM-2 cells, a human multiple myeloma cell line. The libraries used represent a boutique collection of genes

Leonie A. Cluse and Iva Nikolic contributed equally to this work.

Brendan J. Jenkins (ed.), *Inflammation and Cancer: Methods and Protocols*, Methods in Molecular Biology, vol. 1725, https://doi.org/10.1007/978-1-4939-7568-6_17, © Springer Science+Business Media, LLC 2018

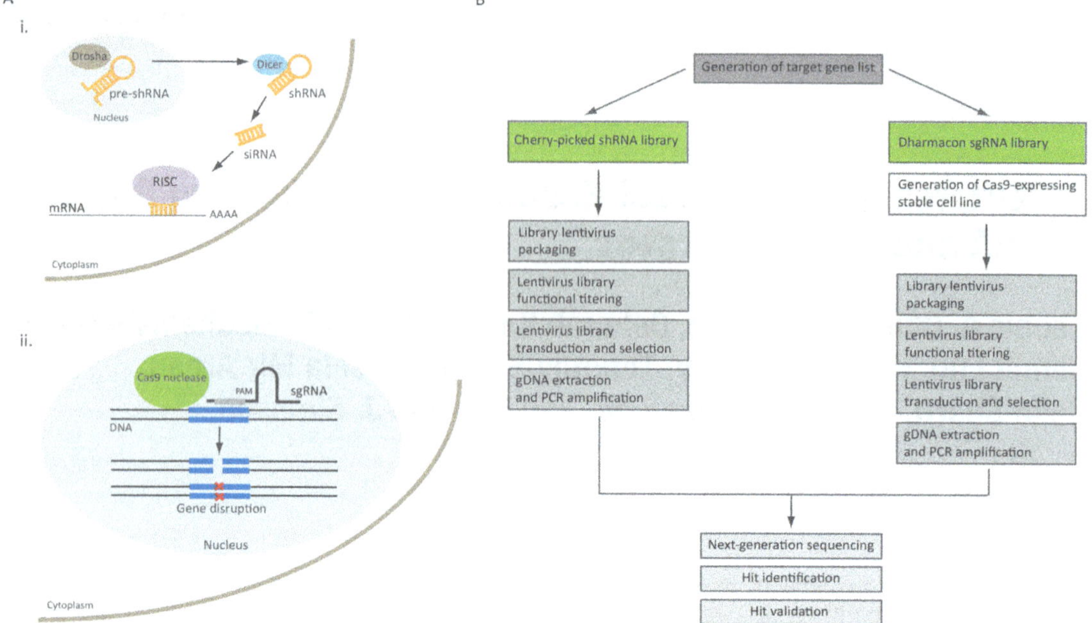

Fig. 1 Basic principles of shRNA and CRISPR screening. (**a**) shRNA and CRISPR are complementary technologies with fundamentally different mode of action. (*i*) Upon transcription in the nucleus a short hairpin RNA (shRNA) undergoes a series of enzymatic steps until it is processed into a short double stranded molecule (siRNA). The sense (passenger) strand is degraded, and the antisense (guide) strand is loaded into the RNA-induced silencing complex (RISC) and directed to mRNA that has a complementary sequence. RISC either cleaves the mRNA or represses its translation. (*ii*) CRISPR system, in contrast, operates directly on target DNA locus. Target specific single-guide RNA (sgRNA) navigates the CAS9 nuclease to the DNA locus of interest, which subsequently introduces a double-stranded break 3 bp upstream of its recognition site (PAM sequence). The cell then launches a double-stranded break repair mechanism, which in most cases introduces short insertions and deletions (indels) in the target locus thus subsequently disrupting gene translation. (**b**) The scheme outlines a workflow of performed pooled shRNA and CRISPR screens

the research team had identified through their own work, through association of pathways with the disease model and through reviews of the literature.

We chose to screen both shRNA and CRISPR resources as the implications of gene depletion versus complete gene deletion were unknown (Fig. 1a). In addition, recent publications suggest that CRISPR screens lead to less biological variation thus simplifying hit calling [1], but also that CRISPR and shRNA technologies act in a complementary manner revealing different aspects of cell biology [2].

The basic steps in setting up a pooled screen (Fig. 1b) include (1) obtaining/designing a pooled library; (2) lentivirus packaging and titration of pooled library; (3) lentivirus library transduction and selection; (4) genomic DNA (gDNA) extraction and PCR amplification; (5) next-generation sequencing (NGS) of amplified DNA libraries; (6) bioinformatics analysis of sequencing data for hit identification; and (7) hit validation. Here we describe in detail each of the steps and provide associated protocols together with extensive notes and discussion on issues we encountered.

Conceptual considerations for setting up an shRNA screen and a CRISPR screen are largely the same (Fig. 1b), with an added step of creating Cas9 expressing cells in CRISPR screens. We therefore structured the Subheading 3 accordingly: key considerations and basic protocols are described through setting up an shRNA screen with additional steps and/or differences pertaining to the CRISPR arm of the experiment. As CRISPR technology is advancing rapidly, the CRISPR screening-associated protocols have been further optimized and improved compared with the earlier shRNA screening pipeline, which is described in detail in the Subheading 4.

Finally, key to any successful screen is the choice of cell line(s). This set of protocols is focused on screening OPM-2 cells, a human myeloma line that grows in suspension [3]. The protocols provided are equally adaptable to cells grown in adherent culture. It is important to note here that cell lines display varying levels of transducibility, and difficult-to-transduce cell lines may not be the best choice for performing a pooled screen, especially at a genome-wide level. The aim of this compendium is to guide you through these considerations to design the most effective screen for your experimental conditions and biological question asked.

2 Materials

2.1 General Cell Culture

All cells are grown under standard incubator conditions of 37 °C with 5% CO_2 unless otherwise indicated. We recommend undertaking short-tandem repeat (STR) profiling of the cell line(s) used for screening to ensure you are working with the correct genetic line from the outset. We also recommend routine mycoplasma testing of the cell lines. When producing virus or transducing cells from commercial virus, you must ensure you are working under appropriate Institute Biosafety guidelines for the safe and effective work and virus disposal.

1. HEK293T complete medium: Dulbecco's Modified Eagle's Medium (DMEM), 20 mM HEPES, 10% Tet-free fetal bovine serum (FBS).
2. OPM-2 complete medium: Roswell Park Memorial Institute (RPMI) 1640, 10% FBS, 1× sodium pyruvate, 1× penicillin-–streptomycin, 1× GlutaMAX.

2.2 Pooled shRNA and sgRNA Libraries

1. GIPZ human whole genome shRNA library (GE Dharmacon).
2. Generation of plasmid DNA (single shRNA construct or pooled) for virus production: grow bacteria taken from glycerol stocks in standard LB-Lennox broth with 100 μg/mL

carbenicillin selection for 21 h at 37 °C in a bacterial shaker at 200 rpm.

3. QIAGEN Plasmid Maxi Kit.
4. Custom Edit-R lentiviral sgRNA pooled lentivirus library (GE Dharmacon).

2.3 Virus Production Reagents

1. 1 mg/mL polyethylenimine (PEI) stock: Heat ultrapure water to 80 °C and add 50 mg of PEI powder in 50 mL of water. Stir until all powder is dissolved. Set pH to 7.4 using drops of concentrated HCl and store at −20 °C in 10 mL aliquots. Keep a working stock at 4 °C. If the 4 °C stock or the freshly thawed stock precipitates, place the solution at 37 °C to redissolve. Stock can be maintained at 4 °C indefinitely provided no precipitation occurs. We recommend testing every new batch before using it in an actual experiment.
2. Lenti-X HTX Packaging Mix 2.
3. Sequa-brene.
4. The nontargeting control in the pGIPZ backbone sequence: 5′-ATCTCGCTTGGGCGAGAGTAAG-3′.

2.4 Screening Reagents

1. Annexin V/PI staining solution: 1:100 dilution of Annexin V-APC and Propidium Iodide (PI) in Annexin binding buffer.
2. Annexing binding buffer: 10 mM HEPES, 140 mM NaCl, 5 M $CaCl_2$.
3. Puromycin dihydrochloride.
4. DNeasy Blood & Tissue kit.

2.5 Next-Generation Sequencing Associated Reagents

1. Phusion HSII Polymerase.
2. Taq Polymerase.
3. UltraPure DNase/RNase-Free Distilled Water.
4. 5 M Betaine solution, PCR grade.
5. NucleoSpin Gel and PCR clean-up kit.
6. Agencourt AMPure XP.
7. HiSeq® Rapid SR Cluster Kit v2.
8. HiSeq® Rapid SBS Kit v2.
9. NextSeq® 500 High Output v2 Kit.
10. D1000 Screen Tape (Agilent Genomics).
11. D1000 Reagents (Agilent Genomics).
12. Qubit dsDNA HS Assay Kit.

2.6 Consumables/ Equipment

1. 96-well cell culture multiwell plate.
2. 24-well cell culture multiwell plate.

3. 6-well cell culture multiwell plate.
4. 96-well PCR plates.
5. 96-well deep well plate.
6. T175 cm^2 and T75 cm^2 tissue culture flasks.
7. Flow cytometry tubes.
8. Polycarbonate bottles with cap assembly, 26.3 mL volume.
9. Optima L-100XP Ultracentrifuge, rotor 70Ti.
10. FACSVerse flow cytometer.
11. FACSAria Fusion cell sorter.
12. TapeStation 2200.
13. NanoDrop 2000 UV-Vis Spectrophotometer.
14. Qubit 2.0 Fluorometer.
15. HiSeq 2500.
16. NextSeq 500.

3 Methods

3.1 Creating a Boutique shRNA Pooled Screening Library or Individual shRNA Constructs

The Victorian Centre for Functional Genomics (VCFG) maintains a pGIPZ-shRNA-miR30 shRNA library as individual constructs in arrayed format to create boutique pooled libraries or work with individual genes. The pGIPZ-shRNA-miR30 vector has a turbo GFP reporter and puromycin selectable marker. The shRNA constructs are maintained as individual glycerol stocks in 96-well plate format and are cherry picked manually using a p200 disposable tip to scrape a small crystal into 96-well deep well plates containing 1 mL of LB-Lennox medium containing carbenicillin. Plates are left shaking for 21 h (200 rpm) in an aerated 37 °C bacterial shaker. To create a pooled library, on a per plate basis, 500 μL of each well is removed and pooled. The remaining 500 μL of culture is used to generate a glycerol stock source plate for future use (rather than returning to the primary library plates) by adding 500 μL of glycerol. The pooled culture is pelleted and DNA extracted using a maxi-prep kit as per manufacturer's recommendations.

3.2 Lentivirus Packaging of Pooled Library

The pGIPZ vector is *tat* dependent, therefore a packaging system that expresses the *tat* gene must be used. For this purpose, we use Lenti-X HTX Packaging Mix, which provides all the necessary lentiviral packaging components in optimized ratios, and enables the generation of high titers of VSV-G pseudotyped lentivirus. It is important to note that the Lenti-X HTX system utilizes Tet-Off transactivation to drive the expression of viral proteins, so medium containing tetracycline-free (Tet-free) serum must be used during viral production.

HEK293T cells must be cultured for at least two passages in Tet-free medium before starting with the virus production to remove all traces of tetracycline.

1. On day 1 (~4:00 pm), seed 12 × 10^6 HEK293T cells per T175 flask in 25 mL of complete medium (*see* Subheading 2.1) and culture overnight at 37 °C with 5% CO_2. Prepare 4× T175 flasks for the pooled shRNA library (*see* **Note 1**).
2. On day 2 (~4:00 pm), prepare a transfection mix for each plasmid, and transfect the cells as follows (volumes are based on each T175 flask): 1.2 mL DMEM with no supplements, 35 μL Lenti-X HTX Packaging Mix, 14 μL of 1 μg/μL pGIPZ construct/pool DNA.
3. Vortex for 10 s at medium speed. Add polyethylenimine solution (PEI; *see* Subheading 2.3) at 4.5 μL per μg of DNA and vortex again for 10 s at medium speed.
4. Incubate at room temperature for 10 min (at this point, a DNA precipitate will form but will not be visible).
5. Add the resulting mixture dropwise to the cells while gently swirling the flasks to evenly distribute the mix.
6. Incubate the cells overnight at 37 °C with 5% CO_2.
7. On day 3 (~9:00 am), aspirate the medium and add 25 mL per T175 cm^2 flask of fresh, complete medium. *At this point live virus is being produced and you must strictly adhere to the viral decontamination rules at your institution until the end of this procedure.*
8. On day 5 (~11:00 am), harvest lentivirus-containing supernatant and concentrate if necessary. Collect the lentivirus-containing supernatant and filter through a 0.45 μm low protein binding filter to remove cell debris. Either aliquot the supernatant and store it at −80 °C, or proceed to concentrate the virus.
9. To concentrate the virus using ultracentrifugation, transfer the supernatant into appropriate ultracentrifuge tubes, weigh carefully and balance them by adding DMEM with no supplements. Use the appropriate rotor and centrifuge the supernatants at 27000 × *g* for 2 h at 20 °C.
10. Slowly decant the supernatant and rest the tubes up-side-down on Kimwipes for 2 min to drain. Try to dry as much medium as possible off the side walls of the tube.
11. Add 600 μL (or sufficient volume to cover the bottom of the tube) of DMEM with no supplements, and incubate for 45 min on a shaker at room temperature. *Make sure to place the tubes on an angle to completely cover the viral pellet.*

12. Complete resuspension by slowly pipetting up and down using a p1000 pipette tip. Virus particles are fragile and should be treated with care.
13. Combine supernatants if working with multiple tubes of same virus and mix well. Aliquot and store at −80 °C (*see* **Note 2**).

3.3 Functional Titering of a Lentiviral Library

Before any screen can commence, you must determine the relative viral titer of the library for each cell line. To be able to deconvolute the screen data and compare the effects of each shRNA, the library must be transduced so that a single hairpin integrates into a single cell. Therefore, the multiplicity of infection (MOI) for cells transduced with a pooled screening approach should be between 0.3–0.5 to ensure that a single integration event occurs in the majority of the cells. Figure 2 shows the relationship between MOI and the % of infected cells carrying a single integrant. The aim of the library functional titering is therefore to determine the amount of virus required to infect ~20–30% of target cells. Below we outline this procedure for OPM-2 cells (suspension cells).

1. On day 1 (~4:00 pm), seed 2×10^4 OPM-2 cells in 100 μL of the complete medium (*see* Subheading 2.1) containing Sequabrene (4 μg/mL final concentration) per well in a 96-well tissue culture plate (*see* **Notes 3–5**). Seed as many wells as needed to test the dilutions outlined below in duplicate.
2. Set up a range of virus dilutions in complete medium: tube one starts at a 1:10 dilution (450 μL media + 50 μL virus) and all

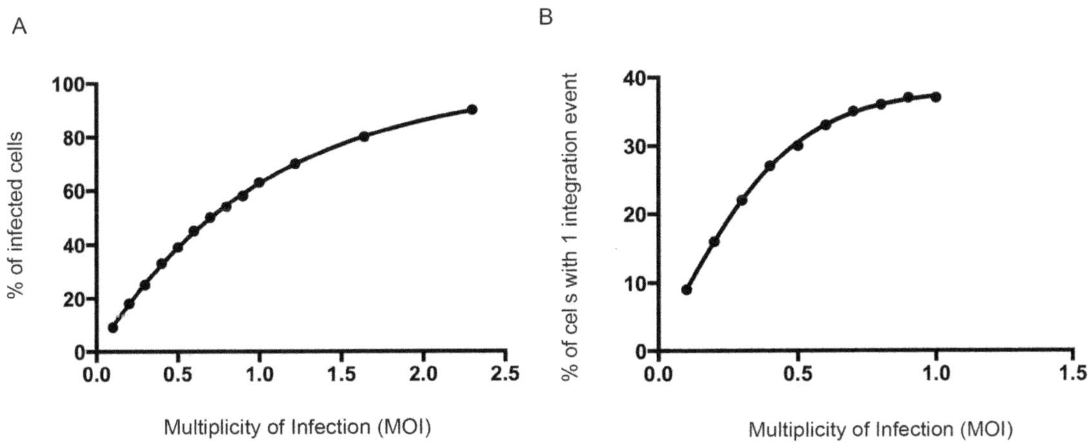

Fig. 2 Pooled library virus transduction and concept of MOI. Multiplicity of Infection (MOI) refers to the ratio of viral particles to the target cells during infection. The actual number of virions transducing the cells, however, is a statistical process: some cells will absorb more than one particle, and some cells will not absorb any virus particles. (**a**) This graph gives a relationship between MOI and % of total cell infection including single-event integration and multiple-event integration. (**b**) This graph gives a relationship between MOI and % of cells infected with a single virus particle. In pooled screens, MOI of 0.3–0.5 is used, which corresponds to 22–30% of cells with a single-integration event

subsequent tubes are serially diluted 1:2 across 11 dilution points.

3. For each dilution, add 100 μL of the virus-containing medium to the cells for a final volume of 200 μL of medium per well (*see* **Note 6**).
4. Incubate the cells for 48 h at 37 °C in 5% CO_2.
5. On day 4, perform FACS analysis. Add propidium iodide (PI—100 ng/mL final concentration) directly in the 96-well plate. Analyze the cells using a FACSVerse plate reader including the following parameters: Forward scatter (FCS), Side-scatter (SSC), GFP expression (FL1), and PI uptake (FL3).
6. Determine the amount of virus required to infect ~20–30% of the cells.

3.4 Performing a Pooled shRNA Screen

In the example of the shRNA and CRISPR screens we outline below, the aim is to identify targets essential for cell viability; these targets therefore should be "lost" over time and statistically lower in representation compared to the starting population. To ensure we can capture the loss of shRNAs or sgRNAs that occur over a defined time frame, we opted to harvest cells at multiple time points post selection (*see* **Note 7**). For the shRNA screen, the cell population carrying the individual hairpins was selected by FACS sorting of GFP positive cells, after which the cells were collected at a T0 time point (4 days post transduction) as well as at three subsequent time points T7, T14, and T21 (Fig. 3). A key factor in performing pooled screens is transducing enough cells to maintain full library representation. In our example, the boutique library contained 1393 shRNAs in total, and we opted to maintain 1000-fold library representation at each step of the screen (*see* **Note 8**). The reason for this is biased library transduction—in reality the representation of the library is not even and the hairpins/guides will not be transduced evenly leaving some overrepresented or underrepresented. To account for this, you should aim to transduce each guide in as many cells as needed to be able to subsequently deconvolute the data and identify true hits. For the same reason, it is important to perform transductions in at least two independent biological replicates. Below we outline a protocol taking into account the above-mentioned factors.

Thaw three vials of the chosen cell line and maintain in culture independently. Passage the cells in T175 cm² flasks to raise sufficient cell numbers for screening.

1. On day 1, perform shRNA library transduction in biological triplicates. Resuspend OPM-2 cells in complete tissue culture medium containing Sequa-brene (4 μg/mL final concentration) at the density of 1×10^5 cells/mL and add 33 mL per T175 cm² flask. For each replicate, plate enough cells to

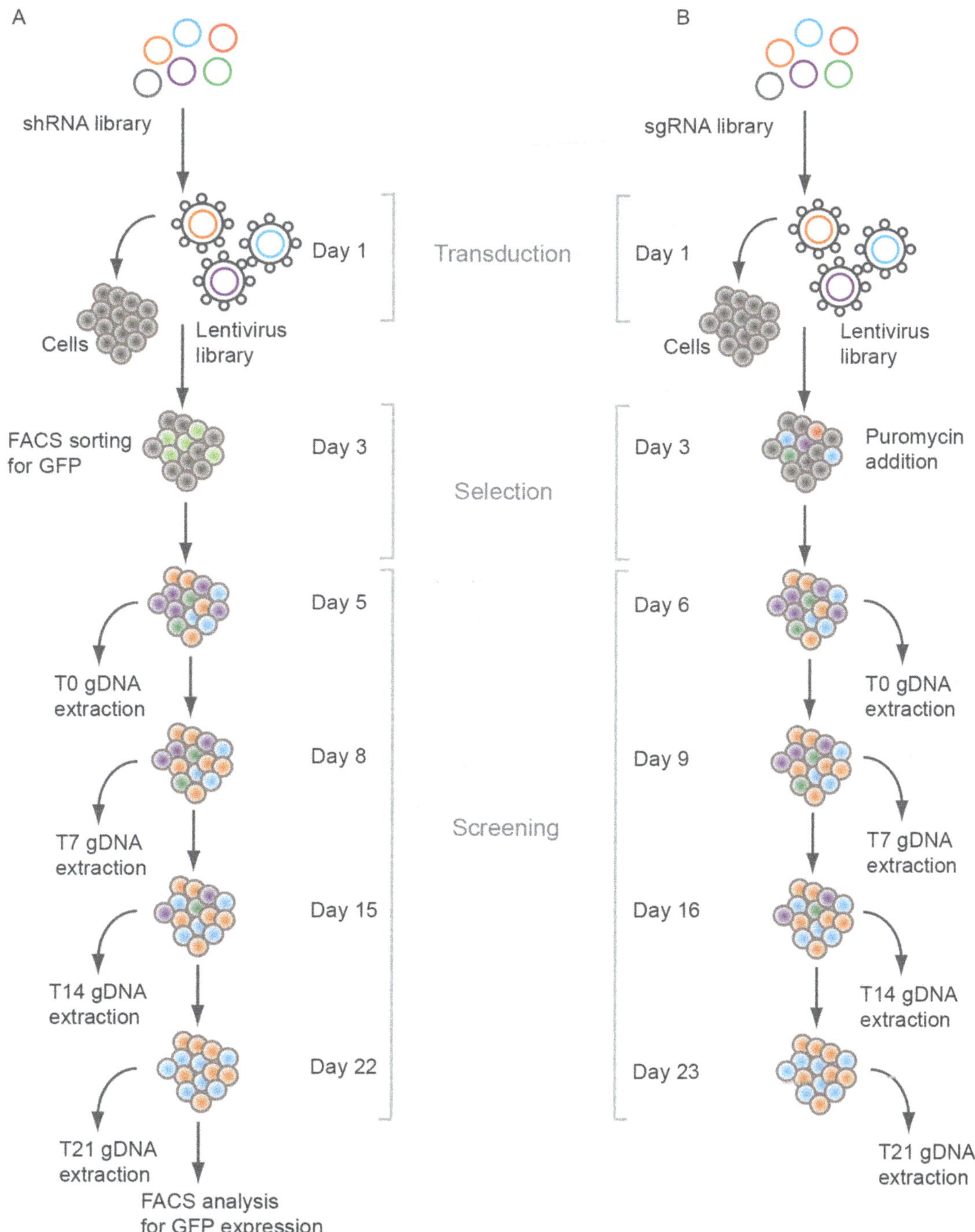

Fig. 3 Overview of sample collection during shRNA and CRISPR screens. (**a**) After shRNA lentivirus library transduction, the infected cells were selected based on GFP expression using FACS sorting and then plated for screening at a cell number equaling 1000-fold library representation. At each collection point (T0, T7, T14, T21), the number of cells collected for gDNA extraction should be equal to 1000-fold library representation and the same number of cells should be plated for further culturing. At the end of the screening process, the remaining cells were FACS analyzed to verify GFP expression. (**b**) The same basic flow was followed for the

achieve 1000-fold library representation taking into account an MOI of 0.3. In our example, the library contained 1393 constructs, requiring ~1.4×10^6 transduced cells. With an MOI of 0.3 (equaling ~22% infection rate), ~6×10^6 of cells were needed per each biological replicate. In each flask, add the amount of virus sufficient to achieve the desired MOI. To calculate this amount, use the data obtained from the functional titration experiment described in Subheading 3.3 and scale up accordingly.

2. Incubate the cells for 48 h at 37 °C in 5% CO_2.
3. On day 3, sort cells for GFP expression using flow cytometry (*see* **Note 9**). Harvest the cells at a density of 2×10^7 cells/mL in complete medium and sort GFP-positive cells, ensuring there are no GFP-negative cells in the final cell population.
4. Count the cells and reseed them in fresh complete medium to expand for further 48 h. This step allows the cells to recover from the sorting process (*see* **Note 10**).
5. On day 5, collect the cells for the T0 time point and seed for subsequent collections. Harvest sufficient cells to ensure 1000-fold representation of the library for the T0 time point (as explained above). Wash the cells with PBS, pellet and store at −80 °C for gDNA extraction.
6. Return the same number of cells to culture until the subsequent harvesting point. If the cells are slow growing, seed 2–3× the required number of cells to ensure sufficient numbers of cells for collection and further culturing at the next time point.
7. Repeat the previous step on days 8, 15, and 22 posttransduction for time points T7, T14, and T21, respectively. It may be necessary to split cultures between these time points depending on the growth characteristics of particular cell lines. *If so, it is important to always keep in culture at least the number of cells required to maintain representation of the library at the chosen level.*
8. At the final time point (T21), analyze the cells not sampled for gDNA extraction by FACS to confirm that the cells still retained GFP expression at the end of the study.
9. Store all cell pellets for gDNA extraction at −80 °C until the screen is finalized and extract simultaneously using the DNeasy

Fig. 3 (continued) CRISPR screen. After library transduction, the infected cells were selected using puromycin and set up for screening adhering to the rules for maintaining library representation at each step of the screen. Please note that the collection points (T0, T7, T14, T21) in the CRISPR screen fall on different days after transduction compared to the shRNA screen

Blood and Tissue kit by strictly adhering to the manufacturer's instructions (*see* **Notes 11** and **12**).

10. Determine the gDNA concentration in each sample by using Qubit Fluorometer (*see* **Note 13**).

3.5 Preparation of gDNA for Next-Generation Sequencing (NGS)

When performing a PCR amplification of the extracted gDNA, it is important to maintain the library representation set at the beginning of the screen. In our example, for each sample, the gDNA extracted from ~1.4×10^6 cells (*see* Subheading 3.4 for detailed calculation) would serve as a PCR template divided over multiple PCR reactions performed according to the protocol below (*see* **Note 14**). Each PCR reaction uses a common forward primer, and a unique reverse primer containing a barcode to allow sample multiplexing and identification of the sample during subsequent sequencing analysis. Forward and reverse primers, in addition, contain the adapter sequence necessary for attaching to the Illumina flow cell allowing for the sequencing library preparation in a single PCR step. The primer sequences are listed in Table 1.

1. For each 50 μL PCR reaction prepare the following mix: 10 μL 5× Phusion buffer, 0.4 μL 2.5 M dNTPs, 5 μL 5 M Betaine, 2.5 μL 50 μM forward (universal) primer, 2.5 μL 50 μM reverse (barcode) primer, 1 μL of 0.8 μg/μL genomic DNA, 2 μL Phusion HSII Polymerase, 26.6 μL UltraPure water.
2. Perform the PCR according to the following cycling conditions over 25 cycles: one initial denaturation cycle of 98 °C, 3 min; 23 denaturation/annealing/extension cycles of 98 °C, 10 s, 60 °C, 15 s annealing, and 72 °C, 15 s extension; one extension cycle of 72 °C, 7 min.
3. Pool the PCR reactions belonging to the same sample and purify using a PCR cleanup kit or AMPure XP beads by following manufacturer's instructions.
4. Quality control-check the libraries by measuring DNA concentration using Qubit and checking DNA size using the agarose gel or a fragment analyzer. In our example, a good quality library displays a sharp peak at 578 bp with no primer dimers when using the DNA1000 assay on a TapeStation 2200 (*see* **Note 15**).
5. Multiplex the samples by pooling the samples together in equimolar ratios. Sequence the pools on a HiSeq 2500 or NextSeq depending on availability or the number of reads needed for true hit identification (*see* **Note 16**). As in the previous steps, library representation must be maintained, so 1000 reads per shRNA is recommended in this example. It is important to note that pooled libraries are low-complexity libraries, and different strategies can be employed to enable their successful sequencing. We used a custom sequencing and

Table 1
shRNA PCR and sequencing primer design for NGS

Primer ID	Index sequence	Complement	Full primer sequence (5′–3′)
Universal forward			aatgatacggcgaccaccgagatctacaccggtgcctgagtttgtttgaa
Reverse index 1	ATCACG	CGTGAT	caagcagaagacggcatacgagatCGTGATggcattaaagcagcgtatccac
Reverse index 2	CGATGT	ACATCG	caagcagaagacggcatacgagatACATCGggcattaaagcagcgtatccac
Reverse index 3	TTAGGC	GCCTAA	caagcagaagacggcatacgagatGCCTAAggcattaaagcagcgtatccac
Reverse index 4	TGACCA	TGGTCA	caagcagaagacggcatacgagatTGGTCAggcattaaagcagcgtatccac
Reverse index 5	ACAGTG	CACTGT	caagcagaagacggcatacgagatCACTGTggcattaaagcagcgtatccac
Reverse index 6	GCCAAT	ATTGGC	caagcagaagacggcatacgagatATTGGCggcattaaagcagcgtatccac
Reverse index 7	CAGATC	GATCTG	caagcagaagacggcatacgagatGATCTGggcattaaagcagcgtatccac
Reverse index 8	ACTTGA	TCAAGT	caagcagaagacggcatacgagatTCAAGTggcattaaagcagcgtatccac
Reverse index 9	GATCAG	CTGATC	caagcagaagacggcatacgagatCTGATCggcattaaagcagcgtatccac
Reverse index 10	TAGCTT	AAGCTA	caagcagaagacggcatacgagatAAGCTAggcattaaagcagcgtatccac
Reverse index 11	GGCTAC	GTAGCC	caagcagaagacggcatacgagatAAGCTAggcattaaagcagcgtatccac
Reverse index 12	CTTGTA	TAGCTT	caagcagaagacggcatacgagatTACAAGggcattaaagcagcgtatccac
Read 1 sequencing primer			gaaggctcgagaaggtatattgctgttg
Index read sequencing primer			ctccttttacgctatgtggatacgctgct

indexing primer as well as a custom sequencing recipe with the steps outlined below (*see* **Note 17** and Table 1).

6. Start sequencing with custom primer hybridization and seven cycles of sequencing with no imaging.
7. Start imaging in cycle 8 and continue for 16 cycles for cluster identification and mapping.
8. Proceed with template denaturation, rehybridization of the sequencing primer, and sequencing for 22 cycles with imaging.
9. Proceed with template denaturation, indexing primer hybridization and six cycles of sequencing with imaging.
10. Demultiplex the samples with bcl2fastq software using Read 2 for the sequence and Read 3 for the index.

3.6 CRISPR Screen

As mentioned in Subheading 1, the considerations for conducting an shRNA screen vs a CRISPR screen are essentially the same, the most important being transducing the library at a low MOI and maintaining optimal library representation at each step of the screen. In our OPM-2 screening example, we modeled the CRISPR screen based on the shRNA screen described above in detail. Below we outline the key differences introduced in the CRISPR screening protocol:

(a) Library origin.

(b) Generation of the Cas9 expressing cells and testing their editing efficiency.

(c) Performing a puromycin kill curve.

(d) Functional titration of the sgRNA lentivirus library.

(e) Performing the screen.

(f) gDNA PCR amplification and sequencing.

3.6.1 sgRNA Library Origin

To conduct a CRISPR screen in OPM-2 cells, we obtained a custom Dharmacon library containing ~10 different sgRNAs against each of the previously selected targets, as well as additional 100 nontargeting and 33 positive control guides, amounting to 2913 constructs in total. The sgRNA sequences were generated using a proprietary Dharmacon algorithm optimized to select for highly functional sgRNAs. Unlike the shRNA library, the vector backbone of the sgRNA library only contains a puromycin selection marker. The majority of commercially available sgRNA libraries are based on the puromycin selection. This requires an additional step to determine the optimal puromycin dose for the cell line of interest (*see* **Note 18**).

3.6.2 Generation of Cas9 Expressing Cell Lines

Before starting the screening process, the stable Cas9-expressing cell line needs to be created and tested for its editing efficiency. The most important factors for successful editing are the cell line of choice and the level of Cas9 protein expression in the cell population. Ensuring that your Cas9-expressing cells are able to efficiently edit a gene of interest prior to the screen is crucial for the success of the screen (*see* **Note 19**).

Generate the Cas9-mCherry lentivirus as described in Subheading 3.2 and determine the viral titer (see **Note 20**).

1. Transduce the cells of interest at a low MOI (0.3–0.5) to ensure single copy integration per cell. In Subheading 3.3, the transduction of OPM-2 cells is described.
2. 48 h posttransduction, FACS sort the cells based on mCherry expression and select the top 10% of cells with the highest level of mCherry expression. Expand the cells and freeze down for future use.

3. To confirm integration and editing efficiency, transduce the Cas9 stable cells with a virus encoding a sgRNA against the mCherry protein or a gene of choice (*see* **Note 21**), and maintain the cells in culture for 7–14 days.
4. After sufficient time has elapsed for editing to be complete, analyze the cells using FACS and determine the loss of mCherry expression in edited cells compared to the control cells (*see* **Note 22**).

3.6.3 Generating a Puromycin Kill Curve

Prior to screening, it is necessary to generate a puromycin kill curve for selecting the optimal puromycin dose to kill all cells not harboring the resistance gene within a 3–5 day period. Below we describe this procedure for OPM-2 cells.

1. On day 1, seed the cells at 2×10^5/mL density in 1 mL of complete medium in a 24-well tissue culture plate. Add media containing a range of puromycin doses. For mammalian cells, a 1–20 μg/mL final concentration of puromycin is sufficient for optimal killing. Culture the cells for at least 5 days and refresh puromycin every second day.
2. On day 3–5, harvest the cells into microfuge tubes and centrifuge them for 3 min at 955 ×*g* using a table-top centrifuge.
3. Discard the supernatant and resuspend cells in 1 mL of PBS. Centrifuge for 3 min at 955 ×*g*.
4. Resuspend the cells in 200 μL of Annexin/PI staining solution (*see* Subheading 2.3) and incubate for 15 min at room temperature.
5. Analyze the cells using FACS by measuring APC and PI uptake (FL-3). Determine the percentage of dead cells compared to nontreated cells.
6. Based on results, select a minimum dose of puromycin sufficient to kill the cells within 3–5 days (*see* **Note 23**).

3.6.4 Functional Titering of the sgRNA Library

Functional titering of the sgRNA library is performed as described in Subheading 3.3 but with puromycin selection instead of sorting for GFP reporter.

1. On day 1 (~4:00 pm), seed 2×10^4 OPM-2 cells in 100 μL of the complete medium containing Sequa-brene (4 μg/mL final concentration) per well in a 96-well tissue culture plate. Seed as many wells as needed to test the dilutions outlined below in duplicate.
2. Set up a range of virus dilutions in complete medium: tube one starts at a 1:10 dilution (450 μL media + 50 μL virus) and all subsequent tubes are serially diluted 1:2 across 11 dilution points.

3. For each dilution, add 100 μL of the virus-containing medium to the cells for a final volume of 200 μL of medium per well.
4. Incubate the cells for 48 hours at 37 °C in 5% CO_2.
5. On day 3, for each virus dilution, split the cells into two wells of a 96-well plate in 100 μL of complete medium.
6. Add complete medium with puromycin into one of the wells (as determined in Subheading 3.6.3), and medium without puromycin in the other well.
7. On day 6, add propidium iodide (PI) at 100 ng/mL final concentration directly in the 96-well plate to be able to distinguish between viable and nonviable cells.
8. Analyze the cells on FACSVerse plate reader including the following parameters: Forward scatter (FCS), Side-scatter (SSC), and PI uptake (FL3).
9. For each virus dilution, calculate the following:

% infection = (# infected with puromycin/ # infected without puromycin – # uninfected with puromycin/ # uninfected without puromycin).

10. Determine the amount of virus required to infect ~20–30% of the cells.

3.6.5 Performing a CRISPR Screen

As mentioned earlier, considerations for the CRISPR screen were based largely on the shRNA screening strategy with some modifications. As per the shRNA screen, we performed three biological replicates using the same strategy of starting with three independent vials of cells. Cells were expanded as per the shRNA screen in T175 cm^2 flasks. In order to achieve a 1000-fold representation with the library size of 2913 constructs and an MOI of ~0.3 it was necessary to transduce 1.4×10^7 OPM2 Cas9-mCherry cells per replicate (as described in Subheading 3.3). Viral transduction followed the method described above in Subheading 3.4. The main difference was selection of the infected cell population, which was achieved by puromycin addition instead of cell sorting (Fig. 3).

3.6.6 PCR Amplification of gDNA for Next-Generation Sequencing

Genomic DNA was isolated for each time point using the same method described for the shRNA screen (*see* Subheading 3.4), and PCR-amplified to prepare the libraries for sequencing. As described in Subheading 3.5, all gDNA extracted from the minimum number of cells necessary to maintain representation should be used for PCR amplification (in our experiment, 1000-fold representation amounted to a minimum of 3×10^6 cells, which equals ~20 μg of gDNA per sample). Considering that performing a PCR reaction as described in Subheading 3.5 would require ~24 PCR reactions per sample (~300 reactions in total), we optimized the PCR reaction to increase the amount of gDNA input per each reaction based on the

Table 2
Edit-R Pooled sgRNA Index PCR primers

Primer ID	Index number	Index sequence
Edit-R Pooled sgRNA Reverse Index PCR Primer 2	2	CGATGT
Edit-R Pooled sgRNA Reverse Index PCR Primer 4	4	TGACCA
Edit-R Pooled sgRNA Reverse Index PCR Primer 5	5	ACAGTG
Edit-R Pooled sgRNA Reverse Index PCR Primer 6	6	GCCAAT
Edit-R Pooled sgRNA Reverse Index PCR Primer 7	7	CAGATC
Edit-R Pooled sgRNA Reverse Index PCR Primer 12	12	CTTGTA
Edit-R Pooled sgRNA Reverse Index PCR Primer 13	13	AGTCAA
Edit-R Pooled sgRNA Reverse Index PCR Primer 14	14	AGTTCC
Edit-R Pooled sgRNA Reverse Index PCR Primer 15	15	ATGTCA
Edit-R Pooled sgRNA Reverse Index PCR Primer 16	16	CCGTCC
Edit-R Pooled sgRNA Reverse Index PCR Primer 18	18	GTCCGC
Edit-R Pooled sgRNA Reverse Index PCR Primer 19	19	GTGAAA

protocol developed by the Broad Institute (*see* **Note 24**). Primer sequences, which are specific to the Dharmacon sgRNA vector, are proprietary, and the barcodes for each reverse primer are displayed in Table 2. Custom sequencing and indexing primers are compatible with the Illumina platform and are also provided by Dharmacon.

1. For each 100 μL reaction prepare the following mix: 10 μL 10× ExTaq buffer, 8 μL 2.5 mM dNTPs, 1 μL 50 μM forward (universal) primer, 1 μL 50 μM reverse (barcode) primer, 1 μL of 1.0 μg/μL genomic DNA, 0.75 μL ExTaq Polymerase, 76.25 μL UltraPure water.
2. Perform the PCR according to the following cycling conditions: one initial denaturation cycle of 98 °C, 3 min; 28 denaturation/annealing/extension cycles of 98 °C, 10 s, 60 °C, 15 s annealing, and 72 °C, 15 s extension; one extension cycle of 72 °C, 5 min.
3. For each sample, take 15–30 μL out of each 100 μL PCR reaction and pool into a microfuge tube. Purify the products by using a PCR cleanup kit or AMPure XP beads according to manufacturer's instructions.
4. Quality-control the prepared libraries by measuring the DNA concentration using Qubit and check DNA size using agarose gel or a fragment analyzer. For the Dharmacon library and

primers used, a ~357 bp amplicon should be clearly visible without traces of a primer dimer.

5. Multiplex the samples by pooling the samples together in equimolar ratios. Sequence the samples on NextSeq aiming to achieve 1000 reads per each sgRNA. For the Dharmacon library, proprietary Read1 Primer and Index Primer are used at 0.3 μM, and the libraries are loaded at a concentration of 1.2–2 pM with 10% of PhiX to increase the library diversity (*see* **Note 25**).

3.7 Bioinformatics Analysis of Pooled Screens

There are a number of publications spanning the shRNA and CRISPR pooled screening field that detail bioinformatics approaches to screen analysis. We provide here our in-house protocols that integrate many open sources packages as detailed.

3.7.1 Curation of Sequencing Reads

1. Trim raw sequencing reads corresponding to the shRNA/sgRNA to 20 bp and align trimmed sequences to the reference library. Use the Bowtie 2 algorithm [4] leaving the default parameters and setting tolerated mismatches to zero. Use all the multimapped reads.
2. Save the aligned reads in the Sequence Alignment Map (SAM) format, then convert to a read count table and import into R for downstream analyses (*see* **Note 26**).
3. Before normalizing the data, check the correlation between the replicates by performing hierarchical cluster analysis in R. Define the previously imported data from **step 1** as a matrix object and set it as an input for the “hclust” function [5], using Euclidean distance as the input parameter for the clustering algorithm.
4. Normalize the aligned raw read counts using median normalization and adjust for differences in sequencing depths (also referred to as library size), and generate counts per million of reads per sample (CPM).
5. After data normalization, the next step is to perform representation analysis. The purpose of representation analysis is to identify how many shRNA/sgRNAs are present at T0. This is performed by comparing the read count of each shRNA/sgRNA against a minimum read count threshold (we recommend using at least 50 reads per construct). If the read count for a specific shRNA/sgRNA matches the threshold then it is considered sufficiently represented (*see* **Note 27**).

3.7.2 Hit Selection Strategies

To be able to capture hits that dropped out significantly at final time point as well as hits that displayed modest but consistent dropout over the experimental time points, we performed both dropout trend analysis (*see* **Note 28**) and a fold change analysis as described below.

1. Prepare a sample annotation file including the columns indicating time points (T0, T7, T14, T21) and biological replicates (1A, 1B, 1C, etc.).
2. Import the sample annotation file and normalized data frame into R and combine.
3. Order the samples in the ascending order of time points and the ascending order of replicates, e.g., T0 (1A, 1B, 1C), T7 (2A, 2B, 2C), T14 (3A, 3B, 3C), and T21 (4A, 4B, 4C).
4. Install and load the "SAGx" R package [6].
5. Input data and sample labels to JT.test() function and run command.
6. The JT test command returns a set of statistical measures for each shRNA/sgRNA including rank correlation, median value for each sample, and a p.value. Pass the p.value column from this data frame to the p.adjust function and select "fdr" as the method variable. This data frame can be then exported as an Excel file.
7. In parallel, calculate the fold change (FC) between T0 and T21 by taking the ratio of the normalized read counts at T21 over T0. Targets with $\geq$50% decrease in read counts at T21 are considered significant (*see* **Note 29**).

3.7.3 Aggregation of shRNAs/sgRNAs Data to a Gene Level Summary

Each pooled library has multiple sequences targeting the same gene and a gene level summary of target activity is the ultimate way to determine a hit. Since different shRNAs/sgRNAs targeting the same gene can display varying levels of specificity and knockdown/knockout efficiency, it is important to factor in the aggregated outcome for each gene target:

1. Aggregate multiple shRNAs/sgRNAs to the gene level and determine the percentage of shRNA/sgRNAs per gene showing a significant dropout trend, and percentage showing $\geq$50-fold decrease of T21/T0 read counts.
2. Select hits based on combining the trend and fold change analysis (*see* **Note 30**). Combine both trend analysis and fold-change methods to select the hits using a significant *p*-value $\leq$ 0.05 for the trend analysis and $\geq$50% decrease of T21 compared to T0.

3.8 Target Validation

After completing the primary shRNA or CRISPR screen and obtaining a list of hits, it is necessary to validate each of the hits in an individual shRNA/sgRNA construct format. Depending on the number of hits to follow up, this step can be more labor intensive than the primary screen itself, and developing methods for high-throughput viral preparation and transduction becomes essential. Below we outline a protocol for virus production in a 6-well tissue culture plate, transduction of individual shRNA/sgRNA constructs in a 96-well plate and further approaches toward hit validation.

1. On day 1, seed 1.5×10^6 HEK293T cells per well of a 6-well plate in 5 mL of RPMI medium with supplements (*see* **Note 31**).
2. On day 2, for each well of a 6-well plate prepare the transfection mix as follows: 170 μL of RPMI with no supplements, 5 μL of Lenti-X HTX Packaging Mix, and 2 μL of 1 μg/μL DNA construct.
3. Vortex for 10 s at medium speed. Add 20.3 μL of 1 mg/mL polyethylenimine (PEI) and vortex again for 10 s at medium speed.
4. Incubate for 10 min at room temperature.
5. Vortex for 10 s at medium speed and add transfection mix dropwise to each well in a spiral pattern to distribute evenly.
6. Incubate the cells overnight at 37 °C in 5% CO_2.
7. On day 3, remove transfection media and replace with 3 mL of RPMI with supplements and incubate for 48 h at 37 °C in 5% CO_2.
8. On day 5, harvest the viral supernatant and filter through a 0.45 μm low protein binding filter. Aliquot the supernatant and store at −80 °C.

Transduction of individual shRNA/sgRNA constructs

9. Seed 2×10^4 OPM-2 cells in 100 μL of the complete medium containing Sequa-brene (4 μg/mL final concentration) per well in a 96-well tissue culture plate.
10. Thaw an aliquot of the virus prepared in the previous step, and add 100 μL of the virus-containing medium to the cells for a final volume of 200 μL of medium per well (*see* **Note 32**).
11. Create a replicate plate by transferring 50 μL of cell suspension from the source plate and adding 150 μL of fresh medium for a final volume of 200 μL. Use the rest of the cells in the source plate for FACS analysis, which should be repeated every 3–4 days.
12. Add PI at 100 ng/mL final concentration directly in the 96-well plate to label dead cells.
13. Analyze the cells using a FACSVerse plate reader. For shRNA constructs, measure GFP expression and determine a dropout of fluorescence compared to cells infected with a negative control virus (*see* Subheading 3.3 and **Notes 33** and **34**). For sgRNA constructs, perform annexin V staining to determine the % of cell death compared to the negative control cells (*see*

Subheading 3.6.3). If verifying increase in cell proliferation/viability, perform a cell viability assay such as alamarBlue or Cell-Titer Glo assay according to the manufacturer's instructions.

3.9 Summary of Additional Steps for Hit Validation

We have outlined strategies toward identifying targets from a screen; however, identifying a target list is, in one respect, just the starting point to a screen. Identifying statistically significant targets and triaging the target list toward a workable number requires integration of existing genomic datasets, pathway information and other bioinformatics strategies. We highly recommend performing transcript profiling on your cell lines of choice in parallel with the screen, thereby identifying off-target effects by only selecting genes that are expressed in the cell line and under the experimental conditions screened. Target specificity can be evaluated at the transcript and protein levels using standard approaches and the specific gene editing events should be confirmed by sequencing. Priorities are generally placed on genes for which multiple constructs have a statistically significant outcome and often for which the known biological pathways have some impact. The thresholds a researcher will set at this point is guided largely by their downstream investment energy and to some extent their willingness to take a risk. Some great discoveries have come from unknown targets identified in a screen! Ultimately, each screen is unique and there is no "one size fits all" process that can be undertaken once a target list has been defined.

4 Notes

1. Critical for the production of high-titer virus is maintenance of HEK293T cells; they should not reach over 80% confluency at any point during regular passaging or virus production. We typically split the cells every 72 h by seeding 2.5×10^6 cells in a T175 cm^2 flask or 1.2×10^6 cells in a T75 cm^2 flask and passage a maximum of ten times before thawing a fresh vial of cells.
2. Viral aliquots should be frozen in workable volumes. We do not recommend multiple freeze–thaw cycles for the same aliquot as virus titers will drop at least 10% after a freeze–thaw. We recommend using a fresh aliquot of virus for every experiment to maintain consistent results.
3. When setting up this assay, optimize the seeding cell number required for your cell line. If the cells are dividing fast, make sure the cells in the negative control wells are not overgrown at the point of cell harvest for FACS analysis, or, if the cells are

slow dividing, ensure there are sufficient cells for a robust readout.

4. The transduction efficiency can often be enhanced by the addition of Sequa-brene, a cationic polymer that reduces the electrostatic repulsion between the negatively charged surfaces of both the viral particles and the target cell membranes. We compared the transduction of OPM-2 cells with and without Sequa-brene and showed that at 4 μg/mL Sequa-brene enhances transduction efficiency. We recommend performing a similar experiment and determining the optimal Sequa-brene concentration for your cell lines of interest.
5. Always ensure that the external rows and columns in a 96-well plate have media in them but no experimental cells to reduce any possibility of edge effects. We recommend either replicate plates or replicate wells.
6. In some cases, transduction of cells by the method of spinoculation can enhance transduction efficiency. We recommend testing this method with your cell lines of interest. Add virus and centrifuge the plates at 1200 × *g* for 30–120 min (test for optimal results) at 32 °C before returning the cells to the incubator for overnight culturing. In the case of OPM-2 cells this did not enhance their transduction efficiency.
7. Collection of cells at different time points during the screen helps identify the optimal time point for harvesting cells and analyzing the screen. This may be particularly important for positive selection screens where resistant clones compete amongst each other within a cell population.
8. The decision on the level of library representation in your screen will depend on multiple factors including the type of the screen (negative or positive selection), size of the library and growth characteristic of your cell lines. Generally, for negative selection (drop out) screens, such as the example we describe, 500- to 1000-fold library representation is sufficient to identify true hits at the end of the screen. In this case, the cells carrying shRNA or sgRNA that constitute hits gradually disappear from the population, but occasionally false hits will occur due to random sampling effects as well as variable transduction and integration site issues. To be able to distinguish between true and false hits, enough cells have to be transduced with each of the constructs. In the case of positive selection screens, where shRNAs or sgRNAs enable cells to grow out in response to a pressure (e.g., drug treatment), it is easier to capture true hits and therefore 100- to 300-fold library representation is typically sufficient.

9. Cell sorting instruments should have a laser compatible with the fluorophore marker being used and should have aerosol containment for sorting virus infected cells.
10. How well the cells recover from the sorting process depends on the cell line and we recommend testing this in advance. The challenge is that there has to be enough cells at the T0 time point for both gDNA extraction as well as further culturing of the cells at the desired library representation. In our example, OPM-2 cells did not proliferate well after the sorting process, and at the T0 and T7 time points there were not enough cells to harvest at 1000-fold representation. Instead, our representation dropped to 500-fold, which was still within the recommended limits for a negative selection screen. If your cell line does not recover well from sorting, consider switching to puromycin selection (described below for the CRISPR screen) instead of sorting for GFP. Alternatively, transduce a larger number of cells at the beginning of the screen to compensate for the cell loss/reduced proliferation and to achieve sufficient cell number at T0 and subsequent time points.
11. We highly recommend testing the gDNA extraction protocol before screening to ensure the anticipated number of cells and subsequent gDNA yield is sufficient for the library amplification steps. We recommend eluting the gDNA from the column in 200 μL of H_2O (or Elution Buffer) for optimal DNA recovery. It is important not to overload to column, and if collecting more cells than the manufacturer's recommendation, divide the cell extract over several columns and combine the eluate at the end.
12. During gDNA extraction, ensure the samples are well mixed at each step of the protocol, particularly during the early resuspension and lysis steps to prevent the solution from becoming overly viscous, which can lead to a partial loss of DNA while extracting from the columns.
13. Using a NanoDrop does not distinguish between DNA and other impurities present in the sample, which can lead to an overestimation of DNA concentration. It is important to use a fluorometric assay such as the Qubit to precisely quantify the amount of DNA in the samples.
14. As mentioned in the Subheading 3.4 and **Note 10**, we did not have enough cells at T0 and T7 time points to maintain 1000-fold representation, and consequently, we also had less gDNA as an input for the PCR amplification step. However, we performed a titration experiment and varied the amount of gDNA in the PCR reaction to determine the lowest amount of gDNA necessary to maintain the representation of the original library. As low as 200 ng of gDNA was sufficient to achieve >98.5%

representation of hairpins and >99% correlation between technical duplicates. We do recommend, however, to carefully plan your experiment and optimize the critical steps, so as to be able to maintain the chosen library representation throughout the screen.

15. When checking the PCR product of a pooled library on a fragment analyzer, it is common to observe a second peak of higher molecular weight adjacent to the "correct" library peak. In our experience, this does not affect the sequencing process. In addition, gDNA is frequently copurified with the PCR amplicon, which can be observed as a peak of much higher molecular weight compared to the amplicon peak. This will not impact the sequencing of the samples but can lead to DNA quantity overestimation when measured by Qubit. In this case, we recommend determining the proportion of total DNA belonging to the PCR amplicon based on the TapeStation trace and adjust the Qubit quantification results accordingly. Alternatively, qPCR can be performed to precisely quantify the PCR product before sequencing.
16. In our example, two pools with 12 samples each were created and loaded at 8 pM on a lane of an Illumina HiSeq Rapid 2500 flow cell using cBot clustering. An Illumina TruSeq Rapid SR Cluster and TruSeq Rapid SBS Kit HS (50 cycles) were used per sequencing run.
17. In our example, the custom sequencing primer is designed to anneal to the conserved region of the pGIPZ vector and start reading at the first base of the shRNA [7]. However, the complexity of the shRNA sequences is very low for the first eight nucleotides and prevents robust cluster mapping. We have customized the sequencing protocol on the HiSeq to include eight dark cycles and start imaging in a far more universally variable region. Once clusters are mapped, the sequence then runs back through to capture the entire sequence. This results in a much higher readout performance without the need to spike in >30–40% of PhiX in each run.
18. In most of our CRISPR experiments we use a two-vector CRISPR system consisting of a Cas9-expressing vector, which is initially introduced into the cells to generate a Cas9 stable cell line, and a sgRNA-expressing vector, which is subsequently transduced into the Cas9 stable cells to enable sgRNA expression and the actual genome editing. All-in-one vectors encoding for both Cas9 and sgRNA in the same backbone are also available commercially through Addgene. Due to their size, however, the lentiviral packaging is less efficient and the resulting titers are typically very low, making the entire screen far more difficult to manage.

19. According to the literature and our own experience, some cell lines are more difficult to edit, and in this case single cell sorting and selection for individual Cas9 cell clones can help identify a clone with an improved editing efficiency. In most cases, however, we do not select for single cell clones but use a polyclonal pool of Cas9-expressing cells. In addition, the level of Cas9 expression is the most important factor for successful editing, which is why we typically use a Cas9-mCherry (or another fluorescent reporter) construct to identify only the highest Cas9 expressing cells.
20. In a subset of cell lines, high level Cas9 expression is not tolerated resulting in a mixed Cas9 cell population that can contain Cas9 negative cells. In this case, we recommend using a Cas9-blasticidin construct (Addgene), where the Cas9 positive cell population can be maintained by blasticidin selection throughout the screening period.
21. We designed a sgRNA sequence against mCherry to test the cells' editing efficiency (5′-GGCCACGAGTTCGAGATCGA-3′). The caveat of this approach is that the mCherry protein is extremely stable, which is compounded by selecting for mCherry-high expressing cells. This has most likely led to an underestimation of the cells' editing efficiency in our case. If possible, we recommend designing a sgRNA against a gene that serves as a positive control in your assay to assess the editing efficiency of your cell lines. In this case, you can use the same construct to test and optimize different steps in the screen (e.g., optimal time points for cell collection).
22. It is preferred to have at least 50% of the cell population showing efficient editing and functional protein knockout to ensure the success of the screen.
23. It is important to select the minimum dose of puromycin to kill the noninfected cells in the specified timeframe. Higher doses of puromycin and therefore more stringent selection conditions could bias the selection of cells with multiple integrated sgRNAs.
24. This protocol was adapted from the protocol developed by the Broad Genetic Perturbation Platform (Broad Institute) for screening of the genome-wide CRISPR libraries (Broad GPP genome-wide Brunello and Brie library; available through Addgene). We performed a titration experiment with a range of increasing amounts of DNA and compared the performance of the Phusion Polymerase (used for shRNA experiments) and ExTaq Polymerase. We determined that ExTaq performs better, achieving the maximum input of 3 μg gDNA per reaction with the primers used for this vector.

25. In most cases, NextSeq offers the most cost-effective way to sequence samples. The chemistry that NextSeq uses, however, differs compared to HighSeq, which requires caution when sequencing low-complexity libraries. Although we used a custom Read1 sequencing and indexing primer, allowing the reads to start at a variable region and therefore alleviating the issue of low complexity during sequencing, we spiked the libraries with 10% PhiX Control to further increase library complexity.
26. Alternatively, newly developed packages such as MAGeCK, the "Model-based Analysis of Genome-wide CRISPR/Cas9 Knockout" method [8] can be implemented to perform a start-to-end analysis pipeline including alignment and normalization as well as downstream analysis of essential genes and pathways. This method displays robust performance against other computational methods including edgeR, DESeq, and RIGER, in terms of handling sequencing data with different sequencing depths and ranking the number of sgRNAs per gene.
27. Setting the minimum read count threshold should also be considered in the context of the whole screen and the level of construct recovery. It is possible that 50 reads per construct is too stringent and in some cases you may not recover many constructs. We recommend setting your own cutoff for representation analysis.
28. To detect the shRNAs/sgRNAs showing consistent dropout trends over all the time points, a trend analysis can be performed on the normalized data using the Jonckheere–Terpstra (JT) statistical test. For each shRNA/sgRNA, this rank-based nonparametric test provides the median read counts at each time point and assigns a rank correlation value and False Discovery Rate (FDR) corrected p-value of significanceRank correlation indicates the strength of the dropout trend, with −1 indicating a strong dropout trend and 1 indicating strong enrichment. JT-trend analysis is generally more powerful when read counts consistently dropout at each time point, irrespective of the magnitude of change in read counts at each individual time point. The JT test can detect significant strong negative correlation even if a fold-change difference between T0 and T21 is modest. On the contrary, the JT test does not identify those targets that show a strong drop out when comparing T0 and T21 but have inconsistent intermediate time points.
29. It is important to note that the fold-change values between T0 and T21 may not always reflect or correlate with the rank correlation. We have found that selecting the hits based on just the fold change may identify more targets therefore we

recommend considering both rank correlation and fold-change based approaches in parallel to stratify the hits.

30. For genome-wide screens, and if testing whether the read count is significantly different between any two conditions (e.g., treated vs. untreated) we recommend using advanced computational methods such as "Second Best Rank," "Weighted Sum," "RIGER," "RSA," and "MAGeCK." As mentioned earlier, we recommend MAGeCK; however, it may be less sensitive if there are no replicates or small boutique screens.
31. For virus production, use the base medium appropriate for the target cell line. In our case, OPM-2 cells are cultured in the RPMI medium.
32. Unlike the pooled library, transduction of the individual shRNA/sgRNA constructs can be performed at a higher MOI, which will enable a higher infection rate in the cell population. For instance, at MOI = 10 all cells in the population will be infected. For this reason, we typically do not titer the produced virus but keep the production and transduction consistent.
33. For validation experiments using individual hairpins we found it was best to take the first time point at 72–96 h posttransduction as the percentage of GFP expression appeared to be increasing during this time frame. For certain cell lines, FACS analysis was performed only once per week as cells grew too slowly to ensure sufficient cell numbers for more frequent analysis.
34. We have noticed that GFP intensity detected in the FL1 channel can increase over time appearing much brighter at later time points. This seems specific to the pGIPZ vector as it encodes for a turbo GFP reporter. This alert is to ensure you are aware of the possibility and treat cells accordingly.

Acknowledgments

The authors are grateful to James Goldmeyer and Louise Baskin (Dharmacon GE) for technical discussions regarding library design.

The Johnstone laboratory (R.W.J.) is supported by research funding from the Leukaemia Foundation of Australia, The Kids Cancer Project, the Cancer Council Victoria, the National Health and Medical Research Council of Australia (NHMRC) and the Victorian Cancer Agency.

The Shortt laboratory (J.S.) is supported by funding from the Victorian Cancer Agency and Snowdome Foundation Fellowship. Cancer Council Victoria Venture Grant.

The Victorian Centre for Functional Genomics (K.J.S.) is funded by the Australian Cancer Research Foundation (ACRF), the Australian Phenomics Network (APN) through funding from the Australian Government's National Collaborative Research Infrastructure Strategy (NCRIS) program and the Peter MacCallum Cancer Centre Foundation.

References

1. Evers B, Jastrzebski K, Heijmans JP, Grernrum W, Beijersbergen RL, Bernards R (2016) CRISPR knockout screening outperforms shRNA and CRISPRi in identifying essential genes. Nat Biotechnol 34:631–633
2. Morgens DW, Deans RM, Li A, Bassik MC (2016) Systematic comparison of CRISPR/Cas9 and RNAi screens for essential genes. Nat Biotechnol 34:634–636
3. Katagiri S, Yonezawa T, Kuyama J, Kanayama Y, Nishida K, Abe T, Tamaki T, Ohnishi M, Tarui S (1985) Two distinct human myeloma cell lines originating from one patient with myeloma. Int J Cancer 36:241–246
4. Langmead B, Salzberg SL (2012) Fast gapped-read alignment with Bowtie 2. Nat Methods 9:357–359
5. Langfelder P, Zhang B, Horvath S (2008) Defining clusters from a hierarchical cluster tree: the Dynamic Tree Cut package for R. Bioinformatics 24:719–720
6. Bromberg P (2016) SAGx: statistical analysis of the GeneChip. R package version 1480
7. Strezoska Z, Licon A, Haimes J, Spayd KJ, Patel KM, Sullivan K, Jastrzebski K, Simpson KJ, Leake D, van Brabant Smith A, Vermeulen A (2012) Optimized PCR conditions and increased shRNA fold representation improve reproducibility of pooled shRNA screens. PLoS One 7:e42341
8. Li W, Xu H, Xiao T, Cong L, Love MI, Zhang F, Irizarry RA, Liu JS, Brown M, Liu XS (2014) MAGeCK enables robust identification of essential genes from genome-scale CRISPR/Cas9 knockout screens. Genome Biol 15:554

Chapter 18

Immuno-detection of Immature and Bioactive Forms of the Inflammatory Cytokine IL-18

Brendan J. Jenkins and Virginie Deswaerte

Abstract

Gastric cancer (GC) is the third most lethal cancer worldwide, and like many other types of cancers, it is associated with precursory chronic inflammatory responses. In the context of many inflammation-associated cancers such as GC, activation of the innate immune response by infectious microbes and/or host-derived molecules is often characterized by production of the cytokines interleukin (IL)-1β and IL-18, which can often have divergent and opposing (i.e., pro or anti) roles in inflammation and oncogenesis. The processing of these mature bioactive cytokines from their inactive precursor polypeptides is dependent upon the enzyme Caspase-1, which is part of multiprotein complexes called "inflammasomes." Considering the recent mounting evidence for the role of IL-18 in the pathogenesis of GC, here, we describe a Western blotting technique used on genetic mouse models for GC to detect and characterize both pro-Il-18 and mature IL-18 proteins.

Key words Interleukin (IL)-18, Mouse cancer models, Tissue lysates, Western blotting

1 Introduction

Gastric cancer (GC) is one of many cancers (e.g., colon, liver, and lung) for which there is a well-established causal link with chronic inflammation [1, 2]. Activation of the inflammatory response triggered by bacterial infection with *Helicobacter pylori* (*H. pylori*) in GC [3] is associated with activation of the inflammatory Caspase-1 by the inflammasomes [4, 5]. Active Caspase-1 is a cysteine-dependent protease that induces the maturation of pro-inflammatory cytokines interleukin (IL)-1β and IL-18 into mature IL-1β and IL-18 [6], which in addition to chronic inflammatory responses has also been intimately linked to the inflammatory form of lytic cell death known as pyroptosis [7, 8]. In various cancers, it has been shown that IL-18 can display opposing antitumorigenic or protumorigenic effects dependent upon the tissue and cellular context [9]. In GC patients, it has been demonstrated that IL-18 levels are increased [10–12] while experimental data from human GC cell lines also suggest that

Brendan J. Jenkins (ed.), *Inflammation and Cancer: Methods and Protocols*, Methods in Molecular Biology, vol. 1725,
https://doi.org/10.1007/978-1-4939-7568-6_18,

IL-18 may contribute to the malignant progression of tumors [11, 13, 14]. Despite those findings, a definitive role for IL-18 and more specifically mature IL-18 in GC remains unproven. While being able to distinguish between pro-IL-18 (24 kDa) and mature IL-18 (18 kDa) in tumor tissues (in this case, gastric) is a critical parameter in determining a causal role for IL-18 in disease pathogenesis, methods to identify each IL-18 form are currently limited. Indeed, with existing commercial IL-18 ELISA kits it is not possible to discriminate active and nonactive form of the proteins. Here, we describe a Western blot protocol to process stomach tissue from mouse models of GC in order to specifically detect both pro-Il-18 and mature IL-18 proteins.

2 Materials

2.1 Preparation of Tissue Lysates

1. RIPA buffer (2×): 100 mM Tris–HCl, 300 mM NaCl, 1% (v/v) Triton X-100, 1% sodium deoxycholate, 0.2% SDS, 2 mM EDTA, 2 mM EGTA, adjust to pH 7.4 and store at 4 °C. Prior to use, dilute to 1× in Milli-Q water, add one cOmplete Protease Inhibitor Mini Cocktail Tablet and one PhosSTOP Phosphatase Inhibitor Cocktail Tablet per 10 mL RIPA buffer.
2. 10% ammonium persulfate (APS) solution in water (*see* **Note 1**).
3. Laemmli sample buffer (4×): Prior to mixing with the sample, add 100 μL of 2-mercaptoethanol per 900 μL (final concentration of 355 mM) (*see* **Note 2**).
4. Tissue homogenizer.
5. Flat-bottom tubes.
6. Standard 1.5 mL microcentrifuge tubes.
7. Heat block.
8. Microcentrifuge.
9. 1.5 mL microcentrifuge tubes.
10. 37 °C incubator.

2.2 SDS-PAGE

1. Running buffer (10×): 250 mM Tris, 1.92 M glycine, 1% SDS. Store at room temperature (RT) and prior to use dilute to 1× in Milli-Q water.
2. Transfer buffer (10×): 250 mM Tris, 1.92 M glycine. Store at 4 °C prior to use. To obtain 1× transfer buffer, dilute 100 mL of 10× transfer buffer, 800 mL of water, and 100 mL of methanol (*see* **Note 3**).
3. 1.5 M Tris–HCl buffer, adjust pH to 8.8.

4. 15% resolving gel: 2.3 ml Milli-Q water, 5 mL 30% Acrylamide/Bis Solution, 2.5 mL 1.5 M Tris–HCl buffer, 100 μL 10% SDS, 100 μL 10% APS, and 4 μL TEMED.
5. Isopropyl alcohol.
6. 0.5 M Tris–HCl buffer, adjust pH to 6.8.
7. 5% stacking gel: 2.05 mL Milli-Q water, 0.5 mL 30% Acrylamide–Bis Solution, 375 μL 0.5 M Tris–HCl buffer, 30 μL 10% SDS, 30 μL 10% APS, and 3 μL TEMED.
8. Prestained molecular weight standards.
9. SDS-PAGE apparatus and electrophoresis power supply system.
10. Nitrocellulose membrane.

2.3 Immunoblotting

1. Blocking buffer (Odyssey).
2. TBS 10×: 1.4 M NaCl, 0.2 M Tris pH 7.6. Store at RT and prior to use dilute to 1× in Milli-Q water.
3. Washing buffer (T-TBS): 0.1% Tween 20 in 1× TBS.
4. Primary antibodies against mouse IL-18 and tubulin.
5. Secondary (fluorescent-conjugated) antibodies against the species the primary antibody is raised against (e.g., Alexa Fluor® anti-rabbit for anti-IL-18, and IRDye® 800CW anti-rat for tubulin).
6. Infrared imaging system (Odyssey CLx).
7. Tube roller.
8. Rocker.

3 Methods

3.1 Preparation of Tissue Lysates

1. Transfer frozen tissue samples (*see* **Note 4**) into flat bottom tubes containing 500 μL of RIPA buffer and incubate 20 min at 37 °C (*see* **Note 5**).
2. Homogenize tissue samples using a small probe at RT. Once all samples are homogenized, transfer each homogenate to a fresh 1.5 mL microcentrifuge tube and spin down for 20 min at 14,000 × *g* at RT.
3. Transfer supernatant to fresh 1.5 mL microcentrifuge tubes and incubate 20 min at 37 °C.
4. Proceed with quantification of protein lysates (*see* **Note 6**), store samples at −80 °C for further use or prepare each samples at a concentration of 1 μg/μL of protein into new 1.5 mL microcentrifuge tube with RIPA buffer and Laemmli sample buffer (*see* **Note 7**).

5. Reduce proteins by boiling at 95 °C for 5 min. Briefly microcentrifuge protein samples to collect condensation, put the samples on ice for 5 min and store at −20 °C.

3.2 SDS-PAGE

1. Prepare the 1.5 mm thick, 15% resolving SDS-PAGE gel (*see* **Note 8**) and pour between glass plates (leaving room for stacking gel) (*see* **Note 9**). Overlay with ~1 mL isopropyl alcohol to prevent contact with atmospheric oxygen (which inhibits acrylamide polymerization) and ensure a smooth surface of the resolving gel solution. Leave gel to solidify for 30 min at RT.
2. Remove isopropyl alcohol and carefully dry with Whatman paper.
3. Prepare the 5% stacking gel to use and pour onto resolving gel. Insert combs immediately and leave gel to solidify for 30 min at RT.
4. When gel is fully solidified, remove comb, assemble SDS-PAGE apparatus and fill with running buffer ensuring wells are covered (*see* **Note 10**).
5. Load equal amounts of protein (20–30 μg) into the wells of proteins into each well of SDS-PAGE gel. Include 5 μL of the prestained molecular weight standard in one well.
6. Run the gel at 120 V for 2 h (*see* **Note 11**). Stop running gel just before sample buffer migrate off the bottom of the resolving gel.
7. Following SDS-PAGE separation, separate the gel from the plates with the help of a spatula and remove the stacking gel.
8. Gently lay on top of the gel a nitrocellulose membrane (*see* **Note 12**) preliminarily equilibrated in transfer buffer for 5 min and cut to the shape of the gel. Make sure there are no bubbles between the membrane and the gel. The polyacrylamide gel and nitrocellulose membrane are sandwiched between two filter papers and two sponges, and preliminarily soak in cold transfer buffer. Place this assembly in the SDS-PAGE apparatus and electrophoresis power supply system, add a cooling unit and fill with transfer buffer.
9. Transfer the protein to the nitrocellulose membrane at 45 min at 30 V.

3.3 Western Blotting

1. Following transfer, briefly wash the membrane in T-TBS and place it in a 50 mL Falcon tube (or similar) containing 3 mL of blocking buffer in order to block nonspecific epitopes (*see* **Note 13**). Incubate for 1 h at RT on a tube roller.
2. Following blocking, place the membrane in a new 50 mL Falcon tube (or similar) with IL-18 antibody diluted to

1:1000 in 3 mL blocking buffer, for overnight incubation at 4 °C on a tube roller (*see* **Note 14**).

3. Remove membrane from Falcon tube and store primary antibody at 4 °C (*see* **Note 15**). Wash membrane three times in T-TBS for a minimum of 5 min each wash at RT with gentle rocking, discarding the buffer between each incubation.
4. Place the membrane in a new 50 mL Falcon tube (or similar) with α-tubulin antibody diluted to 1:1000 in 3 mL blocking buffer in order to confirm equal protein loading between samples. Incubate 1 h at RT.
5. Repeat **steps 3** and **4**.
6. In a new 50 mL Falcon tube (or similar), incubate the membrane in Alexa Fluor® 680 goat anti-rabbit antibody and IRDye® 800CW goat anti-rat antibody both diluted to 1:1000 in 3 mL blocking buffer for 1 h at RT on a tube roller and protected from light.
7. Following incubation, discard secondary antibodies and wash membrane three times in T-TBS for a minimum of 5 min each wash at RT with gentle rocking, discarding the buffer between each incubation.
8. Transfer membrane to infrared imaging system (Odyssey® Clx), and capture image at a wavelength of 700 and 800 nm (*see* **Note 16**). Figure 1 shows an example of Western blotting for IL-18 and α-tubulin on mouse stomach samples.

4 Notes

1. APS solution is stable at 4 °C for 2 weeks (freezing is recommended for longer storage).
2. Laemmli sample buffer at 355 mM with 2-mercaptoethanol is stable at RT for 2 weeks.
3. 1× transfer buffer is put in the freezer 2 h prior to use.
4. Proteins can be easily extracted from tissues snap-frozen in liquid nitrogen, such as whole stomachs (washed in PBS first), antrum, or tumor tissue dissected from whole stomach, via homogenization. If the tissue is large (e.g., whole stomach or tumor tissue) small pieces can be excised off the main organ after snap freezing with a scalpel blade in a petri dish on dry ice.
5. This protocol has been tested in cold conditions by keeping the tissues samples on ice or at 4 °C and the mature form of IL-18 couldn't be detected.
6. Protein lysates can be quantified by any method desired, such as the Lowry method.

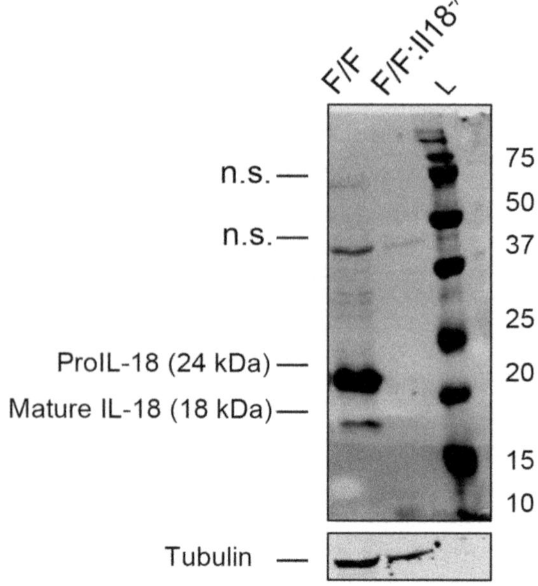

Fig. 1 Western blotting for IL-18 on gastric tumor tissue from mice. The expression of pro-IL-18 and mature IL-18 along with α-tubulin to confirm equivalent protein loading, are shown by Western blotting on gastric tissue extracted from *gp130*$^{F/F}$ (F/F) and *gp130*$^{F/F}$:*Il18*$^{-/-}$ (F/F:Il18$^{-/-}$) mice. The whole blot shows the presence of nonspecific bands (n.s.), as well as the band representative of proIL-18 (at ~24 kDa) and mature IL-18 (at ~18 kDa). L = prestained molecular weight standard

7. Dilute three parts sample with one part 4× Laemmli sample buffer at 355 mM with 2-mercaptoethanol (e.g., add 50 μL of Laemmli sample buffer to 150 μL of protein lysates).
8. The percentage of acrylamide in the resolving gel depends on the molecular weight of your protein of interest. For example, to detect IL-18, knowing that the proform is 24 kDa and the mature form is 18 kDa, a 15% acrylamide gel can be used.
9. Ensure the apparatus is clean, and wipe glass plates with 95% ethanol and air-dry prior to use.
10. The gel can be stored at 4 °C when wrapped with wet pepper towel for 2 days to avoid the gel to dry.
11. Run at low voltage (about 90 V) until proteins enter in the stacking gel.
12. Polyvinylidene fluoride (PVDF) membranes can be used instead of nitrocellulose membranes.
13. After transfer, it is possible to stain the membrane with Ponceau red to assess total protein profile and transfer efficiency.
14. The membrane can be incubated in primary antibody for up to 72 h at 4 °C on the tube roller; however, this may also increase

background staining. Alternatively, the membrane can be incubated in primary antibody for 1–2 h at RT on a tube roller if preferred. This technique may be less sensitive than overnight incubation at 4 °C however.

15. The primary antibody can be stored at 4 °C for reuse in the next 2 weeks (up to three times is recommended) or at −20 °C for longer storage. However, the buffer should be carefully monitored for contamination and discarded if appears.

16. After immunoblotting the membrane can be stripped by sealing in a plastic envelope with ~5 ml membrane stripping buffer (contains the following per 100 mL: 20 mL 10% SDS, 12.5 mL Tris–HCl (pH 6.8), 67.5 mL Milli-Q water and 0.8 mL β-mercaptoethanol) and incubating for ~20 min in a 55 °C water bath. Then, wash the membrane thoroughly in TBS-T and follow method to block and reprobe with another antibody (e.g., IL-1β).

References

1. Fox JG, Wang TC (2007) Inflammation, atrophy, and gastric cancer. J Clin Invest 117:60–69
2. Mantovani A, Allavena P, Sica A, Balkwill F (2008) Cancer-related inflammation. Nature 454:436–444
3. Correa P, Piazuelo MB (2011) Helicobacter pylori infection and gastric adenocarcinoma. US Gastroenterol Hepatol Rev 7:59–64
4. Latz E, Xiao TS, Stutz A (2013) Activation and regulation of the inflammasomes. Nat Rev Immunol 13:397–411
5. Stutz A, Golenbock DT, Latz E (2009) Inflammasomes: too big to miss. J Clin Invest 119:3502–3511
6. Martinon F, Burns K, Tschopp J (2002) The inflammasome: a molecular platform triggering activation of inflammatory caspases and processing of proIL-beta: Mol Cell 10:417–426
7. Chen Y, Smith MR, Thirumalai K, Zychlinsky A (1996) A bacterial invasin induces macrophage apoptosis by binding directly to ICE. EMBO J 15:3853–3860
8. Lamkanfi M, Dixit VM (2010) Manipulation of host cell death pathways during microbial infections. Cell Host Microbe 8:44–54
9. Fabbi M, Carbotti G, Ferrini S (2015) Context-dependent role of IL-18 in cancer biology and counter-regulation by IL-18BP. J Leukoc Biol 97:665–675
10. Haghshenas MR, Hosseini SV, Mahmoudi M, Saberi-Firozi M, Farjadian S, Ghaderi A (2009) IL-18 serum level and IL-18 promoter gene polymorphism in Iranian patients with gastrointestinal cancers. J Gastroenterol Hepatol 24:1119–1122
11. Kang JS, Bae SY, Kim HR, Kim YS, Kim DJ, Cho BJ, Yang HK, Hwang YI, Kim KJ, Park HS, Hwang DH, Cho DJ, Lee WJ (2009) Interleukin-18 increases metastasis and immune escape of stomach cancer via the downregulation of CD70 and maintenance of CD44. Carcinogenesis 30:1987–1996
12. Thong-Ngam D, Tangkijvanich P, Lerknimitr R, Mahachai V, Theamboonlers A, Poovorawan Y (2006) Diagnostic role of serum interleukin-18 in gastric cancer patients. World J Gastroenterol 12:4473–4477
13. Kim KE, Song H, Kim TS, Yoon D, Kim CW, Bang SI, Hur DY, Park H, Cho DH (2007) Interleukin-18 is a critical factor for vascular endothelial growth factor-enhanced migration in human gastric cancer cell lines. Oncogene 26:1468–1476
14. Majima T, Ichikura T, Chochi K, Kawabata T, Tsujimoto H, Sugasawa H, Kuranaga N, Takayama E, Kinoshita M, Hiraide H, Seki S, Mochizuki H (2006) Exploitation of interleukin-18 by gastric cancers for their growth and evasion of host immunity. Int J Cancer 118:388–395

Chapter 19

Optimization Techniques for miRNA Expression in Low Frequency Immune Cell Populations

Victoria G. Lyons, Natalie L. Payne, and Claire E. McCoy

Abstract

In this chapter we outline a RNA extraction method for very low immune cell populations isolated from the central nervous system of mice undergoing experimental autoimmune encephalomyelitis. We compare various normalization and quantification techniques to examine miRNA expression. Our data highlight that employing a mean normalization procedure using a number of well-selected housekeeping miRNA genes, followed by absolute quantification with a standard curve generated from a commercial miRNA oligo, gave the most robust and reproducible miRNA expression results.

Key words microRNA, Experimental autoimmune encephalomyelitis, Immune cells, RT-PCR, Relative quantification, Absolute quantification, Mean normalization, Standard curve

1 Introduction

MicroRNAs (miRNA) are small nucleotide (18–25 nt in length) noncoding RNA molecules that posttranscriptionally regulate coding mRNA molecules. They play an important role in almost all cellular functions to regulate differentiation, proliferation, activation status and effector functions in any given cell type. Due to their involvement in these processes, it is no surprise that their dysresgulation underpins various diseases [1]. Thus, understanding how to reliably measure and quantify miRNAs has immense diagnostic potential, whilst monitoring the changes in expression in models of disease provides insight into complex regulatory networks and the identification of novel biological pathways that play a role in disease pathogenesis. In 2005, a successful real-time RT-PCR quantification technology was developed to detect miRNA molecules in cells and tissues [2]. The technique involves a two-step process and remains the most widely used method for fast, accurate and sensitive miRNA measurement. The first step involves a stem-loop RT primer that hybridizes to the miRNA and is reverse

Brendan J. Jenkins (ed.), *Inflammation and Cancer: Methods and Protocols*, Methods in Molecular Biology, vol. 1725, https://doi.org/10.1007/978-1-4939-7568-6_19, © Springer Science+Business Media, LLC 2018

transcribed using a Multi-Scribe reverse transcriptase. The second step measures the RT products using a conventional TaqMan PCR [2, 3].

Although TaqMan RT-PCR has become the gold standard for miRNA detection in cells and tissues, there are numerous prerequisite considerations. The first consideration is deciding on the method of RNA extraction. Many effective commercial kits and reagents are available for tissues and/or cells (Qiagen miRNeasy kit, Ambion miRVana PARIS, Analytik Jena kit, TRIzol reagent). We have extensively illustrated robust miRNA analysis in RNA extracted from both primary macrophages and macrophage cell lines using a modified protocol from the Qiagen RNeasy kit [4]. This method is ideal for extracting RNA when the starting material has a typical range of 1×10^5–1×10^6 cells per sample. However, this method was no longer appropriate when we performed experiments in vivo, with a need to detect miRNA expression in immune cells with low numbers ranging from 1×10^2–1×10^4. Thus, finding an alternative RNA extraction method became paramount to our studies. We needed to detect miR-155 expression in leukocytes isolated from the central nervous system (CNS) of mice undergoing experimental autoimmune encephalomyelitis (EAE). The CNS is a tissue with notoriously low immune cell numbers, particularly in naïve nontreated mice that are required for comparative analysis. Not only did we need to measure miR-155 expression levels in total CNS-isolated leukocytes, but also in specific immune cell populations, namely macrophages, T and B cells. We compared five methods of RNA extraction in FACS sorted immune cell populations from CNS-isolated leukocytes as follows: (1) Qiagen miRNeasy kit, (2) modified Qiagen RNeasy kit [4], (3) Analytik Jena kit, (4) TRIzol reagent, and (5) TRIzol reagent + carrier protein glycogen. Consistently in our hands, TRIzol reagent alone extracted RNA from as few as 100 cells (1×10^2) cells, giving ranges of 20–200 ng/μl of RNA and robust detection of miR-155.

The second consideration is the normalization method. Traditionally, changes in miRNA expression are determined by normalizing Ct values to an internal control, often called a "housekeeping gene" or in our case a "housekeeping miRNA" [5]. This miRNA should not vary in the tissues or cells under investigation, nor in response to the experimental treatment. Investigators often struggle to determine which housekeeping gene is most appropriate for their experiment in question, due to the divergence of choices that are available. For example, we ourselves have used a range of different housekeeping miRNAs such as RNU6B, snoRNA202, miR-191, and miR-16 depending on the cell type in question and the type of experiment performed [6–8]. We have realized that although certain housekeeping miRNAs may be occasionally constant in one particular immune cell type or experimental condition,

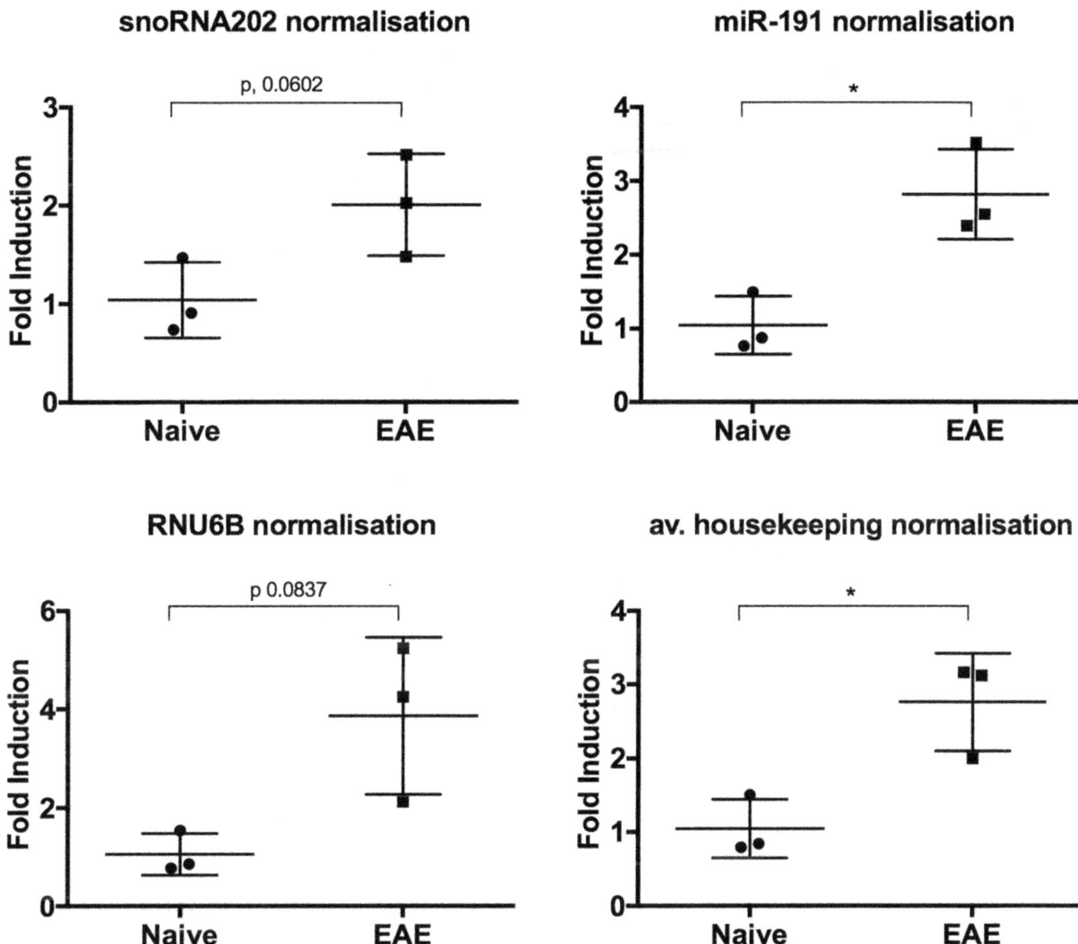

Fig. 1 miR-155 fold induction in CD4$^+$ T cells within the CNS of EAE-induced mice compared to naïve control mice using the ΔΔCt fold method. Data was first normalized to individual housekeeping genes (**a**) sno-202, (**b**) miR-191, (**c**) U6, and (**d**) the average of three housekeeping genes

it may vary considerably in another type of immune cell. Thus, we decided to investigate methods to eliminate these discrepancies by comparing our data when normalizing to the average of three housekeeping genes (RNU6B, snoRNA202, and miR-191) rather than the traditional use of just one (Fig. 1). We found that by averaging three housekeeping genes we obtained more consistent and reliable results between experiments. This is not a surprise and in fact, this method of taking the average of multiple carefully selected housekeeping genes is validated as an accurate normalization method [9, 10]. However, this method is often not sustainable, particularly when samples are precious and cost-burdens are a factor. Yet, by utilizing this method in our preliminary experiments, it gave us the confidence moving forward to choose a single housekeeping miRNA that could reliably reproduce the data obtained when three housekeeping genes were used.

Another important consideration is quantification methods. There are two methods; relative and absolute. Relative quantification describes the change in expression of the target gene (in our case, miR-155) relative to a reference group, often an untreated group or sample at time zero. This method is useful for determining how a given treatment increases the expression of a certain miRNA, where the data is represented as fold-change over non-treated control. The ΔΔCt calculation method is a convenient way to assess the relative expression of miRNAs from RT-PCR experiments [5]. Although this method is popular, it does have drawbacks. The experiment must contain nontreated samples, the PCR efficiency of your target miRNA and housekeeping miRNA must be approximately equal; lastly it cannot accurately determine actual transcript copy numbers in your samples.

In contrast, absolute quantification determines the absolute copy number of the miRNA of interest, by relating the RT-PCR data to a standard curve with known amounts. This method is important for quantifying the actual amount of transcript between different cell types and tissues for example. Using miR-155 as an example, we generated a standard curve using a commercially available miR-155 oligo. Graphing log concentration against Ct generates a slope where we can obtain an equation of the line. Using this equation, we can calculate the concentration of miR-155 in our samples. It also enables the calculation of samples irrespective of a nontreated reference sample that is particularly useful. In addition, we utilized a median normalization method, a method that has been increasing in popularity due to its success in reproducibility [11, 12]. This method removes the doubt that housekeeping genes themselves can be differentially expressed in experimental conditions, and instead relies on normalization by calculating the mean Ct value from all the housekeeping miRNAs. This method is even more robust if three housekeeping genes have been used in the experimental design.

In summary, we outline relative and absolute quantification methods for determining miRNA expression in low number immune cells. The relative method is quick and straightforward for in vitro analysis when, for example, testing agonists and/or drug responses. However, we believe that the absolute quantification method is superior for in vivo analysis where the use of a standard curve and the mean normalization technique ensures accuracy, consistency, and reproducibility.

2 Materials

2.1 EAE Induction

1. 9–10-week-old female C57BL/6J mice.
2. Myelin oligodendrocyte glycoprotein (MOG) 35–55 peptide (lyophilized). Reconstitute lyophilized MOG35–55 peptide in

sterile PBS to a concentration of 20 mg/ml. Aliquot into sterile eppendorf tubes and store at −80 °C.

3. Complete Freund's adjuvant (CFA).
4. *Mycobacterium tuberculosis* H37Ra (killed and desiccated). Reconstitute *M. tuberculosis* in 1 mL sterile water to a concentration of 100 mg/ml. Store at 4 °C for up to 1 month.
5. Pertussis toxin from *Bordetella pertussis* (lyophilized).
6. Sterile Dulbecco's phosphate buffered saline, no calcium or magnesium (PBS).
7. Sterile water.
8. Glass Hamilton syringes (1 × 1 mL, 2 × 10 mL).
9. Three-way stopcock.
10. 1 mL syringe.
11. 25 gauge needle.
12. Insulin syringe.
13. Sterile 1.5 mL eppendorf tubes.
14. Sterile 50 mL tube.

2.2 CNS Dissection

1. CO_2 induction chamber.
2. Surgical instruments: straight dissecting scissors, small blunt curved serrated forceps, hemostats.
3. 25 gauge butterfly needle.
4. 18 gauge needle.
5. 50 and 10 mL syringes.
6. PBS.
7. 60 mm petri dish.
8. Dulbecco's Modified Eagle's Medium (DMEM) with high glucose.
9. 80% ethanol.

2.3 Leukocyte Isolation

1. 60 mm tissue culture treated petri dishes to place CNS after dissection.
2. Sterile stainless steel scalpel blade.
3. Sterile Pasteur pipette.
4. Sterile 70 μm filters.
5. Sterile 15 and 50 mL Falcon tubes.
6. Complete DMEM: 500 mL DMEM supplemented with 10% fetal calf serum (FCS) and 1% penicillin/streptomycin.

7. 70% and 30% Percoll stocks diluted in PBS.
8. Trypan Blue to determine cell viability at a ratio of 1:1.
9. PBS.
10. Digestion buffer: 25 ng/mL DNase, 1 mg/mL Collagenase D in PBS. Digestion buffer needs to be as fresh as possible and prepared within 6 h of carrying out experiment.
11. FACS buffer consisting of PBS, 5–10% FBS, 1 mM Ethylenediaminetetraacetic acid (EDTA), and 0.1% NaN_3 sodium azide.
12. Hemocytometer.

2.4 Fluorescence Activated Cell Sorting (FACS)

1. Corning™ Falcon™ Round-Bottom Polystyrene Tubes.
2. FACS buffer.
3. 1:150 CD16/CD32 (Fc antibody) freshly prepared and diluted in FACS buffer.
4. Compatible flow cytometry cell surface markers as highlighted in Table 1. Make a master mix by diluting all antibodies (1:200) in 100 μL FACS buffer per sample. Generate 1:500 dilution single stains for each antibody in 50 μL FACS buffer.
5. FACS CANTO II flow cytometry machine for sample acquisition and analysis.
6. Cell sorting machine; Beckman Coulter MoFlo XDP.
7. FlowJo Vx 10.0 software for phenotypic analysis.

2.5 RNA Extraction

1. 1.5 mL Eppendorf tubes.
2. 1 mL/sample of TRIzol reagent.
3. 200 μL/sample of chloroform.
4. 500 μL/sample of isopropanol.
5. 1 mL/sample of 80% ethanol.
6. 30 μL/sample of DNase and RNase-free H_2O.

Table 1
Compatible flow cytometry cell surface antibodies

Cell marker	Fluorescent probe	Expression/representative	Location
CD45	PerCpCy5.5	Leukocytes	Cell surface
CD11b	APC	Myeloid cells	Cell surface
F480	FITC	Monocytes/macrophages/eosinophils	Cell surface
CD4	PE	$CD4^+$ cells	Cell surface
CD3	eFluor450	T cells	Cell surface
B220	PE/Cy7	B cells	Cell surface

7. Fume hood (TRIzol contains phenol).
8. Heating block (set at 55–60 °C).

2.6 RT-PCR

1. TaqMan® MicroRNA Reverse Transcription Kit.
2. TaqMan MiRNA Assay. Two components comprised within the assay: 5× primer and 20× FAM-labeled probe per specific miRNA.
3. SensiFAST™ SYBR® Hi-ROX.
4. miR-155 synthetic oligonucleotide with ZEN modifications (5-′-rUrUrA rArUrG rCrUrA rArUrU rGrUrG rArUrA GrGrG rGrU-3′). Reconstitute with DNA/RNase free H_2O to a 100 nM stock according to the material safety data sheet. Generate multiple smaller aliquots at 1 nM and store at −80 °C.
5. 1.5 mL Eppendorf tubes.
6. 8-Strip PCR tube caps (0.2 mL) with flat writing surface.
7. MicroAMP™ Optical 384- or 96-well reaction plate.
8. MicroAMP™ Optical Adhesive Film.
9. 7900HT RT-PCR System with 384- or 96-well block.

2.7 Data Analysis

1. SDS v2.2 software.

3 Methods

3.1 EAE Induction

EAE is induced by subcutaneous injection of 100 μg of the encephalitogenic peptide MOG35–55 (also called antigen) in CFA supplemented with *M. tuberculosis* on day 0. A 1:1 ratio emulsion of MOG35–55 and CFA is prepared and each mouse receives two injections of 100 μl (total of 200 μl per mouse). 200 ng of pertussis toxin is administered intraperitoneally in a volume of 200 μl on day 0 and again on day 2 (*see* **Note 1**).

1. Dilute the 20 mg/ml stock of MOG35–55 1:20 with sterile PBS to achieve a working concentration of 1 mg/ml.
2. Thoroughly vortex the 100 mg/ml stock of *M. tuberculosis* (from **step 4**) and add 400 μl to a 10 ml vial of CFA (*see* **Note 2**). This can be stored at 4 °C for up to 1 month.
3. Calculate the volume of CFA/antigen emulsion required for immunization by multiplying the number of mice to be immunized by 200 μl and then multiplying by 1.5 (*see* **Note 3**). Divide this number by half to give the volume of CFA and the volume of MOG35–55 required. For example: 10 mice × 200 μl per mouse = 2000 μl × 1.5 = 3000 μl total volume required/2 = 1500 μl CFA + 1500 μl MOG35–55.

4. To prepare the emulsion of CFA/antigen, connect 2 × 10 ml glass Hamilton syringes (*see* **Note 4**) to a three-way stopcock and remove the plunger from syringe-1. Secure syringe-2 with tape so that syringe-1 remains upright.
5. Thoroughly vortex CFA prepared in **step 2**. To syringe-1, add equal volumes of CFA and MOG35–55 working solution (prepared in **step 1**) according to the volume calculated in **step 3**.
6. Slowly draw back the plunger of syringe-2 until the entire contents have been drawn into the syringe. Disconnect syringe-2 from the stopcock and expel any air bubbles within the syringe (*see* **Note 5**). Replace the plunger in syringe-1 to the 0 ml mark and then reconnect syringe-2 to the stopcock.
7. Thoroughly mix the contents between the two syringes by alternatively pressing down on the plungers to create an emulsion. Place on ice until required (*see* **Note 6**).
8. Calculate the total volume of Pertussis toxin required by multiplying the number of mice to be immunized by 200 μl and then multiply by 1.2 (to account for loss during loading of syringes).
9. Reconstitute lyophilized Pertussis toxin to a concentration of 100 μg/ml by slowly injecting sterile PBS through the lid with an insulin syringe. Mix gently and allow to dissolve for 5 min. This can be stored at 4 °C for up to 1 month.
10. Dilute the 100 μg/ml stock of Pertussis toxin (from **step 11**) 1:100 with sterile PBS in a 50 ml tube to achieve a working concentration of 1 μg/ml. Place on ice.
11. Immediately prior to immunization, place Pertussis toxin at room temperature and thoroughly mix the CFA/antigen emulsion between the two syringes.
12. Expel the entire emulsion into syringe-1, disconnect syringe-2 and connect a 1 ml glass Hamilton syringe. Slowly load the 1 ml syringe with the emulsion to the 1.2 ml mark (*see* **Note 7**).
13. Disconnect the 1 ml syringe, reconnect syringe-2 and place the emulsion on ice.
14. Attach a 25 gauge needle to the 1 ml syringe, tap gently and expel the emulsion to the 1 ml mark to release any air bubbles.
15. Using the 1 ml syringe, inject each mouse with 100 μl of the CFA/antigen emulsion into each hind limb flank (total of 200 μl per mouse) (*see* **Note 8**).
16. Inject each mouse with 200 μl of Pertussis toxin (prepared in **step 12**) intraperitoneally. Repeat 48 h later.
17. Monitor mice daily for clinical signs of disease from day 8 post immunization (*see* **Note 9**). Clinical scores are assigned according to the scale in Table 2.

Table 2
Clinical grading system for assessment of EAE

Score	Clinical signs
0	Normal. Curling of the tail when the mouse is picked up
0.5	Partial limp tail. The tip of the tail is limp when the mouse is picked up
1	Limp tail. The tail is completely limp when the mouse is picked up
2	Weak hind limbs. The mouse has an abnormal gait and struggles to right itself when placed on its back
2.5	Paralysis of one hind limb. The mouse drags one hind limb and there is no response to toe pinch
3	Paralysis of both hind limbs. There is complete loss of movement in both hind limbs and no response to toe pinch
4	Paralyzed hind limbs and weak forelimbs. Mice are sacrificed for humane reasons
5	Moribund. The mouse is cold to touch and not moving

3.2 CNS Dissection

The below protocol details dissection of the brain and spinal cord separately. Brain and spinal tissue can be processed together for isolation of leukocytes from the entire CNS, separately or if specific regions of the brain or spinal cord need to be examined.

1. Euthanize the mouse by CO_2 asphyxiation, secure the limbs and spray with 80% ethanol.
2. Open the chest cavity to expose the heart (*see* **Note 10**).
3. Insert a 25 gauge butterfly needle attached to a 50 ml syringe prefilled with PBS into the left ventricle of the heart and cut the right atrium of the heart with scissors.
4. Confirm correct placement of the needle be pushing down on the plunger slowly and observing for efflux of blood from the right atrium.
5. Perfuse the mouse with PBS until the blood runs clear and the liver has lost its red color (*see* **Note 11**).
6. To remove the brain, secure the limbs and spray the head and back of the mouse with 80% ethanol.
7. Make an incision through the skin coronally between the eyes and longitudinally to the base of the tail.
8. Hold the head at the base of the skull and cut the skull between the two olfactory bulbs by placing one blade of the dissecting scissors into each eye cavity and cutting coronally.
9. Make a longitudinal cut through the skull along the sagittal suture (*see* **Note 12**). Expose the brain by applying gentle tangential, lateral pressure to tilt back the frontal and parietal

bones on each side with either the blade of the scissors or a pair of curved forceps.

10. Carefully slide forceps under the anterior part of the brain and tilt the brain upward to cut the cranial nerves with scissors.
11. Hold the interparietal bone with forceps and cut on either side to expose the area where the brain and spinal cord meet.
12. Make a cut at the base of the brain where it meets the spinal cord and carefully remove the brain. Place on ice in a 60 mm petri dish with DMEM.
13. To remove the spinal cord, peel back the skin to the base of the tail in order to expose the spinal column.
14. Cut the spinal cord where the spinal column attaches to the pelvis and then cut along the spinal column on each side in order to remove the column.
15. Insert an 18 gauge needle attached to a 10 ml syringe prefilled with PBS into the spinal canal at the caudal end of the spinal column, past the point of resistance.
16. Push down on the plunger to flush the spinal cord into a 60 mm dish containing DMEM with high glucose.

3.3 Leukocyte Isolation

1. Transfer the intact CNS to new 60 mm petri dishes containing freshly prepared digestion buffer.
2. Thoroughly dice the CNS using a carbon steel surgical blade.
3. Incubate the diced CNS for 30 min at 37 °C.
4. Add 2 ml of PBS to each sample to terminate the enzymatic reaction.
5. Within a biological safety cabinet, use a Pasteur pipette to flush the digested CNS through a 70 μm filter into a 15 ml Falcon tube. Continue flushing the CNS with PBS until there is a final volume of 15 ml within the Falcon tube.
6. Centrifuge samples at 4 °C for 5 min at 500 × *g*
7. Decant the supernatant and add 8 ml of 30% Percoll to resuspend the cell pellet.
8. Gently layer the cell suspension at a 45° angle onto the surface of 3 ml of 70% Percoll within a 15 ml Falcon tube.
9. Centrifuge the layered suspension at room temperature for 25 min at 500 × *g* with no brake activation (*see* **Note 13**).
10. A white buffy coat layer will be visible between the will between the 30% and 70% Percoll gradients. This layer contains CNS leukocytes. Using a Pasteur pipette, transfer the buffy coat to a clean 15 ml Falcon tube (*see* **Note 14**).
11. Add PBS to a final volume of 15 ml and centrifuge at 4 °C for 5 min at 1500 rpm.

12. Resuspend the pellet containing the CNS leukocytes in 1 ml of FACS buffer.
13. Count the cells using a hemocytometer in a dilution of 1:1 with Trypan Blue (*see* **Note 15**).

3.4 FACS

1. Centrifuge the CNS leukocytes at 4 °C for 5 min at 150 × *g* and resuspend in 200 μl 1:150 CD16/CD32 for 30 min at 4 °C (*see* **Note 16**).
2. Wash samples with 1 ml of FACS buffer. Remove 2×10^5 cells from each sample into a separate tube. These samples will be used for single stains (i.e., you will need six single stain samples if there are six antibodies in the master mix as highlighted in Table 1). The remaining cells in the original sample will be used for cell sorting.
3. Centrifuge all samples for 5 min at 4 °C at 150 × *g*.
4. Decant supernatants in one swift motion to reduce dead volume within the FACS tube.
5. Add 100 μl of antibody master mix to the cell sorting sample and 50 μl of single stain mix to the single stain samples (*see* **Note 17**).
6. Incubate samples for 30 min in the dark at 4 °C.
7. Wash samples by pipetting 1 ml of FACS buffer into each FACS tube and centrifuging at 150 × *g* for 5 min.
8. Decant supernatants and resuspend cell pellet in 100–150 μl of FACS buffer.
9. Bring samples to the cell sorting machine on ice to prevent cell clumping and death. Most cell sorting machines, i.e., FACS ARIA and MoFlo XDP Cell Sorters, can collect up to four cell populations in four separate fractions.
10. Determine the gating strategy to obtain the desired cell populations. Start by plotting a forward scatter (FS) and side scatter (SC) plot to determine live cells, then gate on $CD45^+$ cells to determine all leukocytes. $F4/80^+CD11b^+$ positive cells will represent macrophages. $CD3^+CD4^+$ positive cells will represent $CD4^+$ T cells and $B220^+$ will represent B cells.
11. Run each sample on the cell sorting machine until there is no sample remaining in the FACS tube.
12. Purified and enriched cell populations are collected into separate fractions within FACS tubes (*see* **Note 18**).
13. Purified populations should be placed on ice until downstream experiments are carried out, i.e., RNA extraction.

3.5 RNA Extraction

The following RNA isolation protocol has been specifically modified to accommodate for low cell numbers using the chemical reagent TRIzol (*see* **Note 19**).

1. Lyse samples in 1 ml of TRIzol Reagent and incubate for 5 min at room temperature within Eppendorf tubes (*see* **Note 20**).
2. Add 200 μl of chloroform to samples and shake vigorously for 30 s to ensure complete mixing between cell lysates, TRIzol, and chloroform.
3. Incubate Eppendorf tubes for 10 min at room temperature.
4. Centrifuge cell lysates at 12,879 × *g* for 15 min at 4 °C.
5. After centrifugation samples are separated into three phases; an organic phase (containing proteins and lipids), an interphase (containing DNA), and most importantly; the desired upper aqueous phase (containing RNA).
6. Carefully pipette 400 μl of the aqueous phase into a clean Eppendorf tube containing 500 μl of Isopropanol. Samples can be placed at −20 °C which has been suggested to increase the yield of RNA or you can proceed directly onto the next step.
7. Centrifuge Eppendorf tubes for 12,879 × *g* for 10 min at 4 °C and carefully decant supernatants (*see* **Note 21**).
8. Resuspend the pellets in 1 ml of 80% Ethanol.
9. Centrifuge Eppendorf tubes at 5031 × *g* for 5 min at 4 °C and decant supernatants.
10. Air-dry samples by inverting Eppendorf tubes onto clean tissue and maintaining this inversion for 5–10 min.
11. Resuspend samples in 30 μl of DNase and RNase free H_2O.
12. Place samples on a heat block set at 55–60 °C.
13. Place samples immediately on ice and measure the RNA concentration by placing 1 μl on a NanoDrop. Typical cell numbers and RNA concentrations from CNS-isolated immune cell populations in a wild-type naïve mouse are shown in Table 3. Store the RNA at −80 °C indefinitely.

Table 3
Cell numbers from immune cell populations enriched by cell sorting with their corresponding RNA concentration yield (ng/μl) within the CNS of a WT naïve C57/Bl6 mouse

Immune cell population	Cell number	RNA concentration (ng/μl)
Macrophages	7600	205.5
$CD4^+$ T cells	745	75
B220 cells	1200	120

3.6 RT-PCR

3.6.1 Sample Preparation

1. Prepare RNA at a stock concentration of 5–10 ng/μl for miRNA expression analysis using DNA/RNase free H_2O (*see* **Note 22**).
2. Thaw all reagents on ice from the TaqMan® MicroRNA Reverse Transcription Kit and the TaqMan® Primer from the TaqMan® MiRNA Assay Kit.
3. Briefly vortex and microcentrifuge dNTPs, 10× buffer, and TaqMan® MiRNA Primers.
4. In a microcentrifuge tube, prepare an RT reaction master mix as outlined in Table 4 comprising of: dNTP, 10× buffer, RNase inhibitor, RT enzyme, and desired primers (*see* **Note 23**). It is essential that at least one housekeeping gene is included such as snoRNA202, RNU6B, and/or miR-191.
5. Add 12 μl of RT reaction master mix into the correct number of thin wall 8-Strip PCR tubes (*see* **Note 24**).
6. Pipette 3 μl of each RNA sample to each labeled corresponding PCR tube and mix gently with a quick flick.
7. Microcentrifuge samples at a low speed for no longer than 5 s to ensure all liquid is gravitated down to the bottom of the PCR tubes.
8. Run the samples on a PCR machine using the following program: 16 °C for 30 min, 42 °C for 30 min, 85 °C for 5 min and 15 °C for ∞.
9. Samples may be kept overnight in a PCR machine at a holding temperature of 15 °C, stored at 4 °C for 1 week or stored at −20 °C for up to 1 year before proceeding (*see* **Note 25**).

Table 4
The reagents and volumes required to generate a 12 μl RT reaction mix for individual miRNA analysis

Reagent	Volume (μl)[a]
dNTP	0.125
10× buffer	1.5
RNase inhibitor	0.18
RT enzyme	1.0
TaqMan primer (5×)	0.375 (per each primer)[b]
H_2O (DNA/RNase free)	Dependent on primer number[c]
Total volume	*12*

[a]These volumes should be multiplied by the number of samples you have (+2 for pipetting error) to create an RT reaction master mix
[b]The reaction can allow multiple miRNA primers (maximum 8) to be accommodated in the one reaction mix
[c]The volume of H_2O will depend on the amount of primers included in the reaction mix

Table 5
The reagents and volumes required to generate a RT-PCR reaction mix for individual miRNA analysis

Reagent	Volume (μl)[a]
2× TaqMan Universal Master Mix	10.0
H_2O (DNA/RNase free)	8.0
20× probe	0.66

[a]These volumes incorporate enough mix to measure one miRNA in duplicate as well as allowing extra for pipetting error, and should be multiplied by the number of samples in your experiment to generate a master mix

10. Thaw newly synthesized cDNA samples if frozen and keep on ice.
11. Prepare individual master mixes for each miRNA intended to be detected. Each master mix comprises of: 2× SensiFAST Probe HiROX buffer, 20× probe, and DNA/RNase-free H_2O made up according to volumes outlined in Table 5 (*see* **Note 26**).
12. Vortex each master mix to ensure that all reagents are thoroughly mixed.
13. Design the experimental layout on a 384- or 96-well RT-PCR plate (*see* **Note 27**).
14. Pipette 8.9 μl of each master mix to appropriate wells (e.g., if there are ten samples and two probes, each master mix would be pipetted into 20 wells (technical duplicates) resulting in a total of 40 wells being used (two probes) in the 384- or 96-well plate).
15. Pipette 1 μl of each cDNA sample into appropriate wells (2 μl of each cDNA sample should be used per probe due to duplicates) (*see* **Note 28**).

3.6.2 Synthetic miRNA Standards Preparation

A miR-155 synthetic oligonucleotide can be used as a method of determining absolute miR-155 expression levels by creating a miR-155 standard curve.

1. Thaw a 1 nM miR-155 synthetic oligonucleotide aliquot on ice.
2. Generate a concentration of 32.8 pM from the 1 nM stock by diluting 4 μl of the 1 nM stock into 118 μl of H_2O.
3. Create a fourfold dilution by diluting 25 μl of the 32.8 pM stock into 75 μl of H_2O, this will be the top standard of the standard curve and contains a concentration of 8.2 pM or 8200 fM.

4. Create 5–7 more serial fourfold dilutions; a final blank template control containing only H_2O must also be included to distinguish background CT noise from the RT-PCR machine.
5. Run these serial dilutions in parallel with experiment samples. For example, following **steps 5–9**, Subheading 3.6.1, add 3 μl of each serial dilution to 12 μl of RT reaction mix. Following **steps 10–15**, Subheading 3.6.1, add 1 μl of the cDNA sample generated onto the appropriate wells of a RT-PCR plate which contains the miR-155 probe.

3.6.3 Loading the Plate

1. Seal the RT-PCR plate with an optical adhesive film. Once the film is sufficiently applied (using applicator provided), tear off the perforated edges.
2. Centrifuge the RT-PCR plate at 150 × *g* for 1 min. This is to ensure there are no droplets trapped at the edge of any wells (the laser within the RT-PCR machine may not identify these drops causing skewed results).
3. On the 7900HT System, start the SDS v2.2 software. In the main menu, select File – New. In the new document dialog box, select the following from the drop-down menu: Absolute Quantification (ΔΔCt) and 384-well format (or 96-well format depending on the plate used).
4. On the right-hand side of the screen, open the New Detector tab; name each miRNA being evaluated within the experiment. Ensure the FAM tab is also highlighted.
5. On the left-hand side of the screen, highlight the wells that contain samples from the experiment and label with the appropriate miRNA detector and sample number.
6. Save as an SDS 7900 Template (.sdt) file.
7. Load and run the RT-PCR plate using the standard default thermal-cycling conditions, changing the reaction volume to 10 μl (*see* **Note 29**). This RT-PCR run takes approximately 1 h 20 min.
8. To retrieve data, go to File and Open saved .sdt file. Click analyze data by pressing the green triangle. Export data as a .txt file to a USB stick.

3.7 Data Analysis

3.7.1 ΔΔCt Method

1. Once the RT-PCR cycle containing all biological experimental samples has completed its run, using Microsoft Excel Spreadsheet, paste the Ct values of the miRNA of interest parallel to the housekeeping miRNA Ct values. The ΔΔCt method is shown in the following equation and described in the following steps.

$$\mathrm{Ct}_{\text{miRNA sample}} - \mathrm{Ct}_{\text{house-keeping miRNA}} = \Delta Ct.$$
$$\Delta Ct_{\text{miRNA sample}} - \Delta Ct_{\text{reference sample}} = \Delta\Delta \mathrm{Ct}.$$
$$\text{Fold Induction} = 2^{-\Delta\Delta \mathrm{Ct}}.$$

2. Subtract the Ct values obtained from experimental miRNA samples away from the chosen housekeeping miRNA Ct values (termed ΔCt). Analysis is possible using one housekeeping gene or the average of multiple house-keeping genes, i.e., snoRNA202, miR-191, U6. Figure 1 illustrates the difference between normalizing the data to three housekeeping genes compared to individual housekeeping genes.
3. Determine the average ΔCt value from your reference group (nontreated group) only, and subtract this value from the ΔCt value of the miRNA sample.
4. The fold change ($2^{-\Delta\Delta Ct}$) is calculated by multiplying ΔΔCt values obtained in the previous step by the power of 2, i.e., POWER(2, ΔΔCt).

3.7.2 Absolute Quantification Method

1. Once the RT-PCR cycle containing all the experimental and standard curve samples has completed its run, using Microsoft Excel Spreadsheet, paste all the Ct values onto an excel sheet.
2. Determine the standard curve first by plotting the Ct values from the serial dilutions against the corresponding concentration expressed in fM. Convert the fM value to a log value, i.e., the top standard of 8200 fM has a log value of 3.9 (*see* Fig. 2). This term is often denoted log copy number.
3. Next, calculate the mean Ct value from the entire set of housekeeping miRNAs used in the experiment. You can calculate this value from the average of one housekeeping miRNA or use the mean value from multiple housekeeping miRNAs.

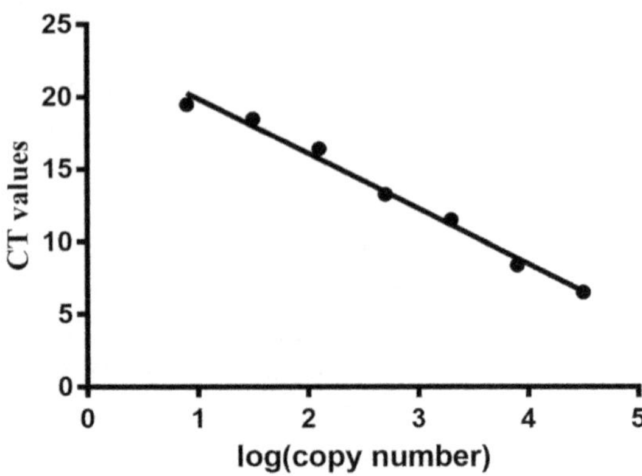

Fig. 2 Standard curve demonstrating Ct values vs log copy number of miR-155 Oligo concentration (fM)

4. Create a Normalization Factor (NF) [12] by subtracting the mean housekeeping Ct value from the sample of interest from the mean Ct value generated in **step 2**.

$$\text{Mean Ct}_{\text{entire house-keeping}} - \text{Mean Ct}_{\text{sample house-keeping}} = \text{NF}$$

5. Add the NF value to the raw Ct value generated for the experimental sample (i.e., the Ct value generated for the miRNA of interest).

$$\text{NF} + \text{Ct}_{\text{miRNA sample}} = \text{normalized Ct value}$$

6. The normalized Ct value is then used to calculate the absolute copy number from the standard curve generated from the synthetic miRNA oligonucleotide (Fig. 2).
7. From the standard curve, determine the equation of the line, i.e., $y = 1.11x \pm 22.22$ (*see* **Note 30**).
8. To solve "x" (log copy number), subtract the numerical value at the end of the equation, i.e., 22.22 from the normalized Ct values obtained in **step 5** and divide this by the numerical value adjacent to x, i.e., 1.11. Therefore, this calculation would resemble the following: (**step 4** − 22.22)/1.11 = x. This gives you a value that equates to log copy number or log fM concentration.
9. Multiply the log value obtained in the previous step by the power of 10, i.e., POWER(10, "x"). The value is often too low to represent on a graph and it is often necessary to multiply the value by the desired exponential factor to represent the data. Figure 3 illustrates the exact same data from Subheading 3.7.1 calculated using the absolute quantification method instead of the ΔΔCt method.

4 Notes

1. Our immunization protocol is sufficient to achieve 100% disease incidence and clinical severity of score 3 (hind limb paralysis) at our facility. A number of factors can influence the incidence and severity of disease, including the age and source of mice, stress, the cleanliness of the animal facility and batch/source of MOG35–55 peptide, *M. tuberculosis* and Pertussis toxin. It is therefore recommended that mice are allowed to acclimatize for 1 week prior to immunization and that the dose of reagents is determined empirically by each investigator.
2. CFA contains 1 mg/ml of heat-killed *M. tuberculosis.*

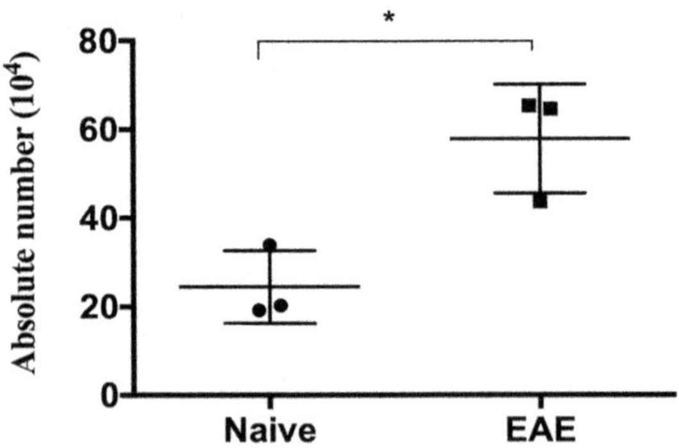

Fig. 3 miR-155 copy numbers in CD4$^+$ T cells within the CNS of EAE-induced mice compared to naïve control mice. Data was calculated using the absolute quantification method and normalized using the mean normalization of three housekeeping miRNAs

3. Due to its consistency there can be a substantial loss of the CFA/antigen emulsion during loading of syringes and thus excess emulsion should be prepared.
4. Additional syringes may be required depending on the number of mice to be immunized.
5. It is critical that no air bubbles are introduced when preparing the emulsion.
6. An emulsion is formed if a drop discharged into room temperature water remains intact on the surface. If the drop disperses additional mixing is required.
7. This is only required the first time the 1 ml syringe is loaded with the emulsion.
8. A bolus mass should form and persist under the skin for the duration of the experiment. Ensure the injection site is not located on the inguinal lymph nodes if they need to be harvested for analysis.
9. The tail can be marked to keep track of individual mice.
10. Hemostats can be used to hold the chest cavity open by clamping the sternum and placing the hemostat over the head.
11. 20 ml is sufficient assuming correct placement of the needle.
12. Ensure the angle of the scissors is as superficial as possible to avoid damaging the underlying brain.
13. Room temperature is important to ensure complete phase separation between Percoll gradients and CNS leukocyte buffy coat layer.
14. It is wise to transfer about 2–3 ml of the buffy coat to maximize the amount of cells that are contained in this fraction.

15. A naïve mouse contains approximately 0.5×10^6 leukocytes in the CNS. This increases to approximately $1–2 \times 10^6$ in a mouse undergoing EAE.
16. Adding CD16/CD32 (Fc antibody) prevents nonspecific binding of FACS antibodies.
17. It is also important to have one sample containing 2×10^5 cells that is unstained and contains no antibody.
18. Confirm with the FACS analyst prior to cell sorting which FACS tubes are compatible for obtaining and collecting samples as compatibilities between cell sorting machines differ.
19. It is possible to investigate both miRNA and gene expression with this optimized TRIzol method. However we only discuss miRNA expression analysis in this chapter.
20. This step must be carried out in a fume hood, due to the presence of phenol in the TRIzol.
21. RNA pellets can become easily dislodged in this step.
22. Keep the RNA samples on ice.
23. As multiple primers can be added to this master mix (maximum 8), the H_2O volume should be determined once all other reagents have been accounted for. For instance, if there is a master mix prepared for 8 samples (+2 for pipetting error) with two primers: $(10)\ 0.125 + (10)\ 1.5 + (10)\ 0.18 + (10)\ 1.0 + [10\ (0.375 \times 2)]$ = total volume of all other reagents. Required total master mix volume of 120 μl (12 μl × 10 samples): total volume of reagents − 120 μl = volume of H_2O.
24. We have found using 8× strip tubes to be the most useful PCR tubes for assessing multiple samples and convenient storage.
25. We have experienced significant degradation and destabilization of cDNA if kept longer than 1 year. It is better to repeat **steps 1–8**, using stored RNA kept at −80 °C rather than reuse stored cDNA for subsequent RT-PCR analysis.
26. Each sample must be run in technical duplicates for each miRNA being assessed.
27. The use of a 384- or 96-well RT-PCR plate depends on the block most frequently used by your gene expression facility and/or the amount of samples you have.
28. We have found that using the same pipette tip between duplicates gives tighter replicates. However, it is necessary to change the pipette tip between samples and when moving onto a new master mix to prevent cross-contamination.

29. It is recommended by the manufacturer's that RT-PCR be performed in a final 20 μl volume. However, we have found a final volume of 10 μl works just as well, thus saving on overall costs.
30. A reliable equation of the lines is generated from standard curves with an R^2 value of 98 or above.

References

1. O'Connell RM, Rao DS, Chaudhuri AA, Baltimore D (2010) Physiological and pathological roles for microRNAs in the immune system. Nat Rev Immunol 10:111–122
2. Chen C, Ridzon DA, Broomer AJ, Zhou Z, Lee DH, Nguyen JT, Barbisin M, Xu NL, Mahuvakar VR, Andersen MR, Lao KQ, Livak KJ, Guegler KJ (2005) Real-time quantification of microRNAs by stem-loop RT-PCR. Nucleic Acids Res 20:e179
3. Schmittgen TD, Lee EJ, Jiang J, Sarkar A, Yang L, Elton TS, Chen C (2008) Real-time PCR quantification of precursor and mature microRNA. Methods 44:31–38
4. Lyons V, McCoy CE (2016) Simple methods to investigate analyse miRNA induction in response to Toll-like receptors. Methods Mol Biol 1390:159–182
5. Livak KJ, Schmittgen TD (2001) Analysis of relative gene expression data using real-time quantitative PCR and the 2(−Delta Delta C (T)) Method. Methods 25:402–408
6. McCoy CE, Sheedy FJ, Qualls JE, Doyle SL, Quinn SR, Murray PJ, O'Neill LA (2010) IL-10 inhibits miR-155 induction by toll-like receptors. J Biol Chem 285:20492–20498
7. Gantier MP, Stunden HJ, McCoy CE, Behlke MA, Wang D et al (2012) A miR-19 regulon that controls NF-kappaB signaling. Nucleic Acids Res 40:8048–8058
8. Fairfax KA, Gantier MP, Mackay F, Williams BR, McCoy CE (2015) IL-10 regulates Aicda expression through miR-155. J Leukoc Biol 97:71–78
9. D'haene B, Mestdagh P, Hellemans J, Vandesompele J (2012) miRNA expression profiling: from reference genes to global mean normalization. Methods Mol Biol 822:261–272
10. Vandesompele J, De Preter K, Pattyn F, Poppe B, Van Roy N, De Paepe A, Speleman F (2002) Accurate normalization of real-time quantitative RT-PCR data by geometric averaging of multiple internal control genes. Genome Biol 3:7
11. Qureshi R, Sacan A (2013) A novel method for the normalization of microRNA RT-PCR data. BMC Med Genet 6:S1–14
12. Kroh EM, Parkin RK, Mitchell PS, Tewari M (2010) Analysis of circulating microRNA biomarkers in plasma and serum using quantitative reverse transcription-PCR (qRT-PCR). Methods 4:298–301

Chapter 20

Assessing the cGAS-cGAMP-STING Activity of Cancer Cells

Geneviève Pépin and Michael P. Gantier

Abstract

DNA sensing by the STING pathway is emerging to be a crucial component of the antitumor immune response. Although it plays a key role in the activation of tumor immune cells, exactly how STING is activated by tumor cells is not fully understood. Recent evidence suggests that cGAS can be directly engaged and produces 2′3′-cyclic-GMP-AMP (cGAMP) within certain tumor cells upon stimulation with DNA damaging agents. Because cGAMP can transfer between adjacent cells, the capacity of tumor cells to produce cGAMP may activate tumor immune cells, even in the absence of functional STING signaling within the tumor. Here we describe a simple coculture protocol allowing for the functional characterization of cGAS/STING activity in tumor cells, together with cGAMP transfer to adjacent cells. This approach will help define how different tumors engage the STING pathway, and whether synthetic STING agonists should be used to potentiate the antitumor effects of chemotherapies.

Key words cGAS, cGAMP, STING, Interferon, Connexin, Cancer, Immunotherapy, Innate immunity

1 Introduction

Stimulator of interferon genes (STING) protein is a key signaling hub in innate immune responses. Anchored to the membrane of the endoplasmic reticulum, STING is activated by several signals, directly sensing bacterial dinucleotides and membranes/lipids trafficking, and indirectly sensing cytoplasmic DNA from bacteria and viruses, via mechanisms explained below (as recently reviewed by Tao et al. [1]). STING activation results in NF-κB and IRF3/7 nuclear translocation, promoting the transcriptional induction of proinflammatory genes and type I Interferons (IFN) [2]. More recently, STING has been shown to play a leading role in the detection of endogenous cytoplasmic DNA leaked from the nucleus after DNA damage [2, 3].

Beyond its role in innate immunity, STING is emerging to be critical to cancer immunity. STING-deficient mice display impaired immune cell infiltration and $CD8^+$ T cell priming, key to a productive immune response against the tumor [4, 5]. Critically, this

Brendan J. Jenkins (ed.), *Inflammation and Cancer: Methods and Protocols*, Methods in Molecular Biology, vol. 1725, https://doi.org/10.1007/978-1-4939-7568-6_20,

observation was restricted to STING and not seen in mice deficient in other innate immune signaling pathway components [5]. Indirect activation of STING by DNA relies first on DNA detection by the cyclic GMP-AMP synthase (cGAS) and its production of the second messenger cGAMP, which subsequently binds to STING [6, 7]. Importantly, cGAMP can activate STING endogenously, i.e. in the cell producing it, but it can also be transferred to adjacent cells through gap junctions, formed by connexins [8]. If these adjacent cGAMP recipient cells express STING, they will activate an immune response, independent of the original response of the donor cell [8]. This unique property was originally exploited by the Hornung laboratory to create a functional assay of cGAMP production, based on cGAMP donor and reporter-recipient cells [8]. Critically, because cGAMP is conserved between humans and mice, coculture strategies relying on cells from the two species facilitate the distinction between donor and recipient immune responses [8, 9] (Fig. 1).

cGAS activation in cancer cells can occur upon sensing of cytoplasmic DNA leaked from the nucleus caused by DNA damage, either spontaneously, or after chemotherapy treatment [10, 11]. Recent evidence suggests that certain tumors can directly produce IFN through activation of cGAS and STING. In line with this, subsets of patients with spontaneous leukocyte infiltration have been reported in ovarian cancer [12], breast cancer [13, 14] and colorectal cancer [15]. Given that IFN production favors

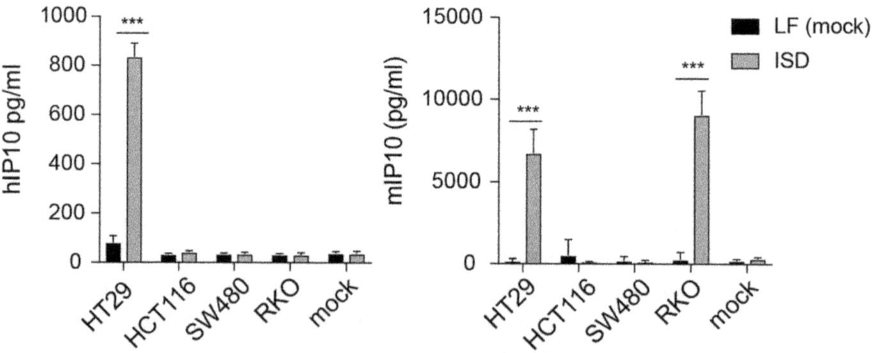

Fig. 1 cGAS-cGAMP-STING activation in human colon cancer cell lines. Human colon cancer cell lines were transfected with ISD and subsequently cocultured with L929 cells. Human and mouse IP-10 were measured separately by ELISA. As described in the literature, HCT116 and SW480 do not express cGAS. As a result, these cells are unable to produce cGAMP under ISD stimulation (and no mIP-10 is produced by L929 cells). Conversely, HT29 cells are cGAS-STING competent, and produce hIP-10 as well as cGAMP-like activity as measured by production of mouse IP-10 by the L929 cells. Finally, according to these results, RKO cells are responsive to cGAS—as seen with mIP-10 production by L929 coculture—but cannot produce human IP-10. Our analysis of STING expression in RKO by western blotting indicates that these cells are indeed deficient for STING. Each treatment was carried out in biological triplicates and the data is average from two independent experiments. Two-tailed unpaired *t*-tests and standard deviation are shown (***$p < 0.001$). *LF* (mock): Lipofectamine 2000 only; *ISD:* interferon stimulating DNA

immune tumor clearance, tumor cells often evolve to escape sensing by the cGAS-STING pathway (through loss of expression of cGAS, STING or downstream signaling components) as seen in melanoma [16] and colorectal cancers [17]. Impaired cell communication, which may inhibit cGAMP horizontal transfer between cells, is also common in cancer cells, where connexin expression is often lost [18, 19].

DNA damaging activities can also potentiate cGAS-STING engagement. DNA binding agents [9, 20, 21], enzymatic cleavage of DNA [22], UV exposure [23], and ϒ-irradiation [24] lead to STING activation and type I IFN production. Relying on a functional assay of cGAMP transfer to reporter cells, we have recently provided the first direct demonstration of cGAS engagement following DNA damage by a DNA binding agent [9]. This assay relied on the treatment of human cells expressing cGAS, later cocultured with a mouse reporter cell line (STING competent) [8, 9]. The following protocol is adapted from this assay to allow for easy characterization of cGAS and STING functionality in human cancer cells, together with their capacity to promote horizontal transfer of cGAMP to adjacent cells. As is shown hereafter, certain cancer cell lines can generate cGAMP, but do not necessarily have the components to sense it and mount an IFN response (Fig. 1). Recent evidence suggests that intratumoral cGAMP administration can stimulate the immune system and tumor clearance [25–29]. This strategy however bears the risk of systemic IFN production and associated "flu-like" symptoms in patients. Making use of the natural capacity of cGAS to be engaged within tumor cells, if functional, would help alleviate such potential systemic effects. Beyond this protocol being of interest to this direct field, the method described here could help stratify cancer patients and their treatment according to the capacity of their tumors to make cGAMP.

2 Materials

2.1 Cell Culture

1. L929 cells, HCT 116, HT-29, SW480, RKO.
2. Dulbecco's Modified Eagle's Medium (DMEM) supplemented with 10% sterile fetal bovine serum (FBS), 1× antibiotic/antimycotic; referred to as complete DMEM.
3. Dulbecco's Phosphate-Buffered Saline (DPBS).
4. Tissue culture plasticware: 100 mm sterile tissue culture dishes, 12-well and 96-well sterile tissue culture plates.
5. Trypsin replacement solution.
6. Hemacytometer.
7. Microscope.

2.2 Cell Transfections

1. Lipofectamine 2000 transfection reagent.
2. Opti-Minimal Essential Medium (Opti-MEM).
3. 1 μg/μL final concentration of naked IFN-stimulating DNA (ISD) made by resuspending 200 μg in 200 μL of endotoxin-free water.

2.3 ELISA

1. Mouse CXCL10/IP-10 ELISA kit.
2. Human IP-10 ELISA kit.
3. Bovine serum albumin solution in DPBS (hereafter assay diluent solution for mouse IP-10).
4. Assay diluent solution (BD optEIA) for human IP-10.
5. DPBS containing 0.05% Tween.
6. 1 N H_2SO_4 0.5 M solution.
7. 0.1 M sodium carbonate, pH 9.5.
8. TMB single solution (Life technologies).
9. Nunc MaxiSorp™ flat-bottom 96-well plates.
10. Microplate reader set at 450 nm with wavelength correction set at 540 or 570 nm.

3 Methods

This section details a method to determine cGAS functionality of human tumor cell lines. Human (h) IP-10 production is used to assess the capacity of the human cancer cell line to make and respond to cGAMP. Mouse (m) IP-10 is used to measure cGAMP transfer to adjacent cocultured Sting competent mouse cells. Collectively, these assays help provide a simple picture of the cGAS functionality of cancer cells, which can also be correlated to cGAS expression by western blotting.

3.1 Cell Culture Maintenance

For each cell line (human cancer cell line and mouse L929 cell line):

1. Grow the cells in complete DMEM at 37 °C in 5% CO_2 incubator until the cells reach an 80–90% confluence (*see* **Note 1**).
2. To split the cells, discard the medium, wash with 10 mL of DPBS. Discard the DPBS.
3. Add 1 mL of TrypLE before incubating for 2–4 min at 37 °C in 5% CO_2 incubator.
4. Gently tap the dish and look under the microscope to make sure the cells are detached. Then, resuspend the cells using 9 mL of complete medium.

5. To passage the cells use 2 mL of the 10 mL cell suspension and transfer it into a new 100 mm sterile tissue culture dish. Keep the rest of the cells and transfer the remaining 8 mL into a 15 mL Falcon tube to perform the reverse transfection.

3.2 Reverse-Transfection of Human Cancer Cell Line with ISD

The protocol and volumes given below are for one human cell line transfected in one 12-well plate and subsequently transferred into three wells of a 96-well plate.

1. Dilute 4 μL of Lipofectamine 2000 in 100 μL of Opti-MEM.
2. Dilute 4 μL of ISD solution at 1 μg/μL in 100 μL of Opti-MEM.
3. Repeat **steps 1** and **2** for the mock solution without adding the ISD (*see* **Note 2**).
4. Incubate the Lipofectamine 2000 and the DNA solutions at room temperature for 5 min.
5. Add the Lipofectamine solution to the DNA solution (resulting in a total of 200 μL of ISD–Lipofectamine mix), and mix by gentle tapping before incubating for 20 min at room temperature. Do the same with the mock solution.
6. During the incubation time, split the cancer cell line as described in Subheading 3.1 and count the cell number in the cell solution with a hemocytometer. Prepare 2 mL of a cell suspension containing 250,000 cells per ml of complete DMEM for each cancer cell line.
7. Add the 200 μL of ISD–Lipofectamine mix directly into one empty well of a 12-well plate. Add 800 μL of the cell suspension on the top of the ISD–Lipofectamine mix, giving a final volume of 1000 μL per well. Do the same for the mock transfection (*see* **Note 3**).
8. Incubate the cells for 6 h at 37 °C in 5% CO_2 incubator.

3.3 Coculture of the Transfected Cells with L929 in the 96-Well Plate

1. Split L929 cells as per Subheading 3.1 and prepare 3 mL of a cell suspension containing 100,000 cells in 1 mL of complete DMEM. Add 200 μL per well of 96-well plate at 37 °C in 5% CO_2 incubator. Let the cells adhere for a minimum of 1 h.
2. Following the 6 h ISD transfection, remove the medium of the transfected cancer cells and wash adherent cells with 1 mL of DPBS. Discard the DPBS.
3. Add 200 μL of TrypLE and incubate at 37 °C in 5% CO_2 until the cancer cells are detached.
4. Resuspend the cancer cells with 1 mL of complete DMEM and transfer the cancer cell solution into a 15 mL Falcon containing 9 mL of complete DMEM. Spin the cancer cells at 350 × *g* for 4 min.

5. Discard the supernatant and repeat the wash step using 10 mL of complete DMEM medium a second time.
6. Discard the supernatant and resuspend the cancer cells in 630 μL of complete DMEM medium (set aside).
7. One condition at the time, discard the supernatant of the adherent L929 cells and replace it with 200 μL of the transfected cancer cell suspension. There should be enough cells to prepare three wells of coculture per well of cancer cell line transfected.
8. Incubate the coculture overnight (approximately 20 h) at 37 °C in 5% CO_2 incubator.
9. Following incubation, transfer the supernatants into a fresh 96-well plate. The supernatants can be directly analyzed by ELISA (*see* **Note 4**), or frozen at −80 °C for later analysis.

3.4 Mouse CXCL10/IP-10 ELISA

1. Day 0: Coat the plate using 100 μL of the capture antibody containing solution diluted in DPBS according to the manufacturer's instructions. Leave the plate sealed with tape at room temperature overnight (*see* **Note 5**).
2. Day 1: Discard the coating solution from the ELISA plate by flipping and tapping the plate on absorbent paper.
3. Wash the wells three-times using 200 μL of DPBS + 0.05% Tween and discard the wash solution by flipping and tapping the plate.
4. Block the plate using 200 μL of a solution containing 1% BSA diluted in DPBS (assay diluent). Incubate at room temperature for 1 h and perform three washes as in **step 3**, immediately above.
5. Freshly prepare the IP-10 standard curve in assay diluent according to the manufacturer's instructions. Standards should range between 62 and 4000 pg/mL.
6. Add 100 μL of neat supernatant per well or 100 μL of each standard to separate wells. Incubate at room temperature for 2 h and then perform three washes as in **step 3**.
7. Add 100 μL of detection antibody in assay diluent according to the manufacturer's protocol. Incubate for 1 h at room temperature and perform three washes as in **step 3**.
8. Add 100 μL of Streptavidin solution in assay diluent according to the manufacturer protocol. Incubate for 30 min at room temperature. Perform five washes as in **step 3**.
9. Add 100 μL of TMB single solution per well and incubate for 30 min at room temperature in the dark.
10. Add 100 μL of 1 N H_2SO_4 per well to stop the reaction.
11. Measure absorbance using a plate reader set at 450 nm.

12. Analyse the data by subtracting the optical density (OD) of the blank to the OD of each samples and determine concentration relying on standard curve projection.

3.5 Human IP-10 ELISA (BD Opt EIA)

1. Day 0: Coat the plate using 100 μL of capture antibody solution diluted in 0.1 M sodium carbonate pH 9.5 solution according to the manufacturer's instructions. Incubate the sealed plate at 4 °C overnight.
2. Day 1: Discard the solution containing the capture antibody from the ELISA plate by flipping and tapping on absorbent paper.
3. Wash the wells three-times using 200 μL of DPBS + 0.05% Tween and discard the last wash by flipping and tapping the plate.
4. Block the plate using 200 μL of assay diluent per well. Incubate at room temperature for 1 h and then perform three washes as in **step 3**.
5. Prepare the standards in assay diluent according to the manufacturer's instructions. Standards should range between 7.5 and 500 pg/mL.
6. Add 100 μL of neat supernatant per well or 100 μL each standard. Incubate at room temperature for 2 h and then perform three washes as in **step 3**.
7. Add 100 μL of the freshly prepared solution containing the detection antibody and the streptavidin diluted in assay diluent according to the manufacturer's instructions. Incubate for 1 h at room temperature and perform five washes as in **step 3**.
8. Add 100 μL of TMB single solution per well and incubate for a maximum of 30 min at room temperature in the dark.
9. Add 100 μL of 1 N H_2SO_4 per well to stop the reaction.
10. Measure the absorbance using a plate reader set at 450 nm.
11. Analyse the data by subtracting the optical density (OD) of the blank to the OD of each samples and determine concentration relying on standard curve projection.

4 Notes

1. Cells should be passaged at least once before use in the assay. The cell proliferation may vary with the different cell lines tested.
2. The mock condition should be prepared the same way as the ISD but by omitting the DNA. This is important since some cells can be activated by Lipofectamine 2000 leading to false positive readings in the interpretation of the results.

3. To control for residual untransfected DNA, a negative transfection control can be used. Here the ISD containing transfection mix is transferred to a well where 800 μL of medium is added without cells. The two washes of the transfected cancer cells prior to the coculture should be enough to get rid of the residual untransfected DNA. This step will control for potential residual DNA when we coculture the transfected cells with the L929 recipient cells.
4. If you intend to do the ELISA the same day, you need to coat your ELISA plate the day before according to the instructions.
5. At this stage, you can keep your coated ELISA plate at 4 °C and perform the rest within a week.

Acknowledgment

We thank Professor Ron Firestein for the gift of the colon cancer cell lines; Dr. Rebecca Smith; Dr. Jonathan Ferrand and Lise Boursinhac for assistance in preparing the manuscript. This work was funded in part by the Australian NHMRC (1022144 to M.P.G.; 1062683 to M.P.G.); the Australian Research Council (140100594 Future Fellowship to M.P.G.); the Canadian Fonds de recherche du Québec – Santé (35071 FRSQ Fellowship to G. P.); and the Victorian Government's Operational Infrastructure Support Program.

References

1. Tao J, Zhou X, Jiang Z (2016) cGAS-cGAMP-STING: the three musketeers of cytosolic DNA sensing and signaling. IUBMB Life 68:858–870
2. Ahn J, Barber GN (2014) Self-DNA, STING-dependent signaling and the origins of autoinflammatory disease. Curr Opin Immunol 31:121–126
3. Hartlova A, Erttmann SF, Raffi FA, Schmalz AM, Resch U, Anugula S, Lienenklaus S, Nilsson LM, Kroger A, Nilsson JA, Ek T, Weiss S, Gekara NO (2015) DNA damage primes the type I interferon system via the cytosolic DNA sensor STING to promote anti-microbial innate immunity. Immunity 42:332–343
4. Klarquist J, Hennies CM, Lehn MA, Reboulet RA, Feau S, Janssen EM (2014) STING-mediated DNA sensing promotes antitumor and autoimmune responses to dying cells. J Immunol 193:6124–6134
5. Woo SR, Fuertes MB, Corrales L, Spranger S, Furdyna MJ, Leung MY, Duggan R, Wang Y, Barber GN, Fitzgerald KA, Alegre ML, Gajewski TF (2014) STING-dependent cytosolic DNA sensing mediates innate immune recognition of immunogenic tumors. Immunity 41:830–842
6. Wu J, Sun L, Chen X, Du F, Shi H, Chen C, Chen ZJ (2013) Cyclic GMP-AMP is an endogenous second messenger in innate immune signaling by cytosolic DNA. Science 339:826–830
7. Sun L, Wu J, Du F, Chen X, Chen ZJ (2013) Cyclic GMP-AMP synthase is a cytosolic DNA sensor that activates the type I interferon pathway. Science 339:786–791
8. Ablasser A, Schmid-Burgk JL, Hemmerling I, Horvath GL, Schmidt T, Latz E, Hornung V (2013) Cell intrinsic immunity spreads to bystander cells via the intercellular transfer of cGAMP. Nature 503:530–534
9. Pepin G, Nejad C, Thomas BJ, Ferrand J, McArthur K, Bardin PG, Williams BR, Gantier MP (2017) Activation of cGAS-dependent antiviral responses by DNA intercalating agents. Nucleic Acids Res 45:198–205

10. Ho SS, Zhang WY, Tan NY, Khatoo M, Suter MA, Tripathi S, Cheung FS, Lim WK, Tan PH, Ngeow J, Gasser S (2016) The DNA structure-specific endonuclease MUS81 mediates DNA sensor STING-dependent host rejection of prostate cancer cells. Immunity 44:1177–1189
11. Lam AR, Le Bert N, Ho SS, Shen YJ, Tang ML, Xiong GM, Croxford JL, Koo CX, Ishii KJ, Akira S, Raulet DH, Gasser S (2014) RAE1 ligands for the NKG2D receptor are regulated by STING-dependent DNA sensor pathways in lymphoma. Cancer Res 74:2193–2203
12. Hwang WT, Adams SF, Tahirovic E, Hagemann IS, Coukos G (2012) Prognostic significance of tumor-infiltrating T cells in ovarian cancer: a meta-analysis. Gynecol Oncol 124:192–198
13. Mahmoud SM, Paish EC, Powe DG, Macmillan RD, Grainge MJ, Lee AH, Ellis IO, Green AR (2011) Tumor-infiltrating CD8+ lymphocytes predict clinical outcome in breast cancer. J Clin Oncol 29:1949–1955
14. Parkes EE, Walker SM, Taggart LE, McCabe N, Knight LA, Wilkinson R, McCloskey KD, Buckley NE, Savage KI, Salto-Tellez-M, McQuaid S, Harte MT, Mullan PB, Harkin DP, Kennedy RD (2017) Activation of STING-dependent innate immune signaling by S-phase-specific DNA damage in breast cancer. J Natl Cancer Inst 109:1–10
15. Galon J, Costes A, Sanchez-Cabo F, Kirilovsky A, Mlecnik B, Lagorce-Pages C, Tosolini M, Camus M, Berger A, Wind P, Zinzindohoue F, Bruneval P, Cugnenc PH, Trajanoski Z, Fridman WH, Pages F (2006) Type, density, and location of immune cells within human colorectal tumors predict clinical outcome. Science 313:1960–1964
16. Xia T, Konno H, Barber GN (2016) Recurrent loss of STING signaling in melanoma correlates with susceptibility to viral oncolysis. Cancer 76:6747–6759
17. Xia T, Konno H, Ahn J, Barber GN (2016) Deregulation of STING signaling in colorectal carcinoma constrains DNA damage responses and correlates with tumorigenesis. Cell Rep 14:282–297
18. Xu N, Chen HJ, Chen SH, Xue XY, Chen H, Zheng QS, Wei Y, Li XD, Huang JB, Cai H, Sun XL (2016) Reduced connexin 43 expression is associated with tumor malignant behaviors and biochemical recurrence-free survival of prostate cancer. Oncotarget 7:67476–67484
19. Danos K, Brauswetter D, Birtalan E, Pato A, Bencsik G, Krenacs T, Petak I, Tamas L (2016) The potential prognostic value of connexin 43 expression in head and neck squamous cell carcinomas. Appl Immunohistochem Mol Morphol 24:476–481
20. Ahn J, Xia T, Konno H, Konno K, Ruiz P, Barber GN (2014) Inflammation-driven carcinogenesis is mediated through STING. Nat Commun 5:5166
21. Luthra P, Aguirre S, Yen BC, Pietzsch CA, Sanchez-Aparicio MT, Tigabu B, Morlock LK, Garcia-Sastre A, Leung DW, Williams NS, Fernandez-Sesma A, Bukreyev A, Basler CF (2017) Topoisomerase II inhibitors induce DNA damage-dependent interferon responses circumventing ebola virus immune evasion. MBio 8(2):pii: e00368-17
22. Pepin G, Ferrand J, Honing K, Jayasekara WS, Cain JE, Behlke MA, Gough DJ, BR GW, Hornung V, Gantier MP (2016) Cre-dependent DNA recombination activates a STING-dependent innate immune response. Nucleic Acids Res 44:5356–5364
23. Kemp MG, Lindsey-Boltz LA, Sancar A (2015) UV light potentiates STING (stimulator of interferon genes)-dependent innate immune signaling through deregulation of ULK1 (Unc51-like kinase 1). J Biol Chem 290:12184–12194
24. Erdal E, Haider S, Rehwinkel J, Harris AL, McHugh PJ (2017) A prosurvival DNA damage-induced cytoplasmic interferon response is mediated by end resection factors and is limited by Trex1. Genes Dev 31:353–369
25. Ohkuri T, Kosaka A, Ishibashi K, Kumai T, Hirata Y, Ohara K, Nagato T, Oikawa K, Aoki N, Harabuchi Y, Celis E, Kobayashi H (2017) Intratumoral administration of cGAMP transiently accumulates potent macrophages for anti-tumor immunity at a mouse tumor site. Cancer Immunol Immunother 66(6):705–716
26. Demaria O, De Gassart A, Coso S, Gestermann N, Di Domizio J, Flatz L, Gaide O, Michielin O, Hwu P, Petrova TV, Martinon F, Modlin RL, Speiser DE, Gilliet M (2015) STING activation of tumor endothelial cells initiates spontaneous and therapeutic antitumor immunity. Proc Natl Acad Sci U S A 112:15408–15413
27. Li T, Cheng H, Yuan H, Xu Q, Shu C, Zhang Y, Xu P, Tan J, Rui Y, Li P, Tan X (2016) Anti-tumor activity of cGAMP via stimulation of cGAS-cGAMP-STING-IRF3 mediated innate immune response. Sci Rep 6:19049

28. Nakamura T, Miyabe H, Hyodo M, Sato Y, Hayakawa Y, Harashima H (2015) Liposomes loaded with a STING pathway ligand, cyclic di-GMP, enhance cancer immunotherapy against metastatic melanoma. J Control Release 216:149–157
29. Corrales L, Glickman LH, McWhirter SM, Kanne DB, Sivick KE, Katibah GE, Woo SR, Lemmens E, Banda T, Leong JJ, Metchette K, Dubensky TW Jr, Gajewski TF (2015) Direct activation of STING in the tumor microenvironment leads to potent and systemic tumor regression and immunity. Cell Rep 11:1018–1030

Chapter 21

Expression and Purification of JAK1 and SOCS1 for Structural and Biochemical Studies

Nicholas P.D. Liau and Jeffrey J. Babon

Abstract

Interferon gamma (IFNγ) is a potent inflammatory and immune cytokine. IFNγ signals via the interferon gamma receptor (IFNGR), which is constitutively bound to Janus Kinase (JAK) 1 and JAK2 via its intracellular domain. These two JAK proteins then initiate the inflammatory signaling cascade. The most potent inhibitor of IFNγ signaling is Suppressor of Cytokine Signaling 1 (SOCS1). SOCS1 negatively regulates IFNγ signaling pathway (and other pathways) by directly inhibiting JAKs. Here, we describe a protocol for the recombinant production and purification of the JAK1 kinase domain and its inhibitor SOCS1, for structural and biochemical studies.

Key words Janus Kinase (JAK), Suppressor of cytokine signaling (SOCS), Protein expression, Protein purification

1 Introduction

1.1 IFNγ Signaling

IFNγ is a proinflammatory cytokine which signals through the IFNGR, a heterodimer consisting of IFNGR1 and IFNGR2 chains [1]. Unlike receptor tyrosine kinases (such as the insulin receptor), the intracellular portion of IFNGR lacks intrinsic kinase activity. IFNGR thus relies on JAK1 and JAK2, which are attached to the intracellular portions of each receptor chain, to phosphorylate downstream substrates and propagate the signal once the receptor is activated [2, 3].

IFNγ signaling is critical to the immune response, and it causes the upregulation of many genes required to respond to infection, such as the major histocompatibility complex class I and II antigen presentation genes [4]. As IFNγ signaling is a potent upregulator of a number of immune cell types, excessive levels of IFNγ signaling can lead to inflammatory and autoimmune diseases [5]. It is thus important that IFNγ signaling is kept in check. The chief negative regulator of IFNγ signaling is SOCS1. SOCS1 knockout mice die neonatally from excessive inflammation characteristic of overactive

Brendan J. Jenkins (ed.), *Inflammation and Cancer: Methods and Protocols*, Methods in Molecular Biology, vol. 1725, https://doi.org/10.1007/978-1-4939-7568-6_21,

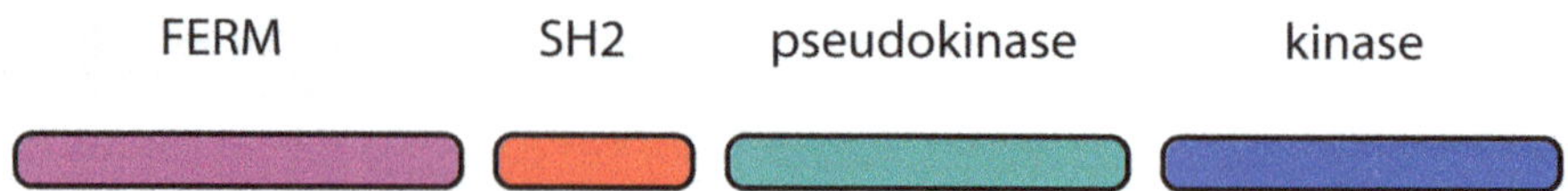

Fig. 1 All JAK family members consist of four domains—The FERM and SH2 domains tether JAK to the cytokine receptor. The pseudokinase domain regulates JAK activity. The kinase domain is the catalytically active domain of JAK

IFNγ signaling and this phenotype is rescued by IFNγ deletion, highlighting the importance of SOCS1 regulation of this pathway [6].

1.2 The JAK Tyrosine Kinases

The JAK proteins are tyrosine kinases, and consist of four family members: JAK1, JAK2, JAK3 and TYK2 [7]. JAKs are found constitutively associated with cytokine receptors. The binding of cytokine to the extracellular portion of the receptor causes JAK to become activated, and it is then able to phosphorylate downstream substrates, especially the Signal Transducers and Activators of Transcription (STAT) transcription factors. Upon phosphorylation, STATs enter the nucleus, where they are able to upregulate the expression of cytokine responsive genes [8]. In addition to their role in IFNγ signaling, JAKs are responsible for signaling in response to a variety of hemopoietic cytokines and mutations in JAK have been associated with a variety of leukemias, lymphomas, and myeloproliferative diseases [9].

All JAK family members consist of four domains (Fig. 1). The N terminal FERM and SH2 domains anchor JAKs to the intracellular portion of the cytokine receptor [10, 11]. The pseudokinase domain is involved in regulation of catalytic activity, and the catalytically active kinase domain is responsible for phosphorylating tyrosine substrate residues. To date, few structural and functional studies have been performed on the full length JAK protein because of the difficulty in purifying and handling the protein [12].

This protocol describes how to produce the kinase domain (also known as the JH1 domain) of JAK1. We have previously shown that JAK1 JH1 produced in such a manner is catalytically active and can be inhibited by SOCS3, a physiological inhibitor of JAK1 [13, 14].

1.3 The Suppressor of Cytokine Signaling (SOCS) Family of Proteins

The SOCS family of proteins has eight members, SOCS1-7 and CIS, each of which possess an SH2 domain, which is responsible for targeting the protein to specific sequences containing a phosphorylated tyrosine residue (Fig. 2). For example, the SOCS3 SH2 domain targets SOCS3 to specific phosphorylated cytokine receptors [13]. In addition, all SOCS proteins contain a SOCS Box domain at their C termini [15, 16]. This motif binds the adapter complex ElonginBC and the ternary SOCS-ElonginB-ElonginC complex (SOCS/BC) then recruits the ubiquitin ligase scaffold

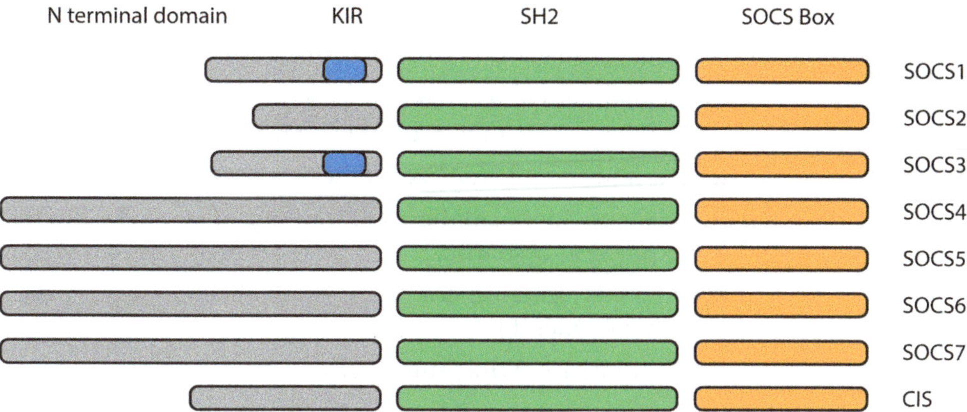

Fig. 2 SOCS family members. All SOCS family members contain an N terminal domain of variable length, an SH2 domain and a SOCS box. SOCS1 and SOCS3 also contain a KIR which is able to directly inhibit JAK1 catalytic activity

protein Cullin5, thereby forming an active E3 ubiquitin ligase which targets substrate proteins for ubiquitination and degradation [17–19]. In addition to their ability to act as E3 ubiquitin ligases, SOCS1 and SOCS3 are unique among SOCS family members in that they contain a kinase inhibitory region (KIR) [20]. This motif allows SOCS1 and SOCS3 to directly inhibit the catalytic activity of JAK1, JAK2, and TYK2 [13, 21–23].

1.4 Overview of Protocol

The tyrosine kinase JAK1 is required for signaling by all interferons. Here, we describe a method for expressing the catalytic domain of JAK1 in *Spodoptera frugiperda* 21 (*Sf*21) insect cells. JAK1 is then purified using a two-step purification process: firstly by nickel affinity purification and then by size exclusion chromatography. The most potent inhibitor of interferon signaling is SOCS1; here we also describe a method for expressing SOCS1 in *E. coli*. SOCS1 is produced as a ternary complex with elonginB and elonginC (its physiological ligands) which greatly assist in stabilizing the purified protein. The SOCS1 construct also lacks part of the N terminal domain, as we have found that its omission significantly improves protein stability. A small molecule phosphotyrosine mimetic, phenyl phosphate, is included during the purification process in order to bind and stabilize the SH2 domain. Once expressed, the SOCS1/elonginB/elonginC ternary complex (SOCS1 B/C) is bound to Glutathione affinity resin, then cleaved from its GST purification tag using TEV protease. SOCS1 B/C is then further purified using size exclusion chromatography. The JAK1 and SOCS1 proteins purified in this way can be used in downstream structural and biochemical studies.

2 Materials

2.1 Cloning

1. General cloning reagents (e.g., PCR reagents, restriction enzymes, *E. coli* DH5α strain, agar plates, antibiotics).
2. Plasmid suitable for bacmid generation (e.g., pFB-LIC-Bse).
3. Reagents for bacmid generation (e.g., Bac-to-Bac Baculovirus Expression System).
4. Plasmids suitable for *E. coli* expression (e.g., pGEX-4T, pACYCDuet-1).
5. *E. coli* BL21 (DE3) tuner cells.

2.2 Generation of JAK1 JH1 Baculovirus and Expression of JAK1

1. *Spodoptera frugiperda* 21 (*Sf*21) insect cell line.
2. Insect cell media (e.g., Insect-XPRESS™ Protein-free Insect Cell Medium with L-glutamine, Lonza).
3. General insect cell culture equipment (e.g., sterile pipettes, 27 °C incubators, flasks for culturing insect cells in suspension, biosafety cabinet, hemocytometer).
4. 15 mL Falcon tubes.
5. 6-well tissue culture plates.
6. 75 cm^2 vented cap tissue culture flasks.
7. Insect cell transfection reagent (e.g., CellFectin II, Thermo Fisher Scientific).
8. Benchtop centrifuge (capable of 1500 × *g* with capacity for 15 mL Falcon tubes).
9. Large centrifuge (capable of 5000 × *g* with capacity for 1 L bottles).
10. 500 mL 0.2 μm sterile disposable filter unit with bottle (e.g., Nalgene Rapid-Flow).

2.3 Expression of JAK1

1. General insect cell culture equipment (e.g., sterile pipettes, 27 °C incubators, flasks for culturing insect cells in suspension, biosafety cabinet, hemocytometer).
2. 50 mL Falcon tubes.
3. Benchtop centrifuge (capable of 1500 × *g* with capacity for 50 mL Falcon tubes).
4. Large centrifuge (capable of 5000 × *g* with capacity for 1 L bottles).
5. Liquid nitrogen.

2.4 Purification of JAK1

1. JAK Lysis Buffer: 10 mM Tris pH 7.5, 150 mM NaCl, 10 mM imidazole, 2 mM tris(2-carboxyethyl)phosphine (TCEP), 1 mM phenylmethanesulfonyl fluoride (PMSF), one EDTA-free

Complete protease inhibitor cocktail tablet per 100 mL, 5 U/mL DNAseI.

2. Sonicator.
3. High speed centrifuge (capable of >40,000 × *g* with capacity for 40 mL tubes).
4. Disposable 0.8 μm syringe filter.
5. Peristaltic pump.
6. 1 mL immobilized metal affinity chromatography (IMAC) cartridge precharged with Ni^{2+} (e.g., HisTrap 1 mL, GE Healthcare).
7. Nickel Buffer A: 20% (v/v) glycerol, 20 mM Tris pH 8.0, 500 mM NaCl, 5 mM imidazole, 2 mM TCEP.
8. Nickel Buffer B: 20% (v/v) glycerol, 20 mM Tris pH 8.0, 500 mM NaCl, 500 mM imidazole, 2 mM TCEP.
9. 2% Nickel Buffer: 9 8% (v/v) Nickel Buffer A, 2% (v/v) Nickel Buffer B.
10. 7% Nickel Buffer: 93% (v/v) Nickel Buffer A, 7% (v/v) Nickel Buffer B.
11. JAK Gel Filtration Buffer: 10% (v/v) glycerol, 20 mM Tris pH 8.0, 500 mM NaCl, 2 mM TCEP.
12. Fast Protein Liquid Chromatography (FPLC) apparatus.
13. Centrifugal concentrator, 10 kDa cutoff.
14. Gel filtration column.
15. Adenosine triphosphate (ATP).
16. $MgCl_2$.
17. SDS-PAGE gels and associated apparatus.
18. Liquid nitrogen.

2.5 Expression of SOCS1 B/C

1. Superbroth: 35 g tryptone, 20 g yeast extract, 5 g NaCl, 2.5 mL 2 M NaOH to 1 L with deionized water.
2. Ampicillin, Chloramphenicol (or other suitable antibiotics for your chosen expression plasmids).
3. Isopropyl thio-β-D-galactoside (IPTG).
4. 50 mL Falcon tubes.
5. 2 L baffled flask.
6. Centrifuge (capable of 5000 × *g* with capacity for 1 L bottles).

2.6 Purification of SOCS1 B/C

1. SOCS1 lysis buffer: Dulbecco's Phosphate Buffered Saline (138 mM NaCl, 2.7 mM KCl, 1.5 mM KH_2PO_4, 8.1 mM Na_2HPO_4 pH 7.2), 1 mM PMSF, 5 mM phenyl phosphate, 5 mM dithiothreitol (DTT), 0.5 mg/mL lysozyme, one

EDTA-free cOmplete protease inhibitor cocktail tablet per 100 mL, 5 U/mL DNAseI.

2. Sonicator.
3. High speed centrifuge (capable of >40,000 × *g* with capacity for 40 mL tubes).
4. Glutathione resin.
5. 30 mL gravity flow column.
6. SOCS1 wash buffer: 10 mM Tris pH 7.5, 150 mM NaCl, 5 mM phenyl phosphate, 5 mM DTT.
7. 50 mL Falcon tubes.
8. Tobacco etch virus protease (TEV).
9. Centrifugal concentrator, 10 kDa cutoff.
10. Gel filtration column.
11. SDS-PAGE gels and associated apparatus.

3 Methods

3.1 Cloning

This section briefly describes the constructs and vectors used to clone JAK1 JH1 and SOCS1 B/C for expression. Standard techniques are used to clone genes of interest into appropriate plasmids for bacmid generation (JAK1 JH1) and *E. coli* expression (SOCS1 B/C). Plasmids encoding SOCS1 B/C are transformed to an appropriate *E. coli* cell line for expression. We have successfully cloned, expressed and purified proteins with the following boundaries:

JAK1 JH1: residues 862-1154 (Uniprot P23458).

SOCS1: residues 52-211 (Uniprot O15524).

Elongin B: residues 1-118 (Uniprot P62829).

Elongin C: residues 17-112 (Uniprot Q15369).

1. Clone JAK1 JH1 into a vector suitable for bacmid generation, containing an N terminal 6× His tag followed by a TEV protease site (e.g., pFB-LIC-BSE).
2. Using Bac-to-Bac Baculovirus Expression System, introduce the JAK1 JH1 gene into a bacmid and purify the bacmid for transformation into *Sf*21 insect cells.
3. Clone SOCS1 into a vector suitable for *E. coli* expression, containing an N terminal glutathione S transferase tag (e.g., pGEX-4T) with an engineered TEV protease site between GST and SOCS1.

4. Clone Elongin B and Elongin C into a vector allowing for dual expression of two proteins simultaneously (e.g., pACYCDuet-1) (*see* **Note 1**).
5. Cotransform both SOCS1 and Elongin B/C containing vectors into *E. Coli* Bl21 (DE3) tuner cells and keep a glycerol stock for later large scale expression.

3.2 Generation of JAK1 JH1 Baculovirus

This section describes the generation of baculovirus in insect cells by the infection of cells with bacmid, which contains the JAK1 JH1 gene, as well as genes required for the generation of virus. Low infectivity first generation baculovirus (P1) is then amplified through two cycles of infection (P2 and P3) to generate a high infectivity virus suitable for liter scale protein expression.

1. In each well of a 6-well tissue culture plate, transfer 2 mL of Sf21 cells at a density of 0.5×10^6 cells/mL. Allow to adhere for 30 min in a humidified 27 °C incubator.
2. Add 1 μg of Bacmid DNA to 200 μL of media and 6 μL of Insect cell transfection reagent in a 1.5 mL Eppendorf tube.
3. Mix gently by tapping and incubate at room temperature for 30–45 min.
4. Add 800 μL media to DNA–media–transfection reagent mix.
5. For each bacmid solution to be transformed, aspirate media from a well of the 6-well plate and replace with bacmid mix (*see* **Note 2**).
6. Incubate for 5–6 h in a humidified 27 °C incubator.
7. Aspirate the supernatant from each cell monolayer and replace with 2 mL media.
8. Incubate for 4 days in a humidified 27 °C incubator.
9. Harvest P1 virus by pipetting the supernatant from each transformed well of the 6-well plate to a 15 mL Falcon tube.
10. Centrifuge to remove debris ($1500 \times g$, 5 min).
11. Transfer supernatant to a new 15 mL Falcon tube and store in the dark at 4 °C (*see* **Note 3**).
12. To prepare P2 virus, add 15 mL *Sf*21 cells at a density of 0.5×10^6 cells/mL to a 75 cm^2 tissue culture flask.
13. Add 200 μL P1 virus.
14. Incubate at 27 °C for 4 days.
15. To harvest P2 virus, decant supernatant into a 15 mL Falcon tube.
16. Centrifuge to remove cell debris ($1500 \times g$, 5 min).
17. Decant supernatant into a new labeled 15 mL Falcon tube and store in the dark at 4 °C.

18. To prepare P3 virus, grow 500 mL *Sf*21 cells in suspension to a density of 1.0×10^6 cells/mL (*see* **Note 4**).
19. Add 5 mL P2 virus.
20. Incubate at 27 °C for 4 days shaking at 90 rpm.
21. To harvest P3 virus, centrifuge to remove cells and cell debris ($6000 \times g$, 45 min, 4 °C) (*see* **Note 5**).
22. Filter-sterilize the supernatant using a 500 mL 0.2 μm sterile disposable filter unit. Be sure to replace the cap inside a biosafety cabinet to maintain sterility.
23. If desired, virus can be titered using standard techniques (*see* **Note 6**).

3.3 Expression of JAK1 JH1

This section describes the expression of JAK1 from P3 baculovirus.

1. Grow 500 mL *Sf*21 cells in suspension to a density of 3.0×10^6 cells/mL (*see* **Note 7**).
2. If P3 virus was titered, infect at a multiplicity of infection of 3.0. If P3 virus was not titered, infect with 150 mL P3 virus (*see* **Note 8**).
3. Incubate for 48 h at 27 °C, shaking at 90 rpm.
4. Pellet cells in a 1 L centrifuge bottle ($4000 \times g$, 30 min, 4 °C).
5. Remove supernatant. Resuspend cell pellet in centrifuge bottle in ~30 mL supernatant. Transfer to a 50 mL Falcon tube (*see* **Note 9**).
6. Repellet cells by centrifugation ($1500 \times g$, 5 min, 4 °C).
7. Discard supernatant. Snap freeze cell pellet on liquid nitrogen. Pellet can be stored at or below −30 °C indefinitely.

3.4 Purification of JAK1 JH1

This section describes the purification of JAK1 JH1 from a frozen cell pellet. JAK1 JH1 has a 6× His tag, which allows the protein to be purified from cell lysate by binding to immobilized Ni^{2+} ions. The protein is then further purified from other impurities using size exclusion chromatography. All steps should be performed at 4 °C to ensure protein stability.

1. Resuspend frozen cell pellet in 10 mL JAK Lysis Buffer for every 100 mL of original cell culture volume (*see* **Note 10**).
2. Sonicate with 18×10 s bursts followed by 10 s rest at a power of 40–60 W. Perform sonication in an ice–water bath to ensure that pellet does not overheat.
3. Pellet the insoluble material by centrifugation in a High speed centrifuge ($40{,}000 \times g$, 60 min, 4 °C) (*see* **Note 11**).
4. Filter the supernatant through a 0.8 μm disposable filter unit using a peristaltic pump (*see* **Note 12**).

5. Equilibrate a 1 mL IMAC cartridge with 5 mL Nickel Buffer A.
6. Apply filtered supernatant to the IMAC cartridge at a rate of not more than 1 mL/min.
7. Wash the IMAC cartridge with 20 mL 2% Nickel Buffer.
8. Wash the IMAC cartridge with 15 mL 7% Nickel Buffer.
9. Elute the protein with 4 mL Nickel Buffer B, keeping the flow through.
10. Optional: if you wish to cleave the 6× His tag from the protein, determine protein concentration by spectrophotometer and add TEV protease at a ratio of 1:100 (w/w) TEV:JAK1 JH1. Allow cleavage reaction to proceed overnight.
11. If required, concentrate the eluted protein in a centrifugal concentrator to an appropriate volume for your chosen gel filtration column (*see* **Note 13**).
12. Separate the protein from impurities (and free tag and protease if cleavage was performed) by running on a Gel filtration column in JAK gel filtration buffer.
13. Immediately add ATP and $MgCl_2$ to fractions suspected of containing JAK1 JH1 to final concentrations of 1 mM and 2 mM respectively (*see* **Note 14**).
14. Analyze fractions by reducing SDS-PAGE.
15. Pool the most pure fractions (as determined by SDS-PAGE, Fig. 3) and concentrate to >5 mg/mL in a 10 kDa centrifugal concentrator.
16. To store protein long term, aliquots may be snap frozen on liquid nitrogen and stored at −80 °C (*see* **Note 15**).

3.5 Expression of SOCS1 B/C

This section describes the expression of SOCS1 B/C from a glycerol stock of *E. coli* Bl21(DE3) tuner cells, containing plasmids encoding for SOCS1, Elongin B, and Elongin C.

1. Take a scraping of glycerol stock and inoculate into 3 mL Superbroth containing 100 μg/mL Ampicillin and 25 μg/mL Chloramphenicol.
2. Incubate overnight at 37 °C with 180 rpm shaking.
3. Inoculate 1 L of Superbroth containing 100 μg/mL Ampicillin and 25 μg/mL Chloramphenicol with the 3 mL overnight culture.
4. Incubate at 37 °C with 180 rpm shaking until A_{600} reaches 0.8–1.0.
5. Induce expression by adding IPTG to a concentration of 25 μM (*see* **Note 16**).
6. Incubate overnight at 18 °C with 180 rpm shaking to express protein.

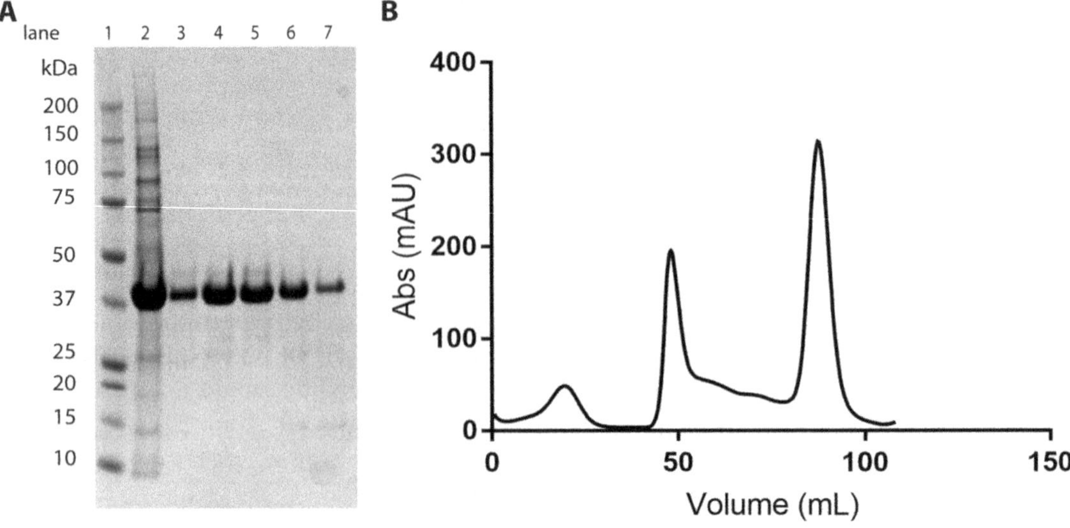

Fig. 3 (**a**) SDS-PAGE gel stained with Coomassie Blue showing crude elution of JAK1 from Ni^{2+} column, (lane 2), and selected fractions across the JAK1 JH1 size exclusion elution peak, as shown in panel **b** (lanes 3–7). (**b**) A_{280} absorbance trace of JAK1 JH1 elution from a Superdex200 16/600 size exclusion chromatography column. The first peak at ~50 mL contains aggregated JAK1 JH1 and contaminants, while the second peak at ~90 mL contains pure JAK1 JH1. Trace represents protein obtained from approximately 1 L of *Sf*21 culture

7. Harvest cells by centrifugation at 6000 × *g*, 20 min, 4 °C.
8. Discard supernatant and transfer cell pellet to a 50 mL Falcon tube.
9. The cell pellet can purified immediately, or it can be snap-frozen on liquid nitrogen and stored at or below −30 °C indefinitely.

3.6 Purification of SOCS1 B/C

All steps should be performed at 4 °C to ensure protein stability.

1. Resuspend cell pellet from 1 L of original culture in 50 mL SOCS1 lysis buffer for 1 hour.
2. Sonicate with 18 × 10 s bursts followed by 10 s rest at a power of 40–60 W. Perform sonication in an ice-water bath to ensure that pellet does not overheat.
3. Pellet the insoluble material by centrifugation in a High speed centrifuge (40,000 × *g*, 20 min, 4 °C).
4. Transfer 2 mL of 50% (v/v) Glutathione resin slurry into a gravity flow column. This will give a packed volume of 1 mL resin.
5. Wash with 20 mL SOCS1 wash buffer (*see* **Note 17**).
6. Pass supernatant over Glutathione resin.
7. Wash Glutathione resin with 50 mL SOCS1 wash buffer.
8. Take a 5 μL sample of beads for later SDS-PAGE analysis.

9. Cap the gravity flow column and resuspend resin in 20 mL SOCS1 wash buffer. Transfer slurry to a 50 mL Falcon tube. Keep the gravity flow column for later use.
10. To cleave SOCS1 B/C from resin, add 0.5 mg TEV. Incubate overnight with gentle rolling to ensure beads do not settle to the bottom of the tube (*see* **Note 18**).
11. Return mixture to the gravity flow column to separate liquid from beads. The flow through contains SOCS1 B/C cleaved from the GST tag, which is still attached to the beads.
12. Take a 20 μL sample of flow through and a 5 μL sample of resin for SDS-PAGE analysis (*see* **Note 19**).
13. Concentrate the flow through to an appropriate volume for your chosen gel filtration column in a 10 kDa concentrator.
14. Separate SOCS1 B/C from impurities by running on a gel filtration column in SOCS1 wash buffer.
15. Analyze fractions by reducing SDS-PAGE.
16. Pool the most pure fractions (as determined by SDS-PAGE, Fig. 4) and concentrate to >5 mg/mL in a 10 kDa centrifugal concentrator.
17. We typically find SOCS1 B/C is stable for several days at 4 °C. To store protein long term, glycerol may be added to 10% (v/v), and aliquots may be snap-frozen on liquid nitrogen and stored at −80 °C.

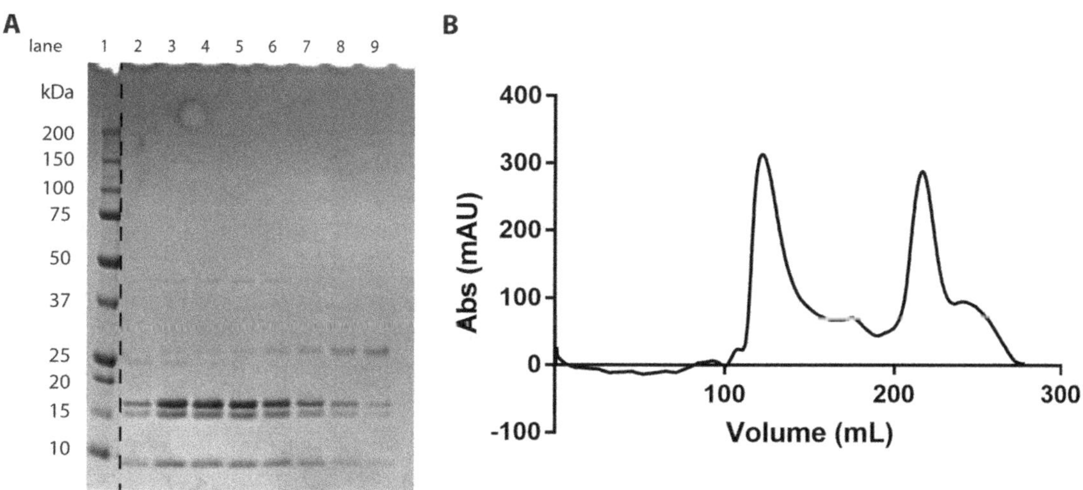

Fig. 4 (**a**) SDS-PAGE gel stained with Coomassie Blue showing selected fractions from size exclusion chromatography peak of SOCS1 B/C, as shown in panel **b** (lanes 2–9). (**b**) A_{280} absorbance trace of SOCS1 B/C elution from a Superdex200 26/600 size exclusion chromatography column. The first peak at ~120 mL contains aggregated SOCS1 B/C and contaminants, while the second peak at ~220 mL contains purified SOCS1 B/C. Trace represents protein obtained from approximately 2 L of *E. coli* culture

18. Optional: Phenyl phosphate may be removed before using SOCS1 B/C for biochemical assays, e.g., by PD-10 desalting column.

4 Notes

1. The vector must have different antibiotic resistance and must contain a different origin of replication to the vector chosen for SOCS1 expression.
2. If performing multiple transformations at once, aspirate and add bacmid mix well-by-well. This prevents the cell monolayers from drying out. Add the bacmid mix by slowly dropping on to the monolayer to avoid detaching the adhered cells.
3. Under these storage conditions, all generations of virus will retain infectivity for >6 months.
4. This protocol can be scaled up or down by adjusting cell culture and P2 virus volumes accordingly.
5. Since virus will be filtered in the next step, the centrifuge bottles need not be sterile.
6. There are a number of protocols for titering baculovirus. We prefer the method outlined in [24], which is less labor-intensive than a plaque assay. It is advisable to titer at least the first few P3 viruses made by this method as quality control.
7. This protocol can be scaled up or down by adjusting cell culture and virus volumes. Accordingly. We typically obtain JAK1 JH1 yields of ~5 mg/L of cell culture. Be sure to allow adequate volume for oxygenation in your chosen culture flask system.
8. Using this method, our mean P3 titer is 7×10^7 PFU/mL. 150 mL of virus ensures that the multiplicity of infection remains at least 3.0 in the majority of cases, without needing to titer each P3 virus. However, titering each virus can potentially yield greater consistency, albeit at the cost of more labor.
9. Insect cell pellets are difficult to transfer in solid form. We have found that resuspension in the used media is the easiest way to transfer the cell mass from a large centrifuge bottle to a vessel more appropriate for storage.
10. This purification procedure can be scaled up to a maximum of approximately two liters of cell culture by increasing buffer volumes accordingly.
11. We have found that centrifugation for less time, or at a lower speed than this, results in a supernatant which contains too much insoluble material for easy purification.

12. **Steps 4–9** can also be performed using a FPLC apparatus with two pumps and an automatic buffer mixing valve (e.g., ÅKTA-prime, GE Healthcare). Supernatant can be injected onto the IMAC column using a Super Loop (GE Healthcare) via appropriate luer lock fittings for a disposable 0.8 μm filter.
13. We typically use a Superdex 200 16/600 size column, which has a maximum sample injection volume of 5 mL. This means that no concentration is required before the gel filtration step.
14. We have found JAK1 JH1 to be unstable and precipitates readily when no compounds are bound to the ATP binding site. ATP and Mg^{2+} stabilize the protein by binding here. The addition of a small molecule ATP analogue JAK inhibitor would very likely have the same (or superior) effect. However be aware that many small molecule inhibitors may affect downstream applications of JAK1, for example, catalytic activity assays.
15. Since the gel filtration buffer includes 10% (v/v) glycerol, no additional cryoprotectant need be added before snap freezing.
16. We have found that the highest SOCS1 B/C yields are obtained when SOCS1 B/C is allowed to express slowly. Overly high expression speed results in the vast majority of SOCS1 B/C forming unfolded aggregate. Tuner cells allow expression levels to be controlled by the addition of variable concentrations of IPTG, and we have found that 25 μM IPTG coupled with overnight expression at low temperature of 18 °C slows down expression enough to result in a higher level of folded and stable SOCS1 B/C.
17. Be careful to pour all solutions slowly down the side of the column to avoid disturbing the packed affinity resin.
18. TEV is generally added at 1/100th of the level of target protein, by mass. However, the concentration of SOCS1 B/C bound to the Glutathione resin cannot be determined spectrophotometrically, so we typically find that 0.5 mg of TEV for every 1 mL resin ensures complete cleavage overnight.
19. Since it is difficult to accurately pipette 5 μL of resin, the different samples cannot be quantitatively compared to one another.

Acknowledgments

This work was supported by the Cancer Council Victoria (Grant-in-aid 1065180) and the National Health and Medical Research Council (NHMRC) Australia (Project grant #112299, Program grant #1113577), an NHMRC IRIISS grant 361646, and a Victorian State Government Operational Infrastructure Scheme grant. J.J.B. is supported by an NHMRC fellowship and NPDL by an Australian Postgraduate Award.

References

1. Schroder K, Hertzog PJ, Ravasi T, Hume DA (2004) Interferon-gamma: an overview of signals, mechanisms and functions. J Leukoc Biol 75:163–189
2. Haan C, Kreis S, Margue C, Behrmann I (2006) Jaks and cytokine receptors—an intimate relationship. Biochem Pharm 72:1538–1546
3. Igarashi K, Garotta G, Ozmen L, Ziemiecki A, Wilks AF, Harpur AG et al (1994) Interferon-gamma induces tyrosine phosphorylation of interferon-gamma receptor and regulated association of protein tyrosine kinases, Jak1 and Jak2, with its receptor. J Biol Chem 269:14333–14336
4. Steimle V, Siegrist CA, Mottet A, Lisowska-Grospierre B, Mach B (1994) Regulation of MHC class II expression by interferon-gamma mediated by the transactivator gene CIITA. Science 265:106–109
5. Pollard KM, Cauvi DM, Toomey CB, Morris KV, Kono DH (2013) Interferon-gamma and systemic autoimmunity. Discov Med 16:123–131
6. Alexander WS, Starr R, Fenner JE, Scott CL, Handman E, Sprigg NS et al (1999) SOCS1 is a critical inhibitor of interferon gamma signaling and prevents the potentially fatal neonatal actions of this cytokine. Cell 98:597–608
7. Ihle JN (1995) Cytokine receptor signalling. Nature 377:591–594
8. Shuai K, Ziemiecki A, Wilks AF, Harpur AG, Sadowski HB, Gilman MZ et al (1993) Polypeptide signalling to the nucleus through tyrosine phosphorylation of Jak and Stat proteins. Nature 366:580–583
9. Jeong EG, Kim MS, Nam HK, Min CK, Lee S, Chung YJ et al (2008) Somatic mutations of JAK1 and JAK3 in acute leukemias and solid cancers. Clin Cancer Res 14:3716–3721
10. Wallweber HJ, Tam C, Franke Y, Starovasnik MA, Lupardus PJ (2014) Structural basis of recognition of interferon-alpha receptor by tyrosine kinase 2. Nat Struct Mol Biol 21:443–448
11. Ferrao R, Wallweber HJ, Ho H, Tam C, Franke Y, Quinn J et al (2016) The structural basis for class II cytokine receptor recognition by JAK1. Structure 24(6):897–905
12. Duhe RJ, Clark EA, Farrar WL (2002) Characterization of the in vitro kinase activity of a partially purified soluble GST/JAK2 fusion protein. Mol Cell Biochem 236:23–35
13. Kershaw NJ, Murphy JM, Liau NPD, Varghese LN, Laktyushin A, Whitlock EL et al (2013) SOCS3 binds specific receptor-JAK complexes to control cytokine signaling by direct kinase inhibition. Nat Struct Mol Biol 20:469–476
14. Babon JJ, Varghese LN, Nicola NA (2014) Inhibition of IL-6 family cytokines by SOCS3. Semin Immunol 26:1–7
15. Hilton DJ, Richardson RT, Alexander WS, Viney EM, Willson TA, Sprigg NS et al (1998) Twenty proteins containing a C-terminal SOCS box form five structural classes. Proc Natl Acad Sci U S A 95:114–119
16. Starr R, Willson TA, Viney EM, Murray LJ, Rayner JR, Jenkins BJ et al (1997) A family of cytokine-inducible inhibitors of signalling. Nature 387:917–921
17. Babon JJ, Sabo JK, Soetopo A, Yao S, Bailey MF, Zhang JG et al (2008) The SOCS box domain of SOCS3: structure and interaction with the elonginBC-cullin5 ubiquitin ligase. J Mol Biol 381:928–940
18. Babon JJ, Sabo JK, Zhang JG, Nicola NA, Norton RS (2009) The SOCS box encodes a hierarchy of affinities for Cullin5: implications for ubiquitin ligase formation and cytokine signalling suppression. J Mol Biol 387:162–174
19. Kershaw NJ, Laktyushin A, Nicola NA, Babon JJ (2014) Reconstruction of an active SOCS3-based E3 ubiquitin ligase complex in vitro: identification of the active components and JAK2 and gp130 as substrates. Growth Factors 32:1–10
20. Kershaw NJ, Murphy JM, Lucet IS, Na N, Babon JJ (2013) Regulation of Janus kinases by SOCS proteins. Biochem Soc Trans 41:1042–1047
21. Yasukawa H, Misawa H, Sakamoto H, Masuhara M, Sasaki A, Wakioka T et al (1999) The JAK-binding protein JAB inhibits Janus tyrosine kinase activity through binding in the activation loop. EMBO J 18:1309–1320
22. Sasaki A, Yasukawa H, Suzuki A, Kamizono S, Syoda T, Kinjyo I et al (1999) Cytokine-inducible SH2 protein-3 (CIS3/SOCS3) inhibits Janus tyrosine kinase by binding through the N-terminal kinase inhibitory region as well as SH2 domain. Genes Cells 4:339–351
23. Babon JJ, Kershaw NJ, Murphy JM, Varghese LN, Laktyushin A, Young SN et al (2012) Suppression of cytokine signaling by SOCS3: characterization of the mode of inhibition and the basis of its specificity. Immunity 36:239–250
24. Harwood S (2007) Small-scale protein production with the baculovirus expression vector system. Methods Mol Biol 388:211–224

Chapter 22

Production of Recombinant Killer Immunoglobulin-Like Receptors for Crystallography and Luminex-Based Assays

Phillip Pymm and Julian P. Vivian

Abstract

The killer immunoglobulin-like receptors (KIR) are a highly diverse family of cell-surface receptors that are of importance to the effector function of Natural Killer cells. KIR have been implicated in the detection and clearance of malignantly transformed cells and in the immune-control of viruses including HIV, HCV and CMV. Recently, the mismatching of donor and recipient KIR has been demonstrated to improve success of hematopoietic stem cell transplantation treatments of leukemias. Due to the high degree of diversity amongst the KIR, a number of strategies are required for the production of recombinant protein for medical, biochemical and structural applications. Each of these strategies has advantages and limitations and is suitable for different subsets of the KIR and their intended use. Here we describe the preparation of these proteins for crystallography and the novel adaptation of tetramer production for this protein family that is suitable for a number of assays including single-antigen bead binding by Luminex. These methods are intended to provide comprehensive details for the production and characterization of each KIR and to be broadly applicable to other cell surface receptors of the immune system.

Key words Recombinant protein expression, HEK 293S, Baculovirus, Inclusion bodies, Tetramer, Luminex, Protein purification, Killer immunoglobulin-like receptors (KIR)

1 Introduction

The killer immunoglobulin-like receptors (KIR) are a family of cell-surface proteins expressed primarily on natural killer (NK) cells, which are central to innate immune function. KIR interact with human leukocyte antigen class I (HLA-I) ligands on target cells and influence NK cell activation and effector function [1–3]. KIR family members have been associated with altered outcome and progression in viral infection [4–6], are important in determining outcome following human stem cell transplants for several leukemias, particularly acute myeloid leukemia (AML), and are also involved in successful placentation during pregnancy [7–10]. The KIR family display a remarkable diversity, being polygenic (14 members) and highly polymorphic within the population, with consequent

Brendan J. Jenkins (ed.), *Inflammation and Cancer: Methods and Protocols*, Methods in Molecular Biology, vol. 1725, https://doi.org/10.1007/978-1-4939-7568-6_22, © Springer Science+Business Media, LLC 2018

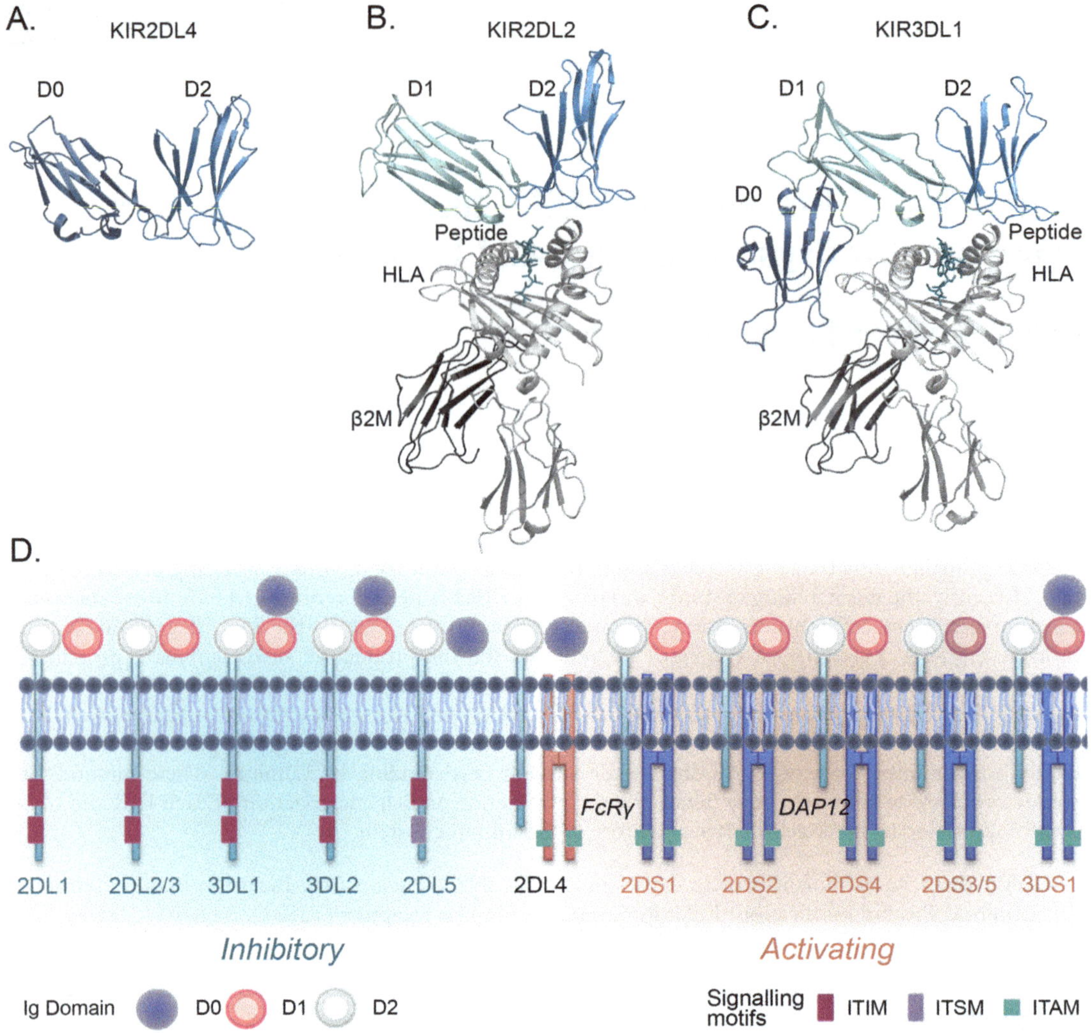

Fig. 1 Structural diversity of the members of the killer cell immunoglobulin-like receptor (KIR) family. Structures showing the arrangement of the KIR extracellular immunoglobulin domains (**a**) KIR2DL4 [12] a D0-D2 arrangement. (**b**) KIR2DL2 in complex with HLA C*03:04 a D1-D2 arrangement [39]. (**c**) KIR3DL1 in complex with HLA B*57:01 a D0-D1-D2 arrangement [13]. (**d**) Schematic representation of the structural features of KIR family members

divergence in structure and function between family members [11]. The extracellular portions of the KIR consist of three different immunoglobulin domains D0, D1, and D2, which can be arranged in three combinations, the two domain (D0–D2) and (D1–D2) KIR or the three domain (D0–D1–D2) KIR (Fig. 1) [12–14].

These differing combinations of extracellular domains give the individual KIR family members diverse properties that have necessitated the use of several strategies for successful expression and purification. The production of high-quality, pure recombinant

KIR proteins has been essential for many scientific and medical applications, including assay development, biochemical and biophysical characterization, protein crystallography, and development of protein-based treatments and drug target identification. This recombinant protein expression has been achieved in a variety of systems, including both bacterial and eukaryotic cell lines.

Bacterial expression, particularly in *E. coli*, is the most common system in use, providing fast expression and high yields for many intracellular proteins [15–17]. The absence of glycosylation machinery in this system also simplifies processing for many crystallographic applications [18]. However, there are many limitations to production of proteins in conventional *E. coli* expression systems, particularly for mammalian proteins and extracellular proteins that require chaperones for correct disulfide formation and folding. Further, correct posttranslational modification can also be essential to create a folded, mature protein in certain cases [18]. Some of these limitations can be overcome in bacterial systems through the expression and purification of insoluble protein in the form of inclusion bodies, which can then be solubilized and refolded in vitro under appropriate conditions [19, 20]. Indeed, this approach has been extremely useful in the production of antigen presenting proteins such as HLA-I, where individual antigens can be introduced in the refolding process to create single species for the investigation of specific immune responses [21]. Indeed, the D1–D2 arranged two-domain KIR can be successfully refolded in vitro following expression as insoluble inclusion bodies. However, this has not been the case for KIR containing a D0 domain. For these we have had greater success with eukaryotic expression systems, with the ultimate application of the recombinant protein further determining the production method.

For the D0-containing KIR, as for proteins that cannot be successfully refolded or where posttranslational modification/glycosylation is desired, expression in eukaryotic systems is the most common option, although modification of prokaryotic expression systems to replicate one or more of these steps has been undertaken [15, 22]. Three well-established approaches for eukaryotic expression are yeast, insect, and mammalian systems. Each of these has distinct advantages and drawbacks in terms of ease and speed, the yield and similarity of the final protein to that found in vivo. While mammalian systems offer the highest physiological relevance for mammalian proteins, particularly with regard to the posttranslational modifications to the protein, these systems can be time-consuming and expensive. The use of the relatively inexpensive polyethylenimine (PEI) as a transfection reagent has somewhat improved this in recent years [23–25]. Insect and yeast systems, while differing in final glycosylation and modification, are often faster approaches with greater final yield [26–28]. Indeed, insect cell expression is the preferred approach for noncrystallographic applications of D0-containing KIR. For crystallographic applications involving D0-containing KIR, glycosylation hinders the formation of regular crystal lattices due to the heterogeneity of attached carbohydrate moieties and their inherent flexibility [18]. Therefore, expression of these D0-contaning KIR is performed in the *N-acetylglucosaminyltransferase I* deficient human embryonic kidney cell line HEK293S [29, 30] which reduces the complexity of the carbohydrate chains and facilitates their enzymatic cleavage prior to crystallization.

Prior biophysical characterization and assaying of ligand interactions by individual KIR has primarily been performed using KIR-Fc fusion proteins [31]. Here, we describe a protocol for the production of tetrameric KIR constructs. These constructs provide an advantage over Fc fusion constructs by increasing avidity. This is particularly useful in light of the relatively low affinity of KIR for their ligands [13, 32]. Further, we describe a Luminex-based assay that has proven invaluable in studies of the KIR family for both ligand discovery and examination of the effects of polymorphism on ligand recognition [31, 33–36]. These assays rely on precisely calibrated fluorescent signatures applied to a latex bead that is conjugated with a specific protein. The bead is then incubated with a fluorescently tagged molecule of interest and both the tag on the bead and analyte are read to assess interaction. The unique fluorescent signature of each bead allows for up to 500 bead conjugates to be assessed simultaneously, creating a highly multiplexed assay. Whilst we have utilized bead-bound HLA to assess KIR binding, the fundamentals of the assay are broadly applicable to protein ligands of immune-receptors.

2 Materials

2.1 Protein Expression Using E. coli BL21 Cells

1. Chemically competent *E. coli* BL21 cells.
2. Luria broth media.
3. 50 mg/ml kanamycin sulfate stock solution.
4. 250 ml to 1 l Erlenmeyer flasks.
5. Plasmid DNA (insert in suitable vector for bacterial expression, e.g., pET30).
6. Luria Broth Agar plates with 50 μg/ml kanamycin sulfate.
7. Isopropyl β-D-1-thiogalactopyranoside (IPTG).
8. Plasmid DNA (Insert in suitable vector such as pET 30b).

2.2 Inclusion Body Purification and Refolding

1. Lysis Buffer: 50 mM Tris–HCl pH 8.0, 100 mM NaCl, 0.5% Triton X-100.
2. Triton Wash Buffer: 50 mM Tris–HCl pH 8.0, 100 mM NaCl, 0.5% Triton X-100, 1 mM EDTA, 1 mM DTT.

3. Resuspension Buffer: 50 mM Tris–HCl pH 8.0, 100 mM NaCl, 1 mM EDTA, 1 mM DTT.
4. Solubilization Buffer: 6 M Guanidine–HCl, 10 mM Tris–HCl pH 8.0, 1 mM DTT.
5. 10 mg/ml lysozyme in dH_2O.
6. 1 mg/ml DNase in 50% glycerol, 75 mM NaCl.
7. Refolding Buffer: 100 mM Tris–HCl pH 8.0, 400 mM L-Arginine, 0.5 mM oxidized glutathione, 5 mM reduced glutathione.
8. Cellulose Membrane Dialysis Tubing.
9. DEAE sepharose resin.
10. 50 ml Econocolumn.
11. Elution buffer: 10 mM Tris pH 8.0, 300 mM NaCl.
12. 10 mM Tris–HCl.
13. 1 l Schott Bottles.
14. Magnetic stirring block.
15. Cell homogenizer.
16. Centrifuge flasks, 50 ml to 1 l volumes.
17. 1 M $MgCl_2$.

2.3 Protein Expression Using Hi5 Cells

1. Hi5™ cells (BTI-TN-5B1–4).
2. Sf9 cells (ATCC® CRL-1711™).
3. Insect expression medium, Insect-XPRESS™ protein-free insect cell medium with L-glutamine.
4. Electrocompetent DH10Bac cells.
5. KGTC Blue-White Selection plates: LB Agar plates containing 50 μg/ml kanamycin, 7 μg/ml gentamycin, 10 μg/ml tetracycline, 50 μg/ml chloramphenicol, 100 μg/ml X-gal, 40 μg/ml IPTG.
6. Cellfectin™ II.
7. T25 tissue culture flask.
8. T175 tissue culture flask.
9. 200 ml to 3 l Erlenmeyer cell culture flasks.
10. Plasmid DNA (Insert in suitable shuttle vector such as pFastBac1).

2.4 Protein Expression Using HEK 293S Cells

1. HEK293S GnTI-cells (ATCC® CRL-3022™).
2. Dulbecco's Modified Eagle's Medium (DMEM).
3. Fetal calf serum (FCS).

4. Nonessential amino acids: 100× MEM Nonessential Amino Acids Solution.
5. 200 mM GlutaMAX™: (L-glutamine, L-alanyl-L-glutamine dipeptide).
6. PSG: Penicillin–Streptomycin–Glutamine (10,000 IU Penicillin, 10 mg/ml Streptomycin, 29.2 mg/ml L-Glutamine).
7. Multi-layer master mix: 40 mM GlutaMAX™, 20× Nonessential amino acids, 200 mM HEPES, 20 mM sodium pyruvate, 1 μM β-mercaptoethanol in DMEM.
8. T300 tissue culture flask.
9. Expanded surface roller bottles or multilayer flasks.
10. Plasmid DNA (Insert in suitable vector such as PhlSec).
11. Polyethylenimine (PEI).
12. Phosphate buffered salt (PBS): 10 mM phosphate buffer, 2.7 mM KCl, 137 mM NaCl, pH 7.4

2.5 Purification of Secreted His-Tagged Proteins from Eukaryotic Cell Lines

1. Tangential Flow Filtration (TFF) unit.
2. 1 l Centrifuge bottles.
3. 0.1 M phenylmethylsulfonyl fluoride (PMSF).
4. Complete™ protease inhibitor cocktail tablets.
5. TFF buffer: 10 mM Tris pH 8.0, 500 mM NaCl.
6. His-Trap FF 5 ml column.
7. Nickel A buffer: 10 mM Tris pH 8.0, 500 mM Nacl, 30 mM imidazole.
8. Nickel B buffer: 10 mM Tris pH 8.0, 500 mM NaCl, 30 mM imidazole, 100 mM EDTA pH 8.0.
9. P1 peristaltic pump.
10. Fast protein liquid chromatography (FPLC) unit.
11. Size exclusion chromatography columns, e.g., G.E® 16/60 Superdex 200 and 26/60 Superdex 200.
12. Centrifugal filter units, e.g., Amicon® Ultra-15.
13. TBS-300, 10 mM Tris pH 8.0, 300 mM NaCl.
14. 500 U/μl Endglycosidase H.
15. 3 M sodium acetate pH 5.5.

2.6 Biotinylation and Tetramerization of BirA Tagged Proteins

1. Avidin, NeutrAvidin®, PE conjugate, Molecular Probes®.
2. 0.5 mg/ml biotin ligase.
3. Biotinylation buffer A: 0.5 M Bicine pH 8.3.
4. Biotinylation buffer B: 100 mM ATP, 100 mM Mg-Acetate, 500 μM d-biotin.

5. TBS-100: 10 mM Tris–HCl, 100 mM NaCl.
   KIR3DL2 buffer: Tris–HCl 10 mM, K-Glutamate 500 mM.
6. 5 ml GE® HiTrap Desalting Columns.
7. Desalting Buffer: 10 mM Tris–HCl pH 8.0, 300 mM NaCl.
8. Streptavidin beads.
9. SDS-PAGE 18% acrylamide gel.
10. 4× SDS loading dye.
11. 1 M DTT.

2.7 Luminex Assay Using OneLambda Single Antigen Bead Assay HLA Class I

1. Staining Buffer: 10 mM phosphate buffer, 2.7 mM KCl, 300 mM NaCl, pH 7.4, 5% FCS.
2. Wash Buffer: 10 mM phosphate buffer, 2.7 mM KCl, 300 mM NaCl, pH 7.4, 0.25% Tween 20.
3. Analysis Buffer: 10 mM phosphate buffer, 2.7 mM KCl, 300 mM NaCl, pH 7.4.
4. LABScreen Single Antigen HLA Class I Beads.
5. PE-Conjugated Goat Anti-Human IgG.
6. Quantiplex reference beads for instrument calibration.

3 Methods

3.1 Expression and Refolding of KIR in E. coli

For expression in *E. coli*, the extracellular domains of KIR genes are subcloned into the pET30b expression vector (Fig. 2). Expression in *E. coli* is suitable only for two domain KIR with a D1-D2 extracellular domain arrangement. Three domain KIR and those containing a D0 domain refold poorly and must be expressed as a secreted soluble protein from a eukaryotic expression system.

1. Thaw one 50 μl aliquot of chemically competent *E. coli* BL21 cells on ice and add 1 μl (10–100 ng) plasmid DNA.
2. Incubate on ice for 5–15 min.
3. Induce uptake of plasmid DNA by heat shocking the cells. Using a water bath or heat block, incubate the cells at 42 °C for 45 s. Immediately return to ice and incubate for 2 min.
4. Add 250 μl sterile SOC media to the cells using aseptic technique and incubate at 37 °C for 1 h with shaking.
5. Plate 10–100 μl of the cells onto a room temperature LB-agar plate containing 50 μg/ml kanamycin.
6. Incubate overnight at 37 °C.
7. Pick a single colony from the plate and add to 150 ml LB media containing 50 μg/ml kanamycin. Incubate for 8 h or overnight at 37 °C with shaking.

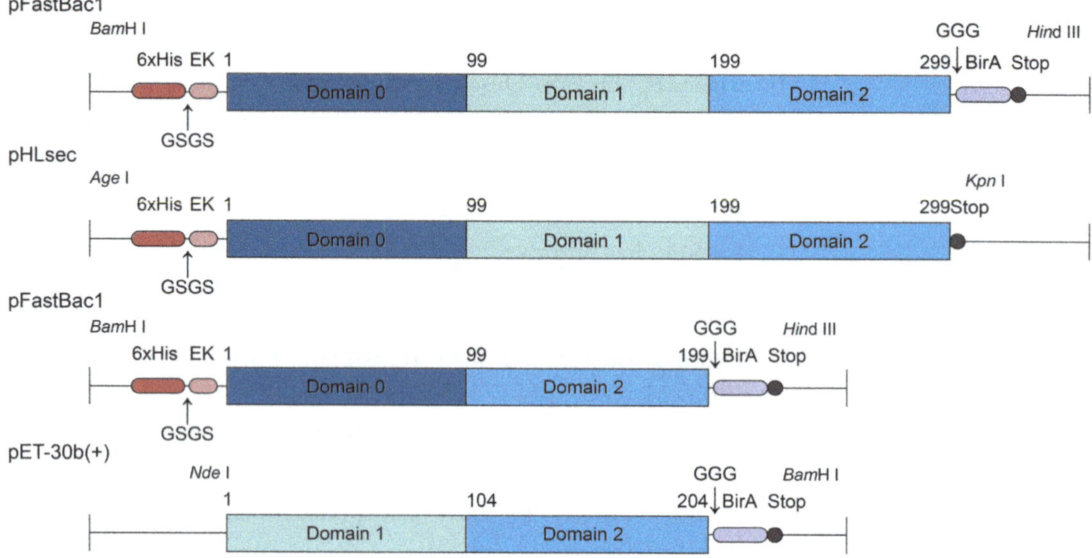

Fig. 2 Insert design for KIR D0-D1-D2, D0-D2, and D1-D2 family members for insertion into their respective vectors. Incorporated restriction sites are shown in italic font. Domain boundaries, tags and linker regions between tags or protein are shown where applicable

8. Measure the optical density of the culture at a wavelength of 600 nm (OD600) with a spectrophotometer and transfer sufficient volume to flasks containing 800 ml LB media (50 μg/ml kanamycin) to give a final OD600 of 0.05. Six flasks totaling 4.8 l provide approximately 0.5–2 g protein for refolding in our experience.
9. Incubate at 37 °C with shaking until an OD600 of 0.5–0.8 is reached. A sample may be taken for comparison of post-induction KIR expression. At this point add IPTG to the flask to a final concentration of 0.5 mM to induce expression of the KIR protein.
10. Incubate for a further 4 h at 37 °C with shaking. A sample may be taken to assess KIR expression by SDS-PAGE.
11. Transfer cultures to 1 l centrifuge flasks and spin for 15 min at 4500 × *g*, 4 °C. Discard the supernatant.
12. Pool cell pellets and resuspend in 100 ml lysis buffer. Freeze overnight to enhance cell lysis or proceed directly to inclusion body purification.
13. Thaw resuspended cell pellets and add 10–30 mg Lysozyme, 2 mg DNase and 5 mM $MgCl_2$. Incubate at room temperature, shaking for 2 h. This should ensure complete lysis of the cells. Following this step, keep sample on ice at all times to reduce degradation of the expressed protein by cellular proteases.

14. Transfer lysed mixture to 250 ml centrifuge tubes and spin at 15,000 × *g*, 4 °C for 15 min.
15. Discard the supernatant and resuspend the cell pellet in 100 ml triton wash buffer using a cell homogenizer.
16. Spin sample at 10000 × *g*, 4 °C for 10 min.
17. Repeat **steps 15** and **16** twice more or until the supernatant is clear and colorless (*see* **Note 1**).
18. Resuspend the cell pellet from the final wash step in 100 ml resuspension buffer. Spin at 10000 × *g*, 4 °C for 10 min and discard the supernatant.
19. Solubilize the pellet in 10–20 ml solubilization buffer. If solubilization is incomplete, incubate overnight at 4 °C on a rotating/roller platform.
20. Transfer the solubilized sample to a 50 ml centrifuge tube and spin at 30,000 × *g*, 4 °C for 20 min. Discard any pelleted material. This is solubilized denatured KIR protein and is now suitable for refolding. If the supernatant is not clear following this step, the sample may be filtered before storage at −80 °C in suitable aliquots.
21. To refold the KIR, cool 500 ml refolding buffer to 4 °C and place on a magnetic stirrer at medium–high speed.
22. Add in 30 mg solubilized KIR dropwise to the buffer.
23. Incubate stirring overnight at 4 °C.
24. Add in 30 mg solubilized KIR dropwise to the buffer and incubate for 8 h before adding a final 30 mg KIR to the refold.
25. Incubate stirring overnight at 4 °C.
26. Prepare 15 l of 10 mM Tris pH 8.0 and cool to 4 °C.
27. Transfer refold into prewetted dialysis tubing and place into the 10 mM Tris for buffer exchange.
28. Leave overnight at 4 °C and replace the 10 mM Tris twice more, incubating 4 h-overnight to allow buffer exchange.
29. Transfer the refold into a 1 l flask and filter excess precipitated material prior to purification

3.2 Expression of KIR in Insect Cells

For insect cell expression, the extracellular domains of KIR genes are subcloned into a modified baculoviral pFastBac-expression vector (Invitrogen, Carlsbad, CA) containing a secretion signal peptide sequence, an N-terminal hexahistidine tag and a C-terminal BirA-tag [37] (Fig. 2).

1. Thaw 100 μl *E. coli* DH10Bac electrocompetent cells on ice. Add approximately 10 ng of plasmid DNA in 1 μl.

2. Transfer to a precooled electrocuvette and electroporate at 1800 V, following the pulse, the time constant should be approximately 5 ms.
3. Immediately add 1 ml LB media and transfer to a sterile eppendorf, incubate at 37 °C for 4 h with shaking.
4. Plate out 10–100 μl cells on KGTC-blue/white selection plates.
5. Incubate at 37 °C for 48 h. Prior to colony selection, place plates at 4 °C for 2 h to increase the color intensity.
6. Select white colonies for colony PCR screening using M13 forward and reverse primers in addition to gene specific primers.
7. Transfer a gene-containing colony into 5 ml LB media containing 50 μg/ml kanamycin, 7 μg/ml gentamycin, and 10 μg/ml tetracycline. Incubate at 37 °C overnight with shaking.
8. Purify the bacmid DNA using a Qiagen plasmid midiprep kit or equivalent. To sterilize the resulting DNA, perform the final ethanol wash of the protocol in a tissue culture cabinet and dissolve the DNA in 50 μl sterile TE buffer or sterile MQ water.
9. In an eppendorf tube, mix 30 μl Bacmid DNA with 300 μl insect expression media. In a separate tube mix 24 μl Cellfectin II with 300 μl insect expression media.
10. Mix the two tubes and incubate for 30 min at room temperature.
11. Transfer 2.5×10^6 Sf9 cells into a T25 tissue culture flask in 5 ml insect expression media. Allow to adhere to the flask for a minimum of 15 min at 27 °C.
12. Remove the media and wash gently with 1–2 ml fresh insect expression media. Do not disturb the cells. Remove the wash and add the 600 μl DNA–Cellfectin mix onto the cells.
13. Incubate the flask at 27 °C for 5 h.
14. Wash the cells with 5 ml insect expression media, remove and replace with 5 ml fresh insect expression media.
15. Incubate the flask at 27 °C for 3 days without shaking.
16. Transfer to a falcon tube and centrifuge at $1000 \times g$ for 10 min at room temperature. Decant the supernatant, this forms the P1 stock. Store in aliquots with 2% FCS at −80 °C until ready for use.
17. Add 2 ml P1 stock to 200 ml Sf9 cells at 2×10^6 cells/ml in insect expression media. Incubate at 27 °C for 3 days with shaking.
18. Transfer to falcon tubes and centrifuge at $1000 \times g$ for 10 min at room temperature. Decant the supernatant into a T75 tissue

culture flask, this forms the P2 stock and can be stored at 4 °C in the dark for future use.

19. Add 5 ml P2 stock to 500 ml Sf9 cells at 2×10^6 cells/ml in insect expression media. Incubate at 27 °C for 3 days with shaking.
20. Transfer to falcon tubes and centrifuge at $1000 \times g$ for 10 min at room temperature. Decant the supernatant into a T175 tissue culture flask, this forms the P3 stock and can be stored at 4 °C in the dark for future use.
21. For expression of KIR, grow 4 l Hi5™ cells to a density of 2×10^6 cells/ml in insect expression media. Add 25 ml P3 stock per liter of Hi5™ cells.
22. Incubate at 27 °C for 3 days with shaking.
23. Transfer cultures to 1 l centrifuge flasks and spin at $4500 \times g$ for 25 min.
24. Pool supernatant for purification. Supernatant can be stored at 4 °C with 0.1 mM PMSF and/or Complete EDTA free protease inhibitor cocktail tablets overnight.

3.3 Expression of KIR in Mammalian Cells

For mammalian expression, the extracellular domains of KIR genes are subcloned into the pHLSec-expression vector containing a secretion signal peptide sequence and an N-terminal hexahistidine tag [38] (Fig. 2).

1. HEK293S cells are grown to 70% confluency using two T300 tissue culture flasks in DMEM supplemented with 10% FCS, 2 mM GlutaMAX™, and 5 ml PSG.
2. Wash the cells using PBS and trypsinize to remove them from the flask. Stop this reaction with 20 ml DMEM containing 10% FCS.
3. Add 10 ml of the DMEM-cell mix to each multi-layer flask (total 4) and fill with 240 ml DMEM supplemented with 10% FCS, 2 mM GlutaMAX™, 2.4 ml PSG, and 15 ml Multi-layer Master mix.
4. Incubate at 37 °C, 5% CO_2 for 48 h.
5. For each flask used, mix 300 μg sterile plasmid DNA with 10 ml serum-free DMEM and add 450 μl PEI (1 mg/ml). Vortex and incubate at room temperature for 15 min.
6. Remove media from multilayer flasks and wash carefully with PBS.
7. Add DNA-PEI mix to the multilayer flask and top up with 240 ml DMEM supplemented with 2% FCS, 2 mM GlutaMAX™, and 15 ml Multi-layer Master mix (*see* **Note 2**).
8. Incubate at 37 °C, 5% CO_2 for 72 h.

9. Prepare 500 ml DMEM supplemented with 2% FCS, 2 mM GlutaMAX™, 5 ml PSG, and 30 ml Multilayer Master mix.
10. Transfer media into 1 l centrifuge flasks. Replace media in flasks with media prepared in **step 9** for a second passage. Incubate at 37 °C, 5% CO_2 for 72 h.
11. Spin collected media at 4500 × *g*, 4 °C for 25 min. Discard pelleted material. Supernatant can be stored at 4 °C with 0.1 mM PMSF and/or Complete EDTA free protease inhibitor cocktail tablets overnight.

3.4 Purification of Refolded Protein

1. Load a clean Econo-Column with 10 ml 50% DEAE slurry and allow to drain.
2. Equilibrate DEAE with 50 ml 10 mM Tris pH 8.0.
3. Load dialyzed refold onto DEAE through gravity flow at 4 °C. Following loading, wash the resin with a further 50 ml 10 mM Tris pH 8.0.
4. Elute captured protein from the DEAE using 50 ml elution buffer.
5. Concentrate the eluted protein to 5 ml total volume using an Amicon centrifugal filter unit with a 10 kDa cutoff for loading onto a size exclusion column.
6. Load protein onto a 16/60 superdex 200 size exclusion column equilibrated in TBS and collect 1 ml fractions for 1 column volume.
7. Run fractions containing peaks at 280 nm on an SDS-PAGE gel to determine fractions containing the KIR protein.
8. Pool these fractions and exchange into 10 mM Tris pH 8.0 using a centrifugal concentrator for anion exchange.
9. Load pooled fractions onto a 5 ml HiTrap Q column equilibrated in Tris pH 8.0. Elute the protein through an increasing salt gradient up to 0.5 M NaCl over 40 min at a 1 ml/min flow rate. Collect 0.5 ml fractions throughout the gradient.
10. Run fractions containing peaks at 280 nm on an SDS-PAGE gel to determine fractions containing the KIR protein. Pool, concentrate and buffer exchange KIR containing fractions as appropriate for downstream applications.

3.5 Purification of His-Tagged Protein

1. Filter supernatant using a 0.8 μm filter and Buffer exchange into TFF buffer using dialysis or through use of tangential flow filtration.
2. Filter buffer exchanged supernatant to remove any precipitated material (0.8 μm pore size maximum) and add Imidazole to a final concentration of 30 mM. Equilibrate a 5 ml HisTrap FF column in Nickel Buffer A.

3. Load sample onto the Nickel column using a P1 peristaltic pump at 4 °C at a 5 ml/min flow rate.
4. Wash nickel column with 100 ml Nickel buffer A.
5. Elute KIR with 50 ml Nickel Buffer B. This buffer will also strip the nickel from the column.
6. Concentrate the eluted protein to 5 ml total volume using an Amicon centrifugal filter unit with a 10 kDa cut-off for loading onto a size exclusion column.
7. Load protein onto a GE 16/60 superdex 200 size exclusion column equilibrated in TBS and collect 1 ml fractions for 1 column volume.
8. Run fractions containing peaks at 280 nm on an SDS-PAGE gel to determine fractions containing the KIR protein.
9. KIR may need further purification using a 26/60 superdex 200 size exclusion column dependent upon contaminants remaining at this stage, otherwise KIR fractions can be pooled, concentrated and buffer exchanged as appropriate for downstream applications.

3.6 Preparation of Protein for Crystallography

KIR produced in 293S cells has glycans suitable for cleavage by Endoglycosidase H. Deglycosylation of the KIR will increase the homogeneity of the sample and increase its suitability for crystallization.

1. Buffer exchange KIR into 10 mM Tris pH 8.0, 300 mM NaCl (TBS-300) using a centrifugal concentrator and concentrate to 5–10 mg/ml.
2. Add 100 mM sodium acetate pH 5.5 to adjust the pH of the sample.
3. Add 100 units endoH per 25 μg KIR and incubate for 5 h at room temperature.

3.7 Biotinylation of Purified KIR Protein

KIR produced with a BirA tag attached at the C-terminus can be biotinylated and subsequently tetramerized for applications including flow cytometry, fluorescent microscopy and Luminex assays (*see* **Note 3**).

1. Buffer exchange KIR into TBS-100 using a centrifugal concentrator and concentrate to 200 μl. Two-domain D1-D2 KIR can be buffer exchanged into 10 mM Tris pH 8.0 only. KIR3DL2 is biotinylated most effectively in KIR3DL2 buffer (*see* **Note 4**).
2. Add 1 part biotinylation buffer A and 1 part biotinylation buffer B to 8 parts KIR (25 μl each buffer if KIR is concentrated to 200 μl). Add 10 μl Biotin ligase (0.5 mg/ml).
3. Incubate at 20 °C overnight or 4 °C for 48 h.

4. Equilibrate a 5 ml HiTrap Desalting column with desalting buffer running at 1 ml/min.
5. Load biotinylation mix onto the desalting column using a 250 μl loop. Collect 0.2 ml fractions from injection, KIR will elute in the first peak with free biotin eluting in a second, large peak (*see* **Note 5**).
6. Pool the KIR containing fractions, and concentrate as required (1 mg/ml for tetramerization).

3.8 Assessment of Biotinylation

A streptavidin pull-down can be run to determine efficiency of the biotinylation reaction. Native gels cannot be run for most three domain KIR due to their high net positive charge (isoelectric point above 9.0).

1. For each sample add 20 μl streptavidin coated sepharose beads to an eppendorf tube. Add 180 μl TBS-300 to beads.
2. Spin at 1000 × *g* for 2 min to pellet beads. Remove buffer carefully and repeat wash.
3. Add 10 μg protein sample to beads with buffer removed and incubate for 10–30 min at room temperature.
4. Add 180 μl buffer and mix briefly. Spin at 1000 × *g*, 2 min as before.
5. Remove buffer and save in a tube marked "wash 1".
6. Repeat **steps 4** and **5** three times, saving buffer from each wash in separate tubes marked washes 2–4.
7. Add 180 μl buffer to beads, mix well and remove 10 μl from this mix for SDS-PAGE.
8. Take 10 μl of saved wash buffers for SDS-PAGE.
9. Samples containing the streptavidin beads should be prepared for a reducing SDS-PAGE gel and incubated at 90 °C for 30 min to remove protein from the beads and dissociate streptavidin from the KIR.
10. Wash samples should be prepared for a reducing SDS-PAGE gel and heated at 90 °C for 5 min.
11. Run bead and wash samples in adjacent wells to compare the ratio of biotinylated to nonbiotinylated protein (Fig. 3).

3.9 Tetramerization of KIR Monomers

For this procedure, all fluorescent conjugates should be kept away from light and incubations should take place in a dark container at room temperature.

1. Adjust the concentration of the KIR to 1 mg/ml of fully biotinylated protein using TBS 300. Unbiotinylated protein may be present in your sample but should not be included when calculating the neutravidin required for tetramerization (*see* **Note 6**).

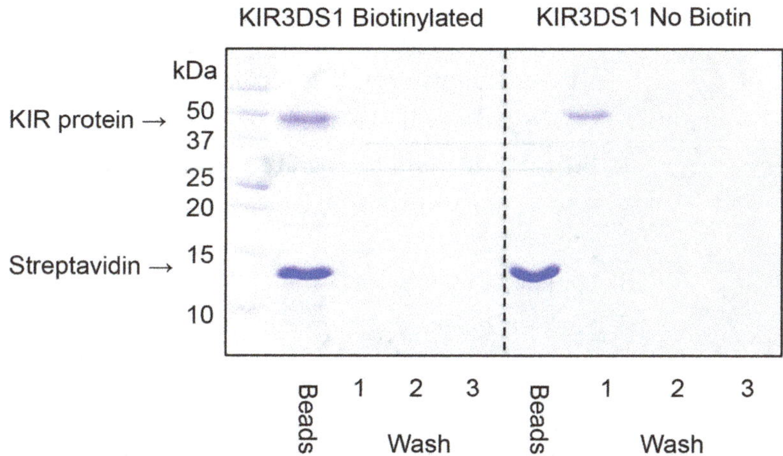

Fig. 3 SDS-PAGE gel visualizing protein bands resulting from streptavidin pull-down. KIR3DS1 is eluted in the bead fraction when biotinylated, indicating binding of the protein to the streptavidin beads through the biotin tag. KIR3DS1 without biotin added is eluted in the first wash fraction, indicating a lack of binding to the streptavidin beads

2. Calculate the amount of neutravidin required to tetramerize the KIR using the following calculation:
   (a) Mw of KIR (including any glycosylation)/Mw neutravidin PE (approx. 308 kDa) = 0.12.
   (b) Amount of KIR in μg/0.12 = volume neutravidin required for a 1:1 molar ratio assuming both KIR and neutravidin are at same concentration (e.g., 1 mg/ml).
   (c) Volume required/4 = to obtain a 4:1 ratio KIR: neutravidin as each neutravidin molecule will bind four KIR.
3. Only for three domain KIR and those with a D0 domain: adjust NaCl concentration in the KIR buffer for a final concentration of 300 mM following tetramerization (as the neutravidin buffer has no NaCl). Lower NaCl concentrations will cause protein precipitation during tetramerization.
4. Divide the total required neutravidin into 10 aliquots and add sequentially to the KIR, follow each addition with an incubation for 10 min at room temperature in the dark.
5. Repeat the addition of the aliquots until all 10 have been added.
6. Store the tetramer at 4 °C until needed (*see* **Note 7**). Spin briefly before use to remove any precipitated protein.

3.10 OneLambda Single Antigen HLA Class I Luminex Assay

1. In a Luminex-compatible 96-well plate add 5 μl of each tetramer in 15 μl Staining Buffer.
2. Add 5 μl vortexed OneLambda Single antigen HLA class I beads to each tetramer mix.

(a) For a negative control, use 5 μl neutravidin-PE or a suitable secondary antibody in place of the tetramer (e.g., anti-human IgG-PE secondary).

3. Cover plate with plastic film and gently vortex.
4. Incubate at room temperature away from light for 30 min.
5. Add 175 μl wash buffer to each well; cover plate in plastic film and vortex.
6. Spin at 1800 × *g* for 5 min.
7. Flick off buffer and blot plate, bead pellets should be visible in the wells following the blotting. Cover the plate with plastic film and dry vortex the beads after this step the pellets should have dispersed and no longer be visible. Resuspend in 200 μl wash buffer and re-cover plate. Repeat vortex.
8. Repeat the wash steps (**6** and **7**) twice.
9. Following the final wash step resuspend the beads in 100 μl resuspension buffer.
10. Run the samples on a pre-calibrated Labscan 100 instrument using a prepared single antigen HLA class I template. Ensure that the bead lot on the template matches the current batch in use.
11. Data is processed using HLAFusion software; both raw and normalized values are outputted in a format for statistical software of choice (e.g., EXCEL) for further analysis. Normalized fluorescence values are obtained by subtracting background values using the following formula.

$$(S\#N - SNC\ bead) - (BG\#N - BGNC\ bead).$$

(S#N = Sample-specific fluorescence value (trimmed mean) for bead #N; SNC bead = Sample-specific fluorescence value for Negative Control (nude) bead; BG#N = Background Negative Control fluorescence value for bead #N; BGNC bead = Background Negative Control fluorescence value for Negative Control bead). Negative control samples were obtained using unconjugated streptavidin-PE in place of the conjugated KIR tetramer.

4 Notes

1. The pellet should be off-white and dry/powdery in consistency. Mucilaginous brown/green pellets through the wash steps may indicate incomplete lysis, DNA contamination or poor protein expression. Repetition of the lysis step (**13**) may be necessary. Ensure complete removal of EDTA from the sample before repeating this step.

2. 3.8 mM valproic acid added to media can enhance expression in a protein dependent manner.
3. KIR containing the D0 domain are often salt-sensitive and precipitate in low salt buffers. However, biotin ligase is inhibited by high salt concentrations. 100 mM NaCl with double the usual amount of ligase is effective for biotinylation of the majority of these KIR, alternatives are noted where they have been found.
4. This buffer has not been suitable in our experience for three-domain KIR other than KIR3DL2, causing precipitation during overnight incubation.
5. Larger injection volumes at this step will reduce separation between the protein and biotin peaks and should be avoided. For larger volume samples consider using a size exclusion column to separate the free biotin from the KIR.
6. If a large percentage of the sample is unbiotinylated, consider adding a size exclusion step following tetramerization.
7. Tetramers should not be frozen and should be used as soon as possible following production. While signal in our assays is detectable for several months, the signal strength drops substantially over a 2-week period.

References

1. Moretta A, Vitale M, Bottino C, Orengo AM, Morelli L, Augugliaro R, Barbaresi M, Ciccone E, Moretta L (1993) P58 molecules as putative receptors for major histocompatibility complex (MHC) class I molecules in human natural killer (NK) cells. Anti-p58 antibodies reconstitute lysis of MHC. J Exp Med 178:597–604
2. Gumperz JE, Litwin V, Phillips JH, Lanier LL, Parham P (1995) The Bw4 public epitope of HLA-B molecules confers reactivity with natural killer cell clones that express NKB1, a putative HLA receptor. J Exp Med 181:1133–1144
3. Litwin V, Gumperz J, Parham P, Phillips JH, Lanier LL (1994) NKB1: a natural killer cell receptor involved in the recognition of polymorphic HLA-B molecules. J Exp Med 180:537–543
4. Martin MP, Gao X, Lee JH, Nelson GW, Detels R, Goedert JJ, Buchbinder S, Hoots K, Vlahov D, Trowsdale J, Wilson M, O'Brien SJ, Carrington M (2002) Epistatic interaction between KIR3DS1 and HLA-B delays the progression to AIDS. Nat Genet 31:429–434
5. Martin MP, Qi Y, Gao X, Yamada E, Martin JN, Pereyra F, Colombo S, Brown EE, Shupert WL, Phair J, Goedert JJ, Buchbinder S, Kirk GD, Telenti A, Connors M, O'Brien SJ, Walker BD, Parham P, Deeks SG, McVicar DW, Carrington M (2007) Innate partnership of HLA-B and KIR3DL1 subtypes against HIV-1. Nat Genet 39:733–740
6. De Re V, Caggiari L, De Zorzi M, Repetto O, Zignego AL, Izzo F, Tornesello ML, Buonaguro FM, Mangia A, Sansonno D, Racanelli V, De Vita S, Pioltelli P, Vaccher E, Berretta M, Mazzaro C, Libra M, Gini A, Zucchetto A, Cannizzaro R, De Paoli P (2015) Genetic diversity of the KIR/HLA system and susceptibility to hepatitis C virus-related diseases. PLoS One 10:e0117420
7. Marra J, Greene J, Hwang J, Du J, Damon L, Martin T, Venstrom JM (2015) KIR and HLA genotypes predictive of low-affinity interactions are associated with lower relapse in autologous hematopoietic cell transplantation for acute myeloid leukemia. J Immunol 194:4222–4230
8. Cooley S, Weisdorf DJ, Guethlein LA, Klein JP, Wang T, Le CT, Marsh SG, Geraghty D, Spellman S, Haagenson MD, Ladner M, Trachtenberg E, Parham P, Miller JS (2010) Donor selection for natural killer cell receptor genes leads to superior survival after unrelated

transplantation for acute myelogenous leukemia. Blood 116:2411–2419

9. Hiby SE, Walker JJ, O'Shaughnessy KM, Redman CW, Carrington M, Trowsdale J, Moffett A (2004) Combinations of maternal KIR and fetal HLA-C genes influence the risk of preeclampsia and reproductive success. J Exp Med 200:957–965
10. Kennedy PR, Chazara O, Gardner L, Ivarsson MA, Farrell LE, Xiong S, Hiby SE, Colucci F, Sharkey AM, Moffett A (2016) Activating KIR2DS4 is expressed by uterine NK cells and contributes to successful pregnancy. J Immunol 197:4292–4300
11. Parham P (2008) The genetic and evolutionary balances in human NK cell receptor diversity. Semin Immunol 20:311–316
12. Moradi S, Berry R, Pymm P, Hitchen C, Beckham SA, Wilce MC, Walpole NG, Clements CS, Reid HH, Perugini MA, Brooks AG, Rossjohn J, Vivian JP (2015) The structure of the atypical killer cell immunoglobulin-like receptor, KIR2DL4. J Biol Chem 290:10460–10471
13. Vivian JP, Duncan RC, Berry R, O'Connor GM, Reid HH, Beddoe T, Gras S, Saunders PM, Olshina MA, Widjaja JM, Harpur CM, Lin J, Maloveste SM, Price DA, Lafont BA, McVicar DW, Clements CS, Brooks AG, Rossjohn J (2011) Killer cell immunoglobulin-like receptor 3DL1-mediated recognition of human leukocyte antigen B. Nature 479:401–405
14. Fan QR, Long EO, Wiley DC (2001) Crystal structure of the human natural killer cell inhibitory receptor KIR2DL1-HLA-Cw4 complex. Nat Immunol 2:452–460
15. Rosano GL, Ceccarelli EA (2014) Recombinant protein expression in Escherichia coli: advances and challenges. Front Microbiol 5:172
16. Baneyx F (1999) Recombinant protein expression in Escherichia coli. Curr Opin Biotechnol 10:411–421
17. Makrides SC (1996) Strategies for achieving high-level expression of genes in Escherichia coli. Microbiol Rev 60:512–538
18. Stevens RC (2000) Design of high-throughput methods of protein production for structural biology. Structure 8:R177–R185
19. Tsumoto K, Ejima D, Kumagai I, Arakawa T (2003) Practical considerations in refolding proteins from inclusion bodies. Protein Expr Purif 28:1–8
20. Burgess RR (2009) Refolding solubilized inclusion body proteins. Methods Enzymol 463:259–282
21. Altman JD, Davis MM (2003) MHC-peptide tetramers to visualize antigen-specific T cells. Curr Protoc Immunol 115:17.3.1–17.3.44
22. Jaffe SR, Strutton B, Levarski Z, Pandhal J, Wright PC (2014) Escherichia coli as a glycoprotein production host: recent developments and challenges. Curr Opin Biotechnol 30:205–210
23. Dyson MR (2016) Fundamentals of expression in mammalian cells. Adv Exp Med Biol 896:217–224
24. Hacker DL, Kiseljak D, Rajendra Y, Thurnheer S, Baldi L, Wurm FM (2013) Polyethyleneimine-based transient gene expression processes for suspension-adapted HEK-293E and CHO-DG44 cells. Protein Expr Purif 92:67–76
25. Pham PL, Kamen A, Durocher Y (2006) Large-scale transfection of mammalian cells for the fast production of recombinant protein. Mol Biotechnol 34:225–237
26. Possee RD (1997) Baculoviruses as expression vectors. Curr Opin Biotechnol 8:569–572
27. Kost TA, Condreay JP, Jarvis DL (2005) Baculovirus as versatile vectors for protein expression in insect and mammalian cells. Nat Biotechnol 23:567–575
28. Luckow VA, Lee SC, Barry GF, Olins PO (1993) Efficient generation of infectious recombinant baculoviruses by site-specific transposon-mediated insertion of foreign genes into a baculovirus genome propagated in Escherichia coli. J Virol 67:4566–4579
29. Reeves PJ, Callewaert N, Contreras R, Khorana HG (2002) Structure and function in rhodopsin: high-level expression of rhodopsin with restricted and homogeneous N-glycosylation by a tetracycline-inducible N-acetylglucosaminyltransferase I-negative HEK293S stable mammalian cell line. Proc Natl Acad Sci U S A 99:13419–13424
30. de Chasseval R, de Villartay JP (1992) High level transient gene expression in human lymphoid cells by SV40 large T antigen boost. Nucleic Acids Res 20:245–250
31. Graef T, Moesta AK, Norman PJ, Abi-Rached L, Vago L, Older Aguilar AM, Gleimer M, Hammond JA, Guethlein LA, Bushnell DA, Robinson PJ, Parham P (2009) KIR2DS4 is a product of gene conversion with KIR3DL2 that introduced specificity for HLA-A*11 while diminishing avidity for HLA-C. J Exp Med 206:2557–2572
32. Pymm P, Illing PT, Ramarathinam SH, O'Connor GM, Hughes VA, Hitchen C, Price DA, Ho BK, McVicar DW, Brooks AG, Purcell AW, Rossjohn J, Vivian JP (2017) MHC-I

peptides get out of the groove and enable a novel mechanism of HIV-1 escape. Nat Struct Mol Biol 24:387–394

33. Moesta AK, Norman PJ, Yawata M, Yawata N, Gleimer M, Parham P (2008) Synergistic polymorphism at two positions distal to the ligand-binding site makes KIR2DL2 a stronger receptor for HLA-C than KIR2DL3. J Immunol 180:3969–3979
34. Hilton HG, Moesta AK, Guethlein LA, Blokhuis J, Parham P, Norman PJ (2015) The production of KIR-Fc fusion proteins and their use in a multiplex HLA class I binding assay. J Immunol Meth 425:79–87
35. Saunders PM, Pymm P, Pietra G, Hughes VA, Hitchen C, O'Connor GM, Loiacono F, Widjaja J, Price DA, Falco M, Mingari MC, Moretta L, McVicar DW, Rossjohn J, Brooks AG, Vivian JP (2016) Killer cell immunoglobulin-like receptor 3DL1 polymorphism defines distinct hierarchies of HLA class I recognition. J Exp Med 213:791–807
36. Hilton HG, Vago L, Older Aguilar AM, Moesta AK, Graef T, Abi-Rached L, Norman PJ, Guethlein LA, Fleischhauer K, Parham P (2012) Mutation at positively selected positions in the binding site for HLA-C shows that KIR2DL1 is a more refined but less adaptable NK cell receptor than KIR2DL3. J Immunol 189:1418–1430
37. Stifter SA, Gould JA, Mangan NE, Reid HH, Rossjohn J, Hertzog PJ, de Weerd NA (2014) Purification and biological characterization of soluble, recombinant mouse IFNbeta expressed in insect cells. Protein Expr Purif 94:7–14
38. Aricescu AR, Lu W, Jones EY (2006) A time- and cost-efficient system for high-level protein production in mammalian cells. Acta Crystallogr D Biol Crystallogr 62:1243–1250
39. Boyington JC, Motyka SA, Schuck P, Brooks AG, Sun PD (2000) Crystal structure of an NK cell immunoglobulin-like receptor in complex with its class I MHC ligand. Nature 405:537–543

Chapter 23

Isolation and Characterization of Mouse Intrahepatic Lymphocytes by Flow Cytometry

Florian Wiede and Tony Tiganis

Abstract

In the field of cellular immunology multicolor flow cytometry is a frequently applied method that allows for the simultaneously detection of multiple parameters on an individual cell basis. Flow cytometry can be used to characterize a wide range of immune cell subsets using fluorophore-conjugated antibodies to a wide range of cellular antigens. The isolation of immune cells from nonlymphoid tissue and their preparation for flow cytometry can be a challenging process with respect to immune cell yields and viability. Here we describe a method for the efficient isolation of viable mouse intrahepatic lymphocytes (IHL) from normal liver tissue and liver cancer and their subsequent characterization by multicolor flow cytometry.

Key words Flow cytometry, Intrahepatic lymphocyte isolation, Liver tumors, Hepatocellular carcinoma, Fluorophore-conjugated antibodies

1 Introduction

Multicolor flow cytometry allows for the simultaneous detection of multiple surface and intracellular proteins on a single-cell level with the help of fluorophore-conjugated reagents [1]. The commercial availability of fluorophore-conjugated monoclonal antibodies for almost any given cell antigen has contributed to flow cytometry being widely used in the biological sciences.

The basic principle of flow cytometry is the transport of particles (usually cells) in a stream of sheath fluid and their interrogation by a beam of monochromatic laser light [2]. When fluorescent cells pass through the laser beam, they simultaneously scatter and emit light. Both events are collected by lenses and passed through a combination of beam splitters and filters that channel the light to detectors. The detectors convert the light into an electronic signal and data is collected on each event. The characteristics of each event are based on its light scattering and fluorescent properties. The scattered light serves to measure cell size and the internal complexity (granularity) [3]. If for example a fluorophore-conjugated

Brendan J. Jenkins (ed.), *Inflammation and Cancer: Methods and Protocols*, Methods in Molecular Biology, vol. 1725, https://doi.org/10.1007/978-1-4939-7568-6_23, © Springer Science+Business Media, LLC 2018

antibody was used to detect an antigen, the intensity of the emitted fluorescent light would be proportional to the level of antigen expression [4, 5].

The introduction of flow cytometry in the 1960s has made an enormous impact in the field of immunology [6–8]. Flow cytometry has become an indispensable method for the phenotypic characterization of immune cells and their subsets [9, 10]. The isolation of immune cells from lymphoid organs such as thymus, lymph nodes and spleen is well established and can be simply done by the mechanical disruption of the tissue. The extraction of immune cells from nonlymphoid tissues however is more challenging as mechanical disruption can result in decreased cell viability and poor immune cell yields [11]. Enzymatic tissue digestion usually improves immune cell recovery, but can alter the phenotype of the immune cells caused by ligand shedding.

Here we describe nonenzymatic and enzymatic methods that allow for the isolation of intrahepatic lymphocytes (IHL) from normal liver tissue (Figs. 1 and 2a, b), liver cancer and tumor adjacent tissue (Fig. 2c) without compromising cellular viability and the immune cell phenotype. The quantification of intrahepatic lymphocyte infiltrates by flow cytometry provides an accurate method to assess immune cell contributions and inflammation in liver diseases such as hepatitis, hepatic steatosis and primary liver cancers such as hepatocellular carcinoma (HCC) [12–14].

2 Materials

2.1 IHL Isolation

1. Isoflurane.
2. 80% (v/v) ethanol.
3. 10× PBS: Dissolve 400 g NaCl, 10 g KCl, 57.5 g Na_2HPO_4, and 10 g KH_2PO_4 in 5 L autoclaved Milli-Q water and stir until chemicals have dissolved. Adjust pH to 7.2.
4. 1× PBS: Dilute 100 mL 10× PBS with 900 mL of autoclaved Milli-Q water.
5. PBS–2% FBS (v/v): Resuspend 20 mL FBS in 980 mL 1× PBS.
6. Heat-inactivated fetal bovine serum (FBS).
7. 33.75% (v/v) isotonic Percoll® in 25 mL: 8.438 mL Percoll®, 0.938 mL 10× PBS, 15.625 mL 1× PBS. Always prepare fresh and use on the same day. Keep working solution on room temperature (*see* **Note 1**).
8. Red blood lysing buffer: 0.83% (m/v) ammonium chloride, 0.01 M Tris (*see* **Note 2**).
9. Sieve made of wire mesh, 200 μM pore size.
10. Petri dish 90 mm.
11. 10 mL syringe.

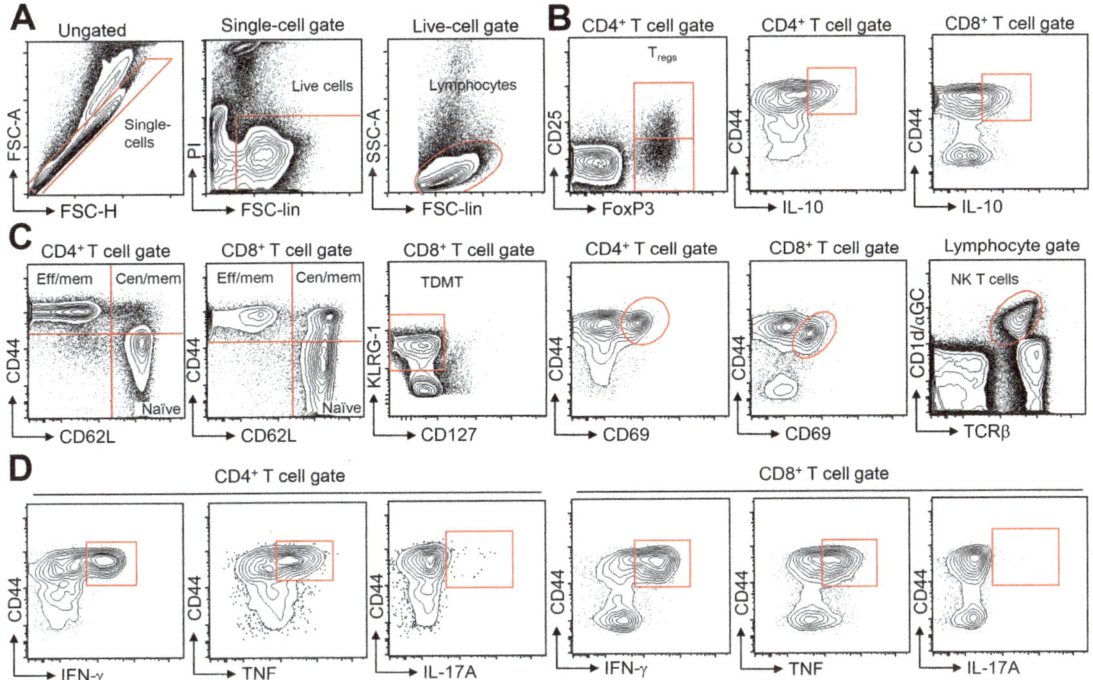

Fig. 1 Percoll® isolated IHL from normal liver tissue acquired with a flow cytometry analyzer and analyzed with flow cytometry analysis software. (**a**) Single-cells were electronically gated for propidium-iodide (PI) negative (live cells). Live lymphocytes were identified according to their FSC/SSC profile. (**b**) Analysis of immunosuppressive T cells. Cells were stained with fluorophore-conjugated antibodies against CD4, CD25 and FoxP3 or CD4, CD8 and IL-10 and $CD4^+CD25^{hi/lo}FoxP3^+$ regulatory T cells or $CD4^+$IL-10- and $CD8^+$IL-10-producing cells were determined. (**c**) Analysis of previously activated memory T cell subsets and natural killer (NK) T cells. Cells were stained with fluorophore-conjugated antibodies against CD4, CD8, CD69, CD44, CD62L, and KLRG-1 and $CD4^+$ and $CD8^+$ naïve ($CD62L^{hi}CD44^{lo}$) central/memory (cen/mem; $CD62L^{hi}CD44^{hi}$) and effector/memory (eff/mem; $CD62L^{lo}CD44^{hi}$) T cells, $CD8^+KLRG\text{-}1^{hi}CD127^{lo}$ terminally differentiated memory T cells (TDMT) and recently activated $CD4^+CD44^{hi}CD69^{hi}$ and $CD8^+CD44^{hi}CD69^{hi}$ memory T cells were determined. Fluorophore-conjugated CD1d/αGC tetramer and anti-TCRβ was used to detect NK T cells ($CD1d/\alpha GC^{hi}TCR\beta^{hi}$). (**d**) Analysis of proinflammatory cytokine producing memory T cells. Cells were stained with fluorophore-conjugated antibodies against CD4, CD8, CD44, IFN-γ, TNF, and IL-17A, and IFN-γ-, TNF-, and IL-17A-producing $CD4^+CD44^{hi}$ and $CD8^+CD44^{hi}$ memory T cells were determined

12. 26 G needles.
13. Curved forceps.
14. Curved scissors.
15. Sharp-tipped scissors.
16. Vacuum pump with trap.
17. Pasteur pipettes.
18. 50 mL Falcon™ tubes.
19. 15 mL Falcon™ tubes.
20. Hemocytometer.
21. Trypan blue.

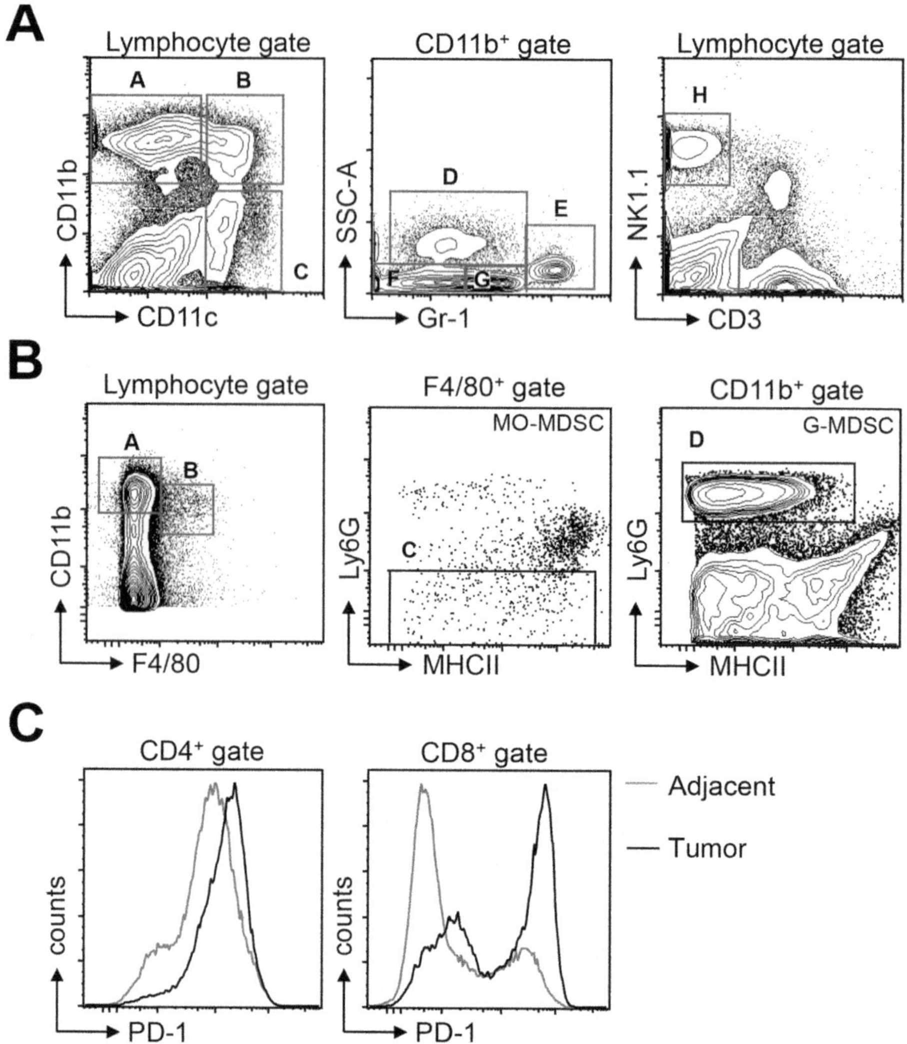

Fig. 2 Percoll® isolated IHL from normal liver tissue (A, B) and tumor versus tumor adjacent tissue (C) acquired with a flow cytometry analyzer and analyzed with flow cytometry analysis software. (**a**) Cells were stained with fluorophore-conjugated antibodies against CD11b, CD11c, Gr-1, NK1.1, and CD3 and $CD11b^{+}CD11c^{-}$ (A) $CD11c^{+}CD11b^{+/-}$ dendritic cells (B, C) and $NK1.1^{+}CD3^{-}$ NK cells (H) were determined. $CD11b^{+}CD11c^{-}$ (A) were further analyzed for eosinophils (D), neutrophils (E), macrophages (F), and monocytes (G) subsets. (**b**) IHL were stained with fluorophore-conjugated antibodies against CD11b, F4/80, Ly6G, and MHC class II and monocytic myeloid-derived suppressor cells (B, C) and granulocytic myeloid-derived suppressor cells (A, D) were determined. (**c**) Cells from tumor and adjacent tissue were stained with fluorophore-conjugated antibodies against CD4, CD8 and PD-1. PD-1 histogram overlays from $CD4^{+}$ and $CD8^{+}$ T cells isolated from tumor versus adjacent tissue are shown. PD-1 is a marker for T cell exhaustion and activation and is increased on tumor-infiltrating T cells compared to T cells isolated from tumor-adjacent tissue

2.2 IHL Isolation from Mouse Tumor Tissue

1. Hank's balanced salt solution (HBSS) containing Ca^{2+} and Mg^{2+}.
2. Liberase™ TM (Enzyme blend made of class I and II collagenases and thermolysin) reconstituted in HBSS (0.05 mg/mL).
3. Shaker at 37 °C.
4. 70 μM cell strainer.

2.3 Flow Cytometry Staining Procedure and Analysis

1. 96-well round bottom polystyrene microtiter plate.
2. Benchtop centrifuge including two plate holders.
3. Vortex mixer.
4. Fridge or ice esky.
5. 12-well multichannel pipette.
6. Incubator at 37 °C/5% CO_2.
7. In vitro T cell activation: Complete RPMI 1640 T cell medium [supplemented with 10% FBS, 2 mM L-glutamine, 100 units/mL penicillin, 100 μg/mL streptomycin, nonessential amino acids, 1 mM Na-pyruvate, 10 mM HEPES, 50 μM 2-mercaptoethanol]; 500× Cell Stimulation Cocktail™ containing phorbol 12-myristate 13-acetate (PMA), ionomycin, brefeldin A, and monensin (eBioscience).
8. Detection of cytosolic proteins: BD Cytofix/Cytoperm™ Fixation/Permeabilization Solution (BD Biosciences).
9. Detection of nuclear proteins: FoxP3 Transcription Factor Staining Buffer Set™ (eBioscience).
10. 5 mL Polystyrene round-bottom tubes with 40 μM cell strainer caps.
11. Flow cytometry cell analyzer.
12. Flow cytometry analysis software.

2.4 Fluorophore-Conjugated Antibodies

1. T cell panel: The following fluorophore-conjugated antibodies were used for flow cytometry: Allophycocyanin (APC)-conjugated TCRβ (H57-597), Pacific Blue (PB)-conjugated, APC-conjugated or phycoerythrin-cyanine 7 (PE-Cy7)-conjugated CD4 (RM4-5), allophycocyanin-cyanine 7 (APC-Cy7)-conjugated or APC-conjugated or PB-conjugated CD8 (53-6.7), phycoerythrin (PE)-conjugated or APC-conjugated CD62L (Mel-14), Fluorescein isothiocyanate (FITC)-conjugated CD44 (IM7), FITC-conjugated CD25 (PC61), PB-conjugated CD69 (H1.2F3), APC-conjugated KLRG-1 (2F1), PE-conjugated CD127 (SB/199), PE-Cy7-conjugated IFN-γ (XMG1.2), Brilliant™ Violet 605 (BV605)-conjugated TNF, PE-conjugated IL-10 (JES5-16E3), Horizon™ V421-conjugated IL-17A (TC11-18H10.1) and PE-conjugated FoxP3 (MF23). Peridinin chlorophyll protein-cyanine 5.5

(PerCP-Cy5.5)-conjugated CD1d/αGC (α-galactosylceramide) tetramer was used to detect NKT cells [15, 16].

2. Macrophage/monocyte panel: The following fluorophore-conjugated antibodies were used for flow cytometry: FITC-conjugated CD11b (M1/70), APC-conjugated CD11c (N418), PE-conjugated Ly-6G/Ly-6C (Gr-1), PB-conjugated NK1.1 (PK136) and PE-conjugated CD3 (145-2C11).
3. Myeloid/granulocyte derived suppressor cell panel: The following fluorophore-conjugated antibodies were used for flow cytometry: PB-conjugated CD11c (N418), FITC-conjugated CD11b (M1/70), PE-conjugated Ly-6G (1A8), APC-conjugated F4/80 (BM8) and PE-Cy7-conjugated MHC class II (M5/114.15.2).

3 Methods

3.1 Isolation of Mouse IHL from Normal Liver Tissue

1. Anesthetize mouse with isoflurane.
2. Euthanize mouse by cervical dislocation.
3. Pin down all four limbs with abdomen facing up and wet with 80% (v/v) ethanol. Use forceps to lift the skin anteriorly to the urethral opening and cut along the ventral midline from the groin to the chin using sharp-tipped scissors. Make two Y-shaped incisions toward the legs and arms and pull the skin back. Open the peritoneal wall and cut the aorta located in the thoracic cavity.
4. Expose the visceral surface of the liver by pushing all four lobes to the upper right and hold the hepatic portal vein with curved forceps. Perform a liver perfusion by injecting 10 mL of ice-cold PBS using a 26 G needle into the hepatic portal vein. The liver will swell up and its color will change from red to straw-brown as the hepatic blood is being cleared (*see* **Note 3**).
5. Remove liver and cut and dispose gallbladder located on the right liver lobe. Store liver in 10 mL PBS–2% (v/v) FBS.
6. Place sieve in 90 mm petri dish and pour liver including 10 mL ice-cold PBS–2% (v/v) FBS storage buffer onto the sieve. Dice liver tissue into 0.5 cm pieces using curved scissors. Using the plunger of a 10 mL syringe mash liver pieces through the wire mesh. Wash with 40 mL ice-cold PBS–2% (v/v) FBS and transfer liver homogenate to a 50 mL Falcon™ tube.
7. Spin at 500 × *g* for 5 min and aspirate supernatant using a Pasteur pipette attached to a vacuum pump.
8. Resuspend cell pellet in 50 mL ice-cold PBS–2% (v/v) FBS and spin at 500 × *g* for 5 min on 4 °C and aspirate supernatant.

9. Resuspend cell pellet in 25 mL isotonic 33.75% (v/v) Percoll® and spin cells at 693 × *g* for 12 min at 20 °C. Set centrifuge acceleration and brakes to 4.
10. Aspirate supernatant (*see* **Note 4**).
11. Resuspend cell pellet in 10 mL ice-cold PBS–2% (v/v) FBS transfer to a 15 mL Falcon™ tube and spin at 340 × *g* for 5 min at 4 °C.
12. Aspirate supernatant and resuspend cells in 1 mL red blood cell lysing solution and incubate for 4 min at room temperature (*see* **Note 5**).
13. Underlay with 1 mL heat-inactivated FBS and spin at 340 × *g* for 5 min at 4 °C.
14. Aspirate supernatant and resuspend cells in 0.5 mL ice-cold PBS–2% (v/v) FBS.
15. Perform cell count using a hemocytometer. Exclude dead cells with trypan blue (*see* **Note 6**).
16. Proceed to *flow cytometry staining and analysis.*

3.2 Isolation of Tumor-Infiltrating and Tumor-Adjacent IHL

1. Isolate liver as described in Subheading 3.1, **steps 1–5** and carefully remove all tumors using sharped-tipped scissors without cutting into adjacent tissue.
2. Remove tumor-adjacent tissue.
3. Wash tumors and tumor-adjacent tissue twice with PBS.
4. *Optional:* Weigh adjacent and tumor tissue (*see* **Note 7**).
5. Place tumors and tumor-adjacent tissue in separate 90 mm petri dishes and add Liberase™ TM buffer dropwise (500 μL to 1 mL per tumor) while mincing the tissue using curved scissors.
6. Transfer to 50 mL Falcon™ tubes and shake for 90 min at 37 °C at 180 rpm.
7. Pass tissue through 70 μM cell strainer and wash with 30 mL PBS–2% (v/v) FBS.
8. Spin at 500 × *g* for 5 min at 4 °C.
9. Aspirate supernatant and resuspend cell pellet in 25 mL isotonic 33.75% (v/v) Percoll®.
10. Perform Percoll® gradient as described in Subheading 3.1, **steps 9–15**.
11. Proceed to next section below.

3.3 Flow Cytometry Staining and Analysis

1. Transfer 1–3 × 10^6 cells to a 96 well Falcon™ round bottom microtiter plate (*see* **Note 8**).
2. Spin at 340 × *g* for 3 min at 4 °C.

3. Surface staining: Flick plate to remove supernatant and resuspend the cell pellet by gently pushing the plate against the rubber cup of a vortex mixer. Resuspend cells by adding 30 μL PBS–2% FBS containing the antibody cocktail (*see* **Note 9**). Push 96 well plate against the rubber cup of a vortex mixer to thoroughly mix the cells (*see* **Note 10**). Incubate cells for at least 20 min on ice or at 4 °C in the fridge in the dark.
4. Resuspend cells in 200 μL PBS–2% FBS using an 12 well multichannel pipette and spin at 340 × *g* for 3 min at 4 °C.
5. Flick plate to remove supernatant and resuspend the cell pellet by gently pushing the plate against the rubber cup of a vortex mixer.
6. Repeat **step 4**.
7. Repeat **step 5**.
8. If in vitro T cell activation and intracellular staining are not required, proceed to **step 13**.
9. In vitro T cell activation: Resuspend cells in 200 μL complete T cell medium supplemented with Cell Stimulation Cocktail™. Incubate for 4 h at 37 °C/5% CO_2 (*see* **Note 11**).
10. Spin at 340 × *g* for 3 min at 4 °C.
11. Flick plate to remove supernatant and resuspend the cell pellet by gently pushing the plate against the rubber cup of a vortex mixer.
12. Intracellular staining of cytoplasmic or nuclear proteins: For the detection of cytoplasmic proteins (IFN-γ, TNF, IL-17A, IL-10) use the BD Cytofix/Cytoperm™ Fixation/Permeabilization Solution and for the detection of nuclear proteins (FoxP3) use the FoxP3 Transcription Factor Staining Buffer Set™. Resuspend cells in 100 μL fixation/permeabilization buffer and incubate for 30 min on ice followed by one wash with 100 μL 1× permeabilization buffer. Resuspend cells in 30 μL 1× permeabilization buffer containing the antibody cocktail and incubate 30 min on ice followed by two washes with 1× permeabilization buffer.
13. Resuspend cells in 200 μL PBS–2% FBS and proceed to sample acquisition (*see* **Notes 12** and **13**).
14. Analyze data with flow cytometry analyzing software (Figs. 1 and 2).

4 Notes

1. It is important to always keep the isotonic Percoll® solution at room temperature and to ensure that the centrifuge is set to

20 °C when spinning cells in isotonic Percoll®. If the isotonic Percoll® solution is used cold, cells can form aggregates and the cell separation will not work efficiently.

2. We use a commercial red blood lysing buffer (Red blood lysing solution, Sigma-Aldrich) as we have noticed fluctuations in the quality of home-made lysis buffers, which can impact on lymphocyte viability.
3. To achieve sufficient yields of certain lymphocyte subsets (e.g., NK T cells) and to reduce the contamination with red blood cells to a minimum, an efficient and successful liver perfusion is essential.
4. At this stage, the hepatocytes float on top and the lymphocytes have formed a loose pellet. Take extra care when taking tubes out of the centrifuge as the floating hepatocytes can easily sink to the bottom when disturbed and the lymphocyte pellet can detach. Start aspirating at the very top of the surface and slowly work your way down to the pellet to prevent the hepatocytes from resuspending with Percoll® solution.
5. Red blood cells interfere with the flow cytometry analysis as they are difficult to discriminate from lymphocytes by size. To remove red blood cells 1 mL of red blood lysing solution and 4 min incubation time at room temperature per perfused liver are sufficient. If there is an unusual high level of red blood cell contamination, buffer volume and incubation time can be increased to 2 mL and 7 min without impacting cell viability.
6. We add a known number of unlabeled beads (e.g., CaliBRITE® beads, BD Biosciences) to each sample before flow cytometry analysis which will provide a more accurate method of quantification when comparing immune cell infiltrates between different mouse genotypes. Unlabeled beads can be easily detected in the forward scatter (FSC) versus side scatter (SSC) during flow cytometry analysis and the total cell number per liver can be calculated with following formula: total cell number/liver = (number of added beads/number of acquired beads) * acquired cell number * (total sample volume/sample volume used for analysis).
7. If absolute cell numbers are required, the number of immune cell infiltrates can be normalized to tissue weight.
8. Using microtiter plates instead of flow cytometry tubes for the staining procedure saves time and reagents and should be the method of choice, if flow cytometry analysis is performed on many samples. Make sure to leave the blank wells around each sample well to avoid spill overs and cross-contaminations in between samples. The sample size should not exceed 24 wells per 96-well plate.

9. We generally add 2% (v/v) FBS to our flow cytometry staining buffers without sodium azide. When biotinylated antibodies together with fluorophore-conjugated Streptavidin are used, we recommend using 0.1% (m/v) BSA instead of FBS to avoid unspecific binding. We also strongly recommend determining the working concentration of each antibody individually before use. We have noticed that many fluorophore-conjugated antibodies can be used in a much lower concentration than recommended by the manufacturers.
10. Our general flow cytometry staining protocol has been optimized for 1×10^6 cells per 10 μL antibody cocktail. This allows for a quick cell resuspension by using the vortex mixer without risking spillages. If the staining volume exceeds 30 μL, we recommend resuspending the samples using a 12-well multichannel pipette to avoid spillages.
11. Incubation with Cell Stimulation Cocktail™ increases the abundance of intracellular cytokines which would be otherwise undetectable by flow cytometry. For the detection of nuclear proteins (e.g., FoxP3) incubation with Cell Stimulation Cocktail™ is not required.
12. We recommend adding a dead cell exclusion marker (e.g., 1 μg/mL propidium iodide, final concentration) to live cells before flow cytometry analysis. For intracellular staining fixable viability dyes from BD Biosciences or eBioscience can be used.
13. We filter the samples by passing the cell suspension through a 40 μM cell strainer prior to sample acquisition. This helps to avoid blockages of the flow cell during sample acquisition.

References

1. Bonner WA, Hulett HR, Sweet RG (1972) Fluorescence activated cell sorting. Rev Sci Instrum 43:404–409
2. Van Dilla MA, Trujillo TT, Mullaney PF (1969) Cell microfluorometry: a method for rapid fluorescence measurement. Science 163:1213–1214
3. Shapiro HM, Schildkraut ER, Curbelo R (1977) Cytomat-R: a computer-controlled multiple laser source multiparameter flow cytophotometer system. J Histochem Cytochem 25:836–844
4. Shapiro HM, Schildkraut ER, Curbelo R (1976) Combined blood cell counting and classification with fluorochrome stains and flow instrumentation. J Histochem Cytochem 24:396–401
5. Shapiro HM (1977) Fluorescent dyes for differential counts by flow cytometry: does histochemistry tell us much more than cell geometry? J Histochem Cytochem 25:976–989
6. Fulwyler MJ (1965) Electronic separation of biological cells by volume. Science 150:910–911
7. Kamentsky LA, Melamed MR Derman H (1965) Spectrophotometer: new instrument for ultrarapid cell analysis. Science 150:630–631
8. Kamentsky LA Melamed MR (1967) Spectrophotometric cell sorter. Science 156:1364–1365
9. Baumgarth N Roederer M (2000) A practical approach to multicolor flow cytometry for immunophenotyping. J Immunol Methods 243:77–97
10. Perfetto SP, Chattopadhyay PK, Roederer M (2004) Seventeen-colour flow cytometry:

unravelling the immune system. Nat Rev Immunol 4:648–655

11. Yu YR, O'Koren EG, Hotten DF (2016) A protocol for the comprehensive flow cytometric analysis of immune cells in normal and inflamed murine non-lymphoid tissues. PLoS One 11:e0150606
12. Li XM, Jeffers LJ, Reddy KR (1991) Immunophenotyping of lymphocytes in liver tissue of patients with chronic liver diseases by flow cytometry. Hepatology 14:121–127
13. Lohr HF, Schlaak JF, Gerken G (1994) Phenotypical analysis and cytokine release of liver-infiltrating and peripheral blood T lymphocytes from patients with chronic hepatitis of different etiology. Liver 14:161–166
14. Shirabe K, Motomura T, Muto J (2010) Tumor-infiltrating lymphocytes and hepatocellular carcinoma: pathology and clinical management. Int J Clin Oncol 15:552–558
15. Matsuda JL, Naidenko OV, Gapin L (2000) Tracking the response of natural killer T cells to a glycolipid antigen using CD1d tetramers. J Exp Med 192:741–754
16. Crowe NY, Uldrich AP, Kyparissoudis K (2003) Glycolipid antigen drives rapid expansion and sustained cytokine production by NK T cells. J Immunol 171:4020–4027

Index

Brendan J. Jenkins (ed.), *Inflammation and Cancer: Methods and Protocols*, Methods in Molecular Biology, vol. 1725, https://doi.org/10.1007/978-1-4939-7568-6, © Springer Science+Business Media, LLC 2018

R

S

T

W

X

Lightning Source UK Ltd.
Milton Keynes UK
UKHW05n1826180418
321296UK00003B/7/P